MEDICAL MINI REVIEW SERIES IN HEPATOLOGY

B. Al-Judaibi and A.B.R. Thomson

www.giandhepatology.com

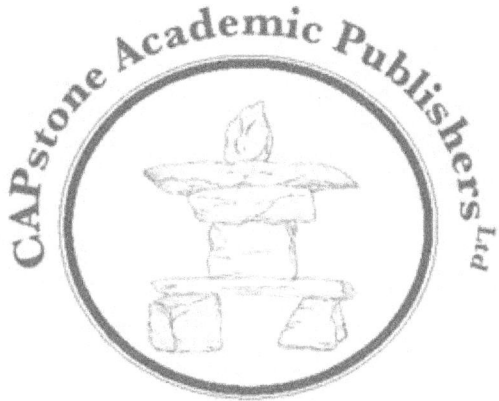

CAPstone (Canadian Academic Publishers Ltd) is a not-for-profit company dedicated to the use of the power of education for the betterment of all persons everywhere.

"The Democratization of Knowledge"

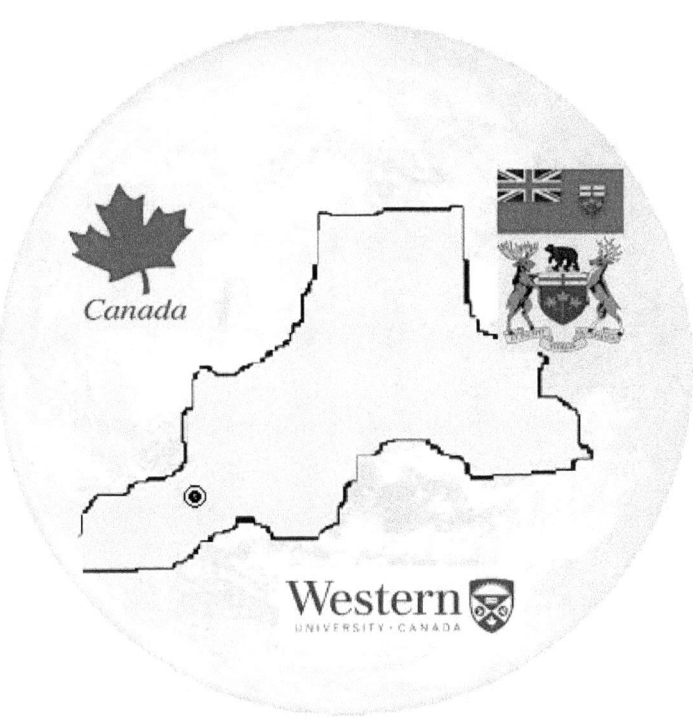

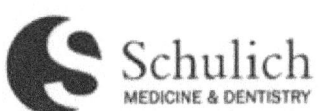
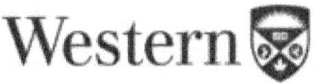

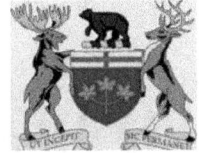

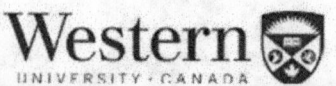

The editors wish to thank the trainee and staff contributors who maintain the excellence of the Division of Gastroenterology at Western University.

LIST OF CONTRIBUTORS

Al Hasan I, MD, FRCP(C)

Al-Judaibi B, MD, FRCP(C)

Alawadh Y, MD, FRCP(C)

Alghanem M, MD, FRCP(C)

Aljawad M, MD, FRCP(C)

Beaton M, MD, FRCP(C)

Beck G, MD, FRCP(C)

Hussain N, MD, FRCP(C)

Levstik MA, MD, FRCP(C)

Malhotra N, MD, FRCP(C)

Marotta P, MD, FRCP(C)

Quang Le NH, MD, FRCP(C)

Qumosani K, MD, FRCP(C)

Rammal A, MD, FRCP(C)

Sandhu A, MD, FRCP(C)

Segal D, MD, FRCP(C)

Sinclair L, MD, FRCP(C)

Tandon P, MD, FRCP(C)

Teriaky A, MD, FRCP(C)

Thomas B, MD, FRCP (C)

Yik D, MD, FRCP(C)

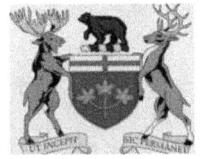

Editor Biographies

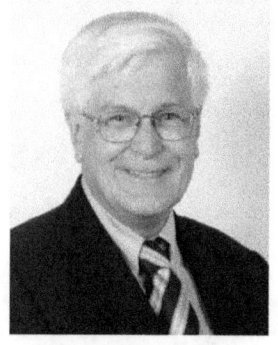

Dr. Alan Thomson has been the President of the Canadian Association of Gastroenterology, a member of the Bockus Society, two–term Governor of Western Canada for the American College of Gastroenterology, winner of the prestigious University Cup in 2001, a recipient of the Gold Medal in Medicine of the Royal College of Physicians and Surgeons (Canada), Chief Royal College examiner in Gastroenterology, Director of the Division of Gastroenterology, three–time Teacher of the Year at the University of Alberta, Award for Excellence in Mentoring Graduate Students and Post–doctoral Fellows, and awarded Distinguished University Professor. Dr. Thomson is a Distinguished Emeritus University Professor at the University of Alberta and is currently an Adjunct Professor at Western University.

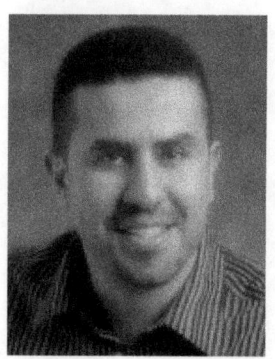

Dr. Bandar Al-Judaibi is an assistant professor at Western and King Saud Universities. He graduated from medical school at King Saud University in 2003 and completed his internal medicine, gastroenterology, clinical pharmacology and hepatology training at Western University. He completed a liver transplantation fellowship at the University of Alberta before he joined the Gastroenterology Division at London Health Sciences Centre in 2013. His research interest is on drug metabolism and liver transplantation. Dr. Al-judaibi has published in peer-reviewed journals such as Gastroenterology, American Journal of Gastroenterology, and Transplantation.

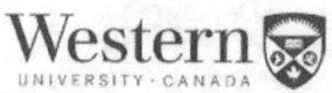

DEDICATION

" As physicians may we help others to walk in Peace"

" انلعل ر رشبلا دعاسن ءابطأك". نيملاس ةايحلا يف اوضمي نا ىل "

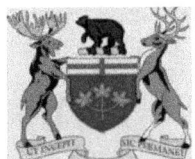

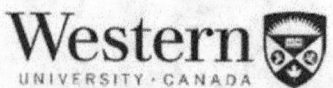

Table of Content

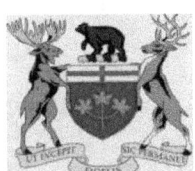

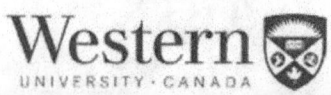

SPECIFIC DIAGNOSES

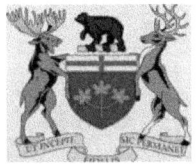

2

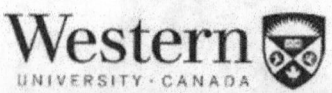

Drug–Induced Liver Injury

Dan Segal

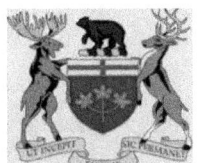

➢ Definition
　o Drug–induced liver injury due to the following:
　　- Prescription drugs
　　- Over the counter drugs
　　- Herbal and dietary supplements

➢ Demography
　o ~ $1/10^5$ exposed
　o Causes: ~ 10% of severe hepatitis that is admitted
　o Most common cause of drug removal from the market (troglitazone, bromfenac)
　o Usually picked–up in post–market surveillance
　o Only 10% of adverse drug reactions are reported
　o Most evidences came from case reports

➢ Types
　o Intrinsic
　　- Potentially affecting all individuals in varying degrees
　　- Dose–dependence and similar picture
　　- Example: acetaminophen, anticancer drugs
　o Idiosyncratic
　　- Affects only rare and susceptible hosts
　　- Less dose–dependent
　　- Varied in latency, presentation and course
　o Ideopathic in ~ 50% of patients

➢ Causes and associations
　o Genetics
　　- Valproic acid and phenytoin have familial predisposition
　　- HLA haplotype may influence the disease pattern
　o Age
　　- Antibiotics and CNS drugs cause more DILI in children
　　- Isoniazid causes more disease in elderly

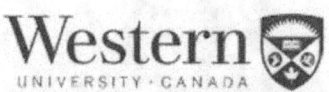

- o Gender
  - – AI type DILI in females with minocycline, methyldopa, diclofenac and nitrofurantoin
- o Pregnancy
  - – IV tetracycline is extremely high risk and should not be used anyway
  - – DILI has high host risk factors
- o Malnutrition
- o Obesity
  - – Obesity creates problems for the liver through the production of NAFLD
  - – DM
    - OR of 2.69 for severity of DILI
- o Comorbid diseases
- o Multiple drugs
  - – Perhaps the altered metabolism leads to toxic products
  - – Differential secretion into bile canaliculi
- o Environmental factors
  - – Smoking
  - – Alcohol consumption
    - Decrease dose threshold for a number of drugs
    - APAP, methotrexate, isoniazid
  - – Infection + Inflammatory episodes
- o Drug–related factors
  - – Daily dose
  - – Metabolic profile
  - – Class effect + cross sensitization
    - If with previous DILI
    - With anaesthetics, TCAs, sulfa products
  - – Drug interactions + polypharmacy
    - Little evidence

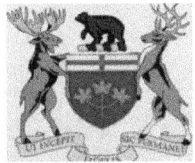

➢ Diagnosis
  o Diagnosis of exclusion
  o Requires thorough history, physical and laboratory testing

➢ Hepatic drug metabolism

SO YOU WANT TO BE A HEPATOLOGIST!

- Define phases I, II and III reactions in hepatic drug metabolism.

➢ Phase I
  o Microsomal drug oxidases and the CYP gene superfamily
    - Involves the hemoproteinof the CYP gene
    - Drugs are converted into a toxic metabolite (i.e. acetaminophen → NAPQI)

➢ Phase II
  o Conjugation
    - Through glucuronic acid or inorganic sulfate by the formation of ester links with the drug

➢ Phase III
  o Secretion of drugs or their metabolites by transporters
    - ATP–binding cassette (ABC) protein
    - MDR1 (multidrug resistance protein C1)
    - MRP1 (multidrug resistance–associated proteins)
      ▪ MRP3 sinusoidal membrane of hepatocytes
      ▪ MRP2 canalicular membrane (CM) of hepatocytes

- Why DILI by drugs metabolized by phase I reactions (i.e. acetaminophen) is localized in zone 3 (around the terminal hepatic venules [THV])?

  o Phase 1 reactions are catalyzed by microsomal drug oxidase, the key component of a hemoprotein of the CYP gene superfamily

  o CYP2E1 is located in hepatocytes forming 1 to 2 hepatocytes with thick rim around the THV

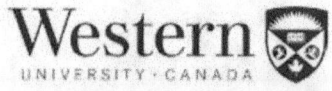

- Give the drugs reported to have an increased risk of hepatotoxicity in patients with chronic liver disease.

Drugs	Underlying liver disease as a risk factor
o Anti–androgens	– Chronic viral hepatitis B and C
o Antiretrovirals (i.e. zalcitabine, saquinavir)	– Hepatitis B and C
o Ibuprofen (NSAIDs)	– Hepatitis C
o Methimazole	– Chronic hepatitis B
o Methotrexate	– Alcoholic liver disease, NAFLD
o Oral contraceptives	– Women with liver tumors or history of jaundice of pregnancy
o Rifampin	– Primary biliary cirrhosis
o Vitamin A (high doses)	– Alcoholic liver disease

Adapted from: Gupta, N.K. and Lewis, J.H. *Aliment Pharmacol Ther* 2008; 28(9):1021-41.

- Give the major **mechanisms** of drug–induced liver injury leading to hepatocyte apoptosis and necrosis.
  - o Direct hepatotoxicity
    - – Injury to the following:
      - Mitochondria
      - Plasma membrane

  - o ROS (reactive oxygen species)
    - – ".....the liver is exposed to oxidative stress by the propensity of hepatocytes to reduce oxygen....."
    - – Some drugs (i.e. acetaminophen) is converted by CYP into pre–oxidant reactive metabolites

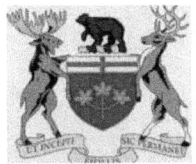

- CYP–mediated metabolism → formation of reactive metabolites → ↓ glutathione → injury to mitochondria → (1) release of cytochrome C and (2) operation of MPT (mitochondrial permeability transition) → activation of caspases → apoptosis
- Formed from injured hepatocytes and kupffer cells
- Reactive metabolites undergo covalent binding to proteins
- Protein–drug adducts
  - Inactive important enzymes
  - May be acted upon by immunodestructive processes
- Glutathione system
  - Pro–oxidants signal Nrf (the redox–sensitive transcription factor)
  - Nrf → ↑ CYP 2E1 expression → ↑ hepatic glutathione synthesis (from cysteine) → ↑ antioxidant effects
  - Cystolic glutathione
    - In the reduced state, resulting from the effect of NADPH and glutathione reductase
    - Glutathione deficiency injures mitochondria, releases cytochrome C and MPT (mitochondrial membrane permeability transition) leading to activation of caspases and apoptosis
- Biochemical pathways of cellular damage
  - Covalent binding of drugs to cellular proteins
  - Oxidation of proteins
  - Post–translational modification of proteins
  - Lipid peroxidation
  - Cleavage of DNA
  - ↑ Ca_i^{2+} (intracellular concentration of Ca^{2+})

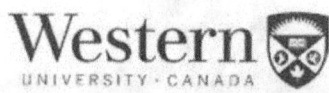

- o Hepatic non–hepatocyte cells
    - Kupffer cells
        - Act as macrophages and antigen–presenting cells
        - Activated Kupffer cells release TNF, ROS and as–L leading to hepatocyte apoptosis and necrosis
    - Endothelial cells
        - Low glutathione context makes them susceptible to vascular injury
    - Stellate cells
        - When activated, will deposit matrix and lead to fibrosis
- o Immunologic mechanisms
    - Formation of ligands with death receptors
    - Porin–mediated introduction of granzyme
    - "altered antigen" of drug metabolites interact with cellular proteins to form drug–protein adducts (haptens)
    - Drug–induced autoimmunity

- In DILI, define Hy law.
    - o In DILI, the findings of clinical jaundice with increased ALT or AST has a mortality rate of ~ 10%

- ➤ Clinical
- Symptoms
    - o Drugs and herbal supplements list
    - o Gender, age, ethnicity (pertinent for competing disorders)
        - PBC, HEV, sarcoids
    - o Concomitant diseases (TPN, shock, anesthesia)
    - o Other drug reactions
    - o Other liver disorders

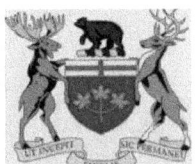

- o Alcohol use (past *vs* present; amount; sporadic *vs* binge)
- o Antibiotics and anti–epileptics account for > 60%
- o Latency
  - – Time pre– and post–exposure to the disease (usually within 6 months)
- o Longer latency
  - – Nitrofurantoin, minocycline, statins
- o Washout history
  - – What happened when drugs are stopped?
- o Rechallenge
  - – What happened if drugs are restarted?
- o Clinical outcomes
  - – Resolution, liver transplantation and timing of each

- Physical
  - o Fever, rash, hepatomegaly, signs of chronic liver disease

- ➤ Investigations
  - o General laboratory results including eosinophil count
  - o Viral hepatitis serology
  - o Autoimmune hepatitis
  - o Imaging
  - o U/S +/- dopplers, CT, or MRI
  - o Histology, if available

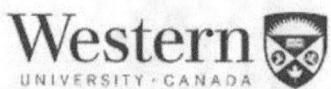

> Drugs commonly associated with drug–induced liver injury (DILI)

		Latency	Typical patterns of injury or identifying features
o	Amoxicillin/ clavulanate	– Short – moderate	Cholestatic injury but can be hepatocellular
			Onset is frequently detected after drug cessation
o	Isoniazid	– Moderate – long	Acute hepatocellular injury is similar to acute viral hepatitis
o	Trimethoprim/ sulfamethoxazole	– Short – moderate	Cholestatic injury but can be hepatocellular and often with immuno–allergic features (i.e. fever, rash, eosinophilia)
o	Fluoroquinolones	Short	Variable hepatocellular, cholestatic or mixed in relatively similar proportions
o	Macrolides	Short	Hepatocellular, but can be cholestatic
o	Nitrofurantoin		
	– Acute form	Short	Hepatocellular
	– Chronic form	Moderate – long (months – years)	Typically hepatocellular, often resembles idiopathic autoimmune hepatitis
o	Minocyclin	Moderate – long	Hepatocellular and often resembles autoimmune hepatitis
o	Anti–epileptic		
	– Phenytoin	Short – moderate	Hepatocellular, mixed or cholestatic often with immuno-allergic features (i.e. fever, rash, eosinophilia) (anti-convulsant hypersensitivity syndrome)

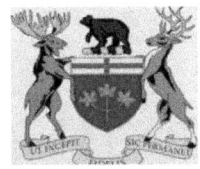

	Latency	Typical pattern of injury or identifying features
– Carbamazepine	Moderate	Hepatocellular, mixed or cholestatic often with immuno-allergic features (anti-convulsan hypersensitivity syndrome)
– Lamotrigene	Moderate	Hepatocellular often with immune-allergic features (anti-convulsant hypersensitivity syndrome)

○ Valproate

	Latency	
– Hyper-ammonemia	Moderate to long	Elevated blood ammonia, encephalopathy
– Hepatocellular	Moderate to long	Hepatocellular
– Reye-like syndrome	Moderate	Hepatocellular, acidosis, microvesicular steatosis on biopsy

○ Analgesics

– Non-selective anti-inflammatory agents	Moderate – long	Hepatocellular injury

○ Immune modulators

– Interferon–β	Moderate – long	Hepatocellular
– Interferon–α	Moderate	Hepatocellular, autoimmune hepatitis–like
– Anti–TNF agents	Moderate – long	Hepatocellular but can have autoimmune hepatitis features
– Azathioprine	Moderate – long	Cholestatic or hepatocellular but can present with portal hypertension (veno–occlusive disease, nodular regenerative hyperplasia)

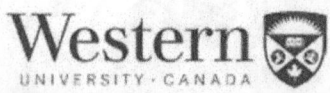

	Latency	Typical pattern of injury or identifying features
○ Herbal and dietary supplement		
– Anabolic, steroids	Moderate – long	Cholestatic; likely contained as adulterants in performance– enhancing
– Flavocoxib	Short – moderate	Mixed hepatocellular and cholstatic
– Green tea extract	Short – moderate	Hepatocellular
– Pyrrolizidine alkaloids	Moderate – long	Sinusoidal obstruction syndrome or veno– occlusive disease; contained in some teas
○ Miscellaneous		
– Allopurinol	Short – moderate	Hepatocellular or mixed; often with immuno–allergic features; granulomas often present on biopsy
– Amiodarone (oral)	Moderate – long	Hepatocellular, mixed or cholestatic; macrovesicular steatosis and steatohepatitis on biopsy
– Androgen– containing steroids	Moderate – long	Cholestatic but can present with peliosis hepatis, nodular regenerative hyperplasia or hepatocellular carcinoma
– Inhaled anesthetics	Short	Hepatocellular may have immuno–allergic features $\pm$ fever
– Methotrexate (oral)	Long	Fatty liver, fibrosis
– Proton pump inhibitors	Short	Hepatocellular, very rare
– Sulfasalazine	Short to moderate	Mixed, hepatocellular or cholestatic; often with immune–allergic features

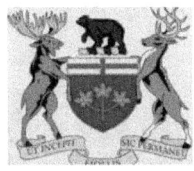

Herbs and OTC Supplements
- o Extremely a common cause of DILI
- o Usual culprits are weight loss and bodybuilding products
- o In Canada, these are mostly regulated under the Natural Health Products Regulation
- o These products have to get license to be sold
- o Safety and efficacy evidences must be provided
  - - Burden of proof is much smaller than a pharma drug
- o Variable batch–to–batch product
  - - Location or condition of growth
  - - Manufacture of product
- o Ingredients are not identified on label
  - - Microbials and heavy metals
  - - Drugs are meant to provide the expected benefit
- o Issues with causality
  - - i.e. RUCAM score incorporates with label warnings, which do not exist

Abbreviations: OTC, over–the–counter; RUCAM, Roussel Uclaf causality assessment method

➤ Laboratory
- o Tools used to suspect DILI
  - - Pattern of injury (R value)
  - - Cause of injury (RUCAM)
- o DILI pattern of injury
  - - R value = (ALT/ULN) / (ALP/ULN)
  - - R = 5 + is hepatocellular pattern
  - - R < 2 is cholestatic pattern
  - - R of > 2 – < 5 is mixed pattern
  - - Note: same drug can present with different pattern

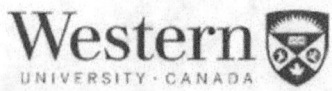

- o Hepatocellular pattern
    - – Viral hepatitis
        - ▪ 3% of those with DILI in 1 registry had HEV IgM
            - – Test if there is recent travel to endemic areas (i.e. third world countries)
    - – Autoimmune hepatitis
        - ▪ Minocycline, nitrofurantoin mimic the disease
    - – Ischemic injury
    - – Acute Budd–Chiari syndrome
    - – Wilson's disease
- o Cholestatic pattern
    - – Pancreatobiliary disease
    - – Extrahepatic *vs* intrahepatic
        - ▪ Includes sepsis, TPN

Abbreviations: ALP, alkaline phosphatase; ALT, alanine aminotransferase; ULN, upper limit of normal

➢ Pathology
- o Liver biopsy is not mandatory!
- o Useful for competing diagnosis with different treatments
    - – Autoimmune hepatitis *vs* DILI
- o Useful in non–resolving injury during washout
    - – Cholestatic slower to resolve than washout
    - – Lack of 50% decline in ALT by day 30
    - – Lack of 50% decline in ALP/bilirubin by day 180
- o Earlier if enzymes are going up
- o Useful if planning in continuing the drugs that may be suspected, i.e.:
    - – Isoniazid, methotrexate
- o Useful if enzymes are never completely normalized

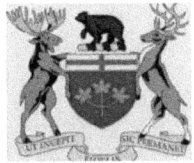

- Give the histopathological changes seen in DILI.
  - Asymptomatic liver disease
  - Acute hepatitis
    - ALT/AST or serum bilirubin may be increased as Hy's law stated, when aminotransferases and serum bilirubin are increased, prognosis is poor (mortality rate is ~ 10% in zonal area and non–zonal necrosis mortality rate is ~ 5%)
  - Acute and chronic steatosis ↓ beta–oxidation → microvesicular steatosis (acute) → macrovesicular (fat droplet occupies > ½ of cytoplasm) steatosis (chronic) histologically resembles NAFLD, NASH and ALD (alcoholic liver disease)
    - Examples of causative drugs are as follows:
      - Ibuprofen
      - Sulindac
  - Acute liver failure (ALF) or fulminant hepatic failure
    - Mortality rate is ~ 50%, especially if the serum bilirubin is > 3x ULN
  - Chronic hepatitis
    - Occurs in 5 – 10% of adverse drug reactions
    - More common with cholestatic or cholestatis with hepatocellular liver injury
    - Autoimmune–like chronic hepatitis (AIH)
      - Female > males
      - Positive ANA, anti–smooth muscle antibody
      - ↑ globulins in serum
    - Histopathologically identical to type 1 autoimmune hepatitis
      - Examples of causative drugs are as follows:
        - Phenytoin
        - Diclofenac
    - Viral hepaititis–like
      - Serology negative
      - Histopathology is similar to chronic viral hepatitis

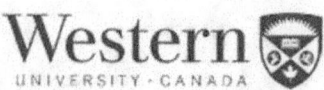

- Examples of causative drugs are as follows:
  - Aspirin
  - Isoniazid
- Chronic granulomatous hepatitis
  - Non–caveating granulomas examples of causative drugs
    - Mesalamine
    - Sulfonamides
    - Periportal hepatitis
    - Hepatocellular injury or cholestasis
    - Not associated with bile ducts
- Phospholipidosis
  - Phospholipids fill the lysosomes, which make hepatocytes appear "foamy" (foamy hepatocytes)
  - Examples are the following of causative drugs:
    - Amiodarone
    - Chlorpromazine
- Cholestasis with or without hepatitis
  - Pure cholestasis
    - Bile plugs in zone 3
    - Minimal hepatocellular inflammation
    - Below are examples of causative drugs
      - OCA (oral contraceptive agents)
      - Anabolic steroids
  - Cholestatic cholestasis
    - Cholestasis surrounded by inflammation
    - Proliferation of bile ducts
    - ↑ ALT/AST, ↑ AP, ↑ GGT
    - Symptoms of hypersensitivity
    - Typical causative drugs are the following:
      - NSAIDs
      - Erythromycin

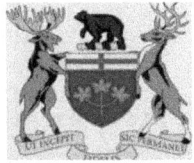

- PBC–like
  - Histopathologically similar to PBC
  - Serologically AMA–negative
  - Typical causative drugs
    - Amitriptyline
    - Erythromycin
  - Ductopenic cholestasis
  - Examples of causative drugs are as follows:
    - Amoxicillin
    - Clindamycin
- Sclerosing cholangitis
  - Diagnostic imaging (ERCP, MRCP) and histopathology results are similar to primary biliary sclerosis

o Fibrosis and cirrhosis
o Vascular disease → endothelial damage → thrombosis
  - NC, HV, PV thrombosis
  - SOS (sinusoidal obstruction syndrome or veno–occlusive disease)
  - Sinusoidal dilation
  - Cavernous hemangioma
  - NRH (nodular regenerative hypertension
  - Peliosis hepatis
o Hepatic vein (HV) thrombosis
  - B–CS (Budd–Chiari syndrome)
  - Associated with the following:
    - Coagulation disorders
    - Myeloproliferative disorders
    - Use of OCA (oral contraceptive agent)
o Autoimmune hepatitis
o Steatohepatitis with or without fibrosis
o Tumor
  - Focal nodular hyperplasia (FNH)
  - Hepatic adenoma
  - Hepatocellular cancer (HCC)
  - Cavernous hemangioma

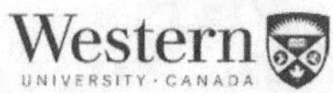

> Risk factors

- Give the risk factors in the development of DILI.
    - Older age
    - Female gender
    - Polypharmacy
    - Past history of adverse drug reaction
    - Alcohol
        - ↓ dose–threshold and ↑ severity of hepatotoxicity of some drugs, i.e. acetaminophen, isoniazid, niacin, methrotrexate
    - Nutritional status
        - Obesity
            - Halothane
        - Malnutrition
            - Methotrexate
            - Tamoxifen
    - Pre–existing liver disease
        - Methotrexate
        - HBV, HCV, HIV/AIDs
            - Anti–TB drugs
            - HAART therapy
            - Anti–cancer drugs
            - Ibuprofen
            - Myeloablation
            - Anti–androgens
            - Sulfonamides
        - HCV
            - Sinusoidal obstruction syndrome

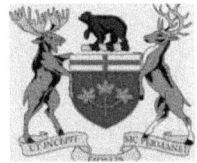

- Give the risk factors in **methotrexate–induced hepatic fibrosis**, clinical importance and the implications for prevention.

Risk factors	Importance	Implications for Prevention
o Age	– Increased risk > 60 years, possibly related to renal clearance and/or biological effect on fibrogenesis	▪ Care in the use of methotrexate in older patients
o Dose	– Incremental dose – Dose frequency – Duration of therapy – Cummulative (total) dose	▪ 5 – 15 mg/week is safe ▪ Weekly bolus (pulse) is safer than daily schedules ▪ Consider liver biopsy every 2 years ▪ Consider liver biopsy after each 2 g of methotrexate
o Alcohol	– Increased risk with daily levels > 15 g (1 – 2 drinks)	▪ Avoid methotrexate use if alcohol intake is not curbed; consider pre–treatment liver biopsy with relevant history of alcohol use
o Obesity	– Increased risk with daily levels > 15 g (1 – 2 drinks)	▪ Avoid methotrexate use if alcohol intake is not curbed; consider pre–treatment liver biopsy with relevant history of alcohol use
o Other diseases	– Increased risk	▪ Consider pre–treatment and interval liver biopsies

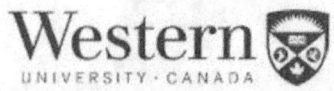

Risk factors	Importance	Implications for Prevention
o Diabetes mellitus	– Increased risk in obese patients (type 2 DM)	▪ Consider pre–treatment and interval liver biopsies
o Pre–existing liver disease	– Greatly increased the risk, particularly related to alcohol, obesity and diabetes (NASH)	▪ Pre–treatment liver biopsy is mandatory ▪ Avoid methotrexate or use at scheduled interval biopsies according to severity of hepatic fibrosis, total dose and duration of methotrexate therapy
o Systemic disease	– Possible risk is greater with psoriasis than rheumatoid arthritis (may depend on pre–existing liver disease, alcohol intake)	▪ None
o Impaired renal function	– Increased risk because of reduced clearance of methotrexate	▪ Reduced dose, greater caution with use
o Other drugs	– NSAIDS, vitamin A and arsenic may increase risk	▪ Greater caution with use ▪ Monitor liver biochemical tests

Printed with permission: *Sleisenger and Fordtran's Gastrointestinal and Liver Disease: Pathophysiology/ Diagnosis/Management.* 9th edition, 2010, Table 86.7, page 1443.

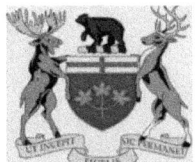

o Other diseases
- Rheumatoid arthritis
  - Salicylates
  - Sulfasalazine
- Diabetes, obesity
  - Methotrexate
- Chronic renal disease
  - Methotrexate → fibrosis
  - Renal transplantation → azathioprine–associated hepatic vascular damage

---

CLINICAL CHALLENGE

Jaw clenching and teeth grinding **(bruxism)** are uncommon extrahepatic manifestations of liver disease. In patients with these signs plus a tender hepatomegaly, sweating, fever and transaminases of > 1000, give the likely diagnosis.

o Acute hepatitis with sweating, fever, jaw clenching and teeth grinding is suggestive of drug–induced liver injury, i.e. from "ecstasy".

• For an extra mark, give the chemical name for ecstasy.

o Ecstasy is **m**ethylene**d**ioxy**m**eth**a**mphetamine.

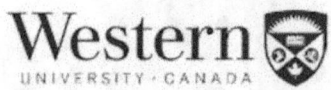

Suggested Algorithm for Patients with Suspected DILI

Abnormal liver enzymes

↓

Thorough history & physical
Complete review of medications and herbals and dietary supplements

↓

Calculate R value*
R value = Serum (ALT/ALT ULN) + (Alk P/Alk P ULN)

R value ≥ 5 (Hepatocellular)	2 < R value < 5 (Mixed)	R value ≤ 2 (Cholestatic)
1st line tests: Acute viral hepatitis serologies, HCV RNA & autoimmune hepatitis serologies: imaging studies (e.g. abdominal ultrasound)	1st line tests: Acute viral hepatitis serologies, HCV RNA & autoimmune hepatitis serologies: imaging studies (e.g. abdominal ultrasound)	1st line tests: imaging studies (abdominal ultrasound) 2nd line tests on a case by case basis: Cholangiography (either endoscopic or MR based), serologies for primary biliary cirrhosis, liver biopsy
2nd line tests on a case by case basis: ceruloplasmin, serologies for less common viruses (HEV, CMV, and EBV), liver biopsy	2nd line tests on a case by case basis: ceruloplasmin, serologies for less common viruses (HEV, CMV, and EBV), liver biopsy	

Assessment of data, causality assessment and diagnosis:
1. Assessment of data:
   a. Completeness: Non-DILI etiologies reasonably excluded
   b. Literature review by use of LiverTox and PubMed
2. Clinical judgement for final DILI diagnosis
3. Expert consultation if doubt persists

Printed with permission: Chalasani, N.P., *et al. Am J Gastroenterol* 2014; 109(7):950-66.

➢ Causation tool: Roussel Uclaf Causality Assessment Method (RUCAM)

  o Tool to help establish the likelihood of DILI

  o Yields score from -9 to +10

  o > 5 is probable

  o Correlation of 0.42 compared to expert opinion

  o Should be used as a guide but not "end all be all"

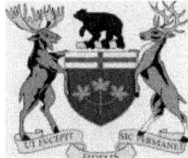

Enzyme pattern	Hepatocellular			Cholestatic or mixed		
Exposure	Initial exposure	Subsequent exposure	Patients	Initial exposure	Subsequent exposure	Patients
o Timing from						
− Drug start	5 – 90 d	1 – 15 d	+2	5 – 90 d	1 – 90 d	+2
	< 5, > 90 d	> 15 d	+1	< 5, > 90 d	> 90 d	+1
− Drug stop	≤ 15 d	≤ 15 d	+1	≤ 30 d	≤ 30 d	+1
Course	Difference between peak ALT and ULN value			Difference between peak AP (or bili) and ULN		
o After drug stop	Decrease ≥ 50% in 8 d		+3	Decrease ≥ 50% in 180 d		+2
	Decrease ≥ 50% in 30 d		+2	Decrease < 50% in 180 d		+1
	Decrease ≥ 50% in >30 d		0	Persistence or increase or no info		0
	Decrease <50% in >30 d		-2			
o Risk factor	Ethanol: yes		+1	Ethanol or pregnancy: yes		+1
	Ethanol: no		0	Ethanol or pregnancy: no		0

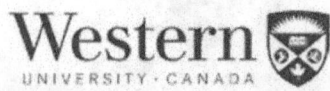

Course	Difference between peak ALT and ULN value		Difference between peak AP (or bili) and ULN	
o Age	≥ 50	+1	≥ 50	+1
	> 50	0	< 50	0
o Other drugs	None or no info	0	None or no info	0
	Drug with suggestive timing	-1	Drug with suggestive timing	-1
	Known hepatotoxin with suggestive timing	-2	Known hepatotoxin w/ suggestive timing	-2
	Drug with other evidence for a role (e.g., + rechallenge)	-3	Drug with other evidence for a role (e.g., + rechallenge)	-3
o Competing causes	All group I[a] and I[b] ruled out	+2	All group I[a] and I[b] rule out	+2
	All group I ruled out	+1	All group I ruled out	+1
	4-5 of group I ruled out	0	4-5 of group I ruled out	0
	< 4 of group I ruled out	-2	< 4 of group I ruled out	-2
	Non-drug cause highly probable	-3	Non-drug cause highly probable	-3

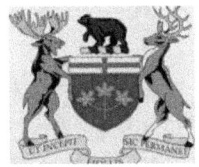

Course	Difference between peak ALT and ULN value		Difference between peak AP (or bili) and ULN	
○ Previous information	Reaction in product label	+2	Reaction in product label	+2
	Reaction, published, no label	+1	Reaction, published, no label	+1
	Reaction unknown	0	Reaction unknown	0
○ Rechallenge	Positive	+3	Positive	+3
	Compatible	+1	Compatible	+1
	Negative	-2	Negative	-2
	Not done or not interpretable	0	Not done or not interpretable	0

Abbreviations: ALT, alanine aminotransferase; AP, alkaline phosphatase; AST, aspartate aminotransferase; D, day; RUCAM, Roussel Uclaf Causality Assessment Method; ULN, upper limit of normal

[a]Group I: HAV, HBV, HCV (acute) biliary obstruction, alcoholism, recent hypotension ("shock liver")

[b]Group II, CMV, EBV, herpes virus infection

Printed with permission: Danan G, et al. *J Clin Epidemiol* 1993; 46: 1323 – 30.

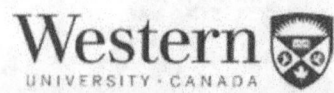

Re–challenge
- o Re–administration of the suspected drug should be avoided due to amnestic response
  - – More rapid, severe injury
- o Desensitization may be undertaken first
- o Only done if there is no suitable alternative drug

➢ Clinicopathological classification
- o Dose–dependent (intrinsic) hepatotoxicity
- o Acute hepatitis
- o Granulomatous hepatitis
- o Chronic hepatitis
- o Acute cholestasis
- o Steatohepatitis
- o Vascular toxicity

➢ Prognosis
- o DILI database
  - – 33% hospitalized
  - – 15% "severe"
  - – 6% died or transplanted
- o Hy Law: for every 10 patients who develop jaundice from DILI, 1 will develop acute liver failure (ALF)
- o Cholestatic disease has better prognosis than hepatocellular
- o If ALF (coagulopathy + encephalopathy) develops
  - – 23% have transplant–free survival
  - – 40% undergo transplantation
  - – UNOS: 7% of indications is idiosyncratic DILI
  - – Prognostic scores of ALF due to DILI are not useful (MELD, APACHE, King's college criteria)

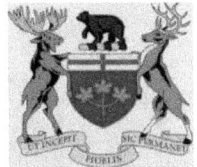

- ➢ Treatment
  - o Remove the offending agent
  - o Exclude other associated liver disorders
  - o Manage complications

- ➢ Long term prognosis
  - o Ensure follow–up of DILI patients
  - o Chronic DILI overlaps with autoimmune hepatitis in ~ 10% of patients
  - o Late cirrhosis is a rare complication of DILI (6%)
  - o DILI in chronic liver disease

- • Drugs that are **relatively contraindicated** and must be used cautiously in patients with liver disease.

o Clonazepam	o Niacin
o Conjugated estrogen and medroxyprogesterone	o Pemoline
o Dantrolene	o Phenelzine
o Felbarnate	o Tacrine (in persons with prior jaundice)
o Gemfibrozil	o Ticlopidine
o Lovastatin and other HMG–CoA reductase inhibitors (statins)	o Tolcapone
o Metformin	o Valproic acid
o Methotrexate	o Zalcitabine
o Naltrexone	

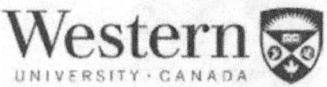

Suggestion from the author: You have better things to do than to memorize this list. In a patient with liver disease, look up this list or look up the dugs to be used.

Adapted from: Gupta, N.K., and Lewis, J.H. *Aliment Pharmacol Ther* 2008; 28(9):1021-41.

- Drugs in lower doses that are recommended in patients with cirrhosis ("**hepatic dosing**").

  - Acetaminophen
  - Benzodiazepines
  - Beta blockers
  - Cetirizine
  - Fluoxetine
  - Indinavir
  - Lamotrigine
  - Losartan
  - Moricizine
  - Narcotics
  - PPIs
  - Repaglinide
  - Risperidone
  - Sertraline
  - Topiramate
  - Tramadol
  - Valproic acid
  - Venlafaxine
  - Verapamil

Adapted from: Gupta, N.K. and Lewis, J.H. *Aliment Pharmacol Ther* 2008; 28(9):1021-41.

- Give the hepatobiliary complications of the **use of oral contraceptive agents** (OCAs).

  - Gallstones
    - Cholestasis
    - Unmasking PBC and other cholestatic diseases

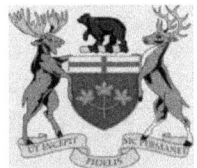

- o Liver
    - – Unmasking porphyria
    - – Tumors
        - ▪ Hepatic adenomas (causative)
        - ▪ ↑ size of FNH (focal nodular hyperplasia)
        - ▪ Hepatocellular carcinoma (rare)
    - – ↑ risk of NASH
    - – Vascular
        - ▪ Budd–Chiari syndrome (hepatic obstruction)
        - ▪ Peliosis hepatis (sinusoidal dilation)

Dose–dependent hepatotoxicity
- o Usually require activation of toxic metabolites
- o Short latency period
- o Examples
    - – Acetaminophen
    - – CAM preparations
    - – Plant and fungal toxins
    - – Methotrexate
    - – Cyclophosphamide
    - – Certain anti–cancer drugs

Acetaminophen
- o Reasons for overdose:
    - – Suicide
    - – Therapeutic misadventure (daily high dose of EtOH misuse)

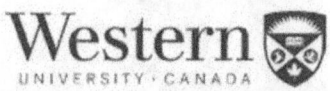

- o Require dose of at least 15 grams but can be as low as 7 grams
- o ↓ toxic threshold that is lowered by:
  - – EtOH
  - – Fasting
  - – Concomitant medication
  - – Induces oxidative metabolism to NAPQI
- o Pathogenesis
  - – Consumption of liver stores of glutathione

➢ Pathology
- o Zone 3 necrosis with minimal inflammation (zone 3 has more CYP2E1 and lower glutathione levels than does zone 1)

Acetaminophen Metabolism

Acetaminophen

Sulfation / Glucuronidation

PAPS

UDP-GA

Detoxification and Elimination

Oxidation CYP450

NAPQI

Glutathione conjugation

Detoxification and Elimination

Interaction with Cellular Macromolecules
TOXICITY

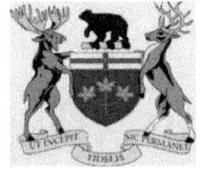

Dose–dependent: Acetaminophen

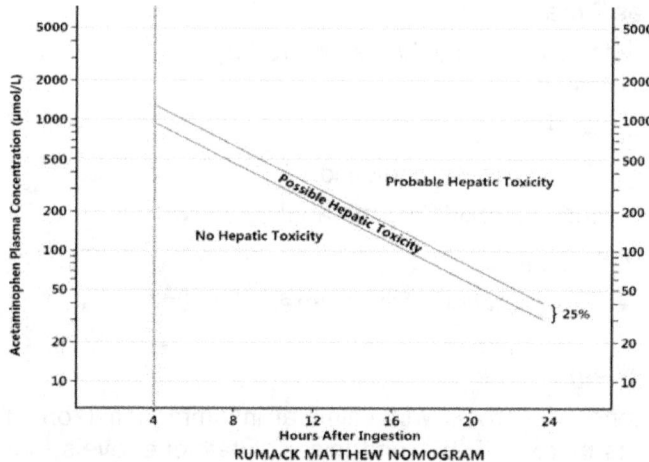

RUMACK MATTHEW NOMOGRAM

Printed with permission: Spiegel, B.M. and Karsan, A.A. Acing the hepatology questions on the GI board exam. Slack Incorporated 2012, Figure 27-1, page 83.

➢ Treatment

• Give the management of patient with acetaminophen (ACM) overdose.

    ○ Suspect acetaminophen overdose if the transaminases are > 1000 IU/mL, and if the serum bilirubin concentrations are normal (in the absence of possible ischemic hepatitis, i.e. hypotension or CV collapse)
       – ABCs
       – Determine the likelihood of hepatotoxicity from nomogram (except in non–intentional cases)
       – Immediately give activated charcoal (1 gm/kg body weight [BW] *po* in a slurry preparation but does not reduce the effect of NAC [N–acetylcysteine]) if presenting within 12 hours
       – Rule out other co–ingestions

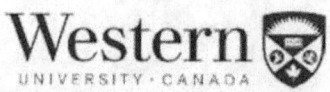

- Serum acetaminophen (ACM) level, urine toxicology screen, LFTs, LEs, INR, arterial lactate
- Stratify the risk for possible need for liver transplantation
- Contact liver transplantation center

CLINICAL PEARL: DILI

The dose of acetaminophen that places the ordinary patient at risk for acute liver failure (ALF) is 8 grams, but the dose level may be lower, especially for smaller patients. It is better to remember the threshold as < 150 mg/kg, rather than 6 – 8 grams.

SO YOU WANT TO BE A HEPATOLOGIST!

A toxic nomogram is available in predicting how long after ingestion will NAC remains effective. The nomogram is **not always strictly followed** because of the relative safety in the use of NAC, and that it may be efficacious even after 48 hours of overdose, or in patients with non–acetaminophen ALF. In addition, the nomogram may have limitations.

• When does the standard acetaminophen toxicity nomogram may not correctly reflect the possible severity of liver disease.

    o Multiple doses of acetaminophen is taken rather than > 4 grams taken at once

    o Unknown time of overdose ingestion

    o Alcoholic patient

    o Fasting patient

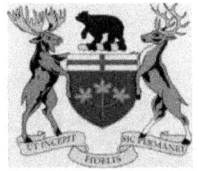

SO YOU WANT TO BE A HEPATOLOGIST!

- Why is drinking alcohol and fasting lower the threshold of acetaminophen hepatotoxicity?

  - Alcohol and fasting → ↑ CYP2E1 expression → ↑ NAPQI (the toxic metabolite) ↓ glutathione stores below a critical level, thereby allowing NAPQI to cause hepatic damage

- Why NAC should be given *po* or IV within 12 – 16 hours of acetaminophen overdose?

  - NAC provides cysteine to stimulate the hepatocytes to synthesize glutathione and to protect against NAPQI

  - After 12 – 16 hours, the NAPQI–associated hepatocyte damage and the cell death pathways cannot be reversed

  - Furthermore, as the hepatocytes are destroyed, there are not enough metabolically healthy cells to convert the cysteine from NAC to glutathione

- If this is true, why is NAC can be given for acetaminophen toxicity even 36 hours after poisoning?

  - NAC will stabilize the vascular reactivity in patients with liver failure, so it may have some benefit beyond the mechanisms of glutathione and NADPQI

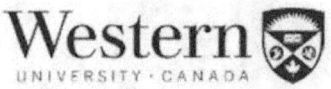

- o **N–acetylcysteine** (NAC), **and other measures**
  - – Oral N–Acetylcysteine (NAC)
    - ▪ Loading dose: 140 mg/kg *po*/NG x 1
    - ▪ 70 mg/kg *q* 4 hours x 17 doses
    - ▪ Stopping rules after 72 hours or when liver chemistry improves
    - ▪ Compazine or Reglan for nausea, *prn*
    - ▪ Cimetidine (P450 inducer)
  - – IV N–Acetylcysteine (NAC)
    - ▪ Dose 1. Loading dose: 140 mg/kg NAC in 200 mL D5W over 1 hr
    - ▪ Dose 2. 50 mg/kg NAC in 500 ml D5W over 4 hr
    - ▪ Dose 3. 125 mg/kg NAC in 1000 ml D5W over 19 hr
    - ▪ Dose 4. 150 mg/kg NAC in 1000 ml D5W over 24 hr
    - ▪ Dose 5. 150 mg/kg NAC in 1000 ml D5W over 24 hr
- o Caution regarding the use of NAC
  - – NAC should be given within 4 hours of overdose, but may still be of value 48 or more hours after ingestion
  - – Do not administer NAC to patients with known sulfa allergy
  - – Administer IV formulation of oral NAC through a leukopore filter in a monitored setting after consent is obtained from the patient or family
  - – IV infusion of NAC leads to anaphylactoid or hypersensitivity reactions in 3 – 5% that is most common during the loading dose
  - – Hold and reduce infusion rate by 50% if rash and nausea occurs; administer fluids, IV benadryl, IV steroids, as needed
  - – For causes of ALF other than acetaminophen, and in patients with stages I or II encephalopathy, NAC may improve outcomes

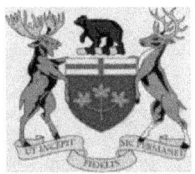

- Give the use of NAC (N–acetylcysteine) in non–acetaminophen ALF.

End points	NAC	No NAC
• Adults		
o Liver transplantation–free survival		
– All patients	40%	27%
– Stages ½ at entry	52%	31%
o MOFS		
– ↑ tissue oxygenation		

- Children

    o ↓ LOS (length of hospital stay)

    o ↑ rate of spontaneous recovery

    o Manage coma (stages III – IV in ALF)
    - Intubation
    - Epidural monitoring of intracerebral pressure (ICP) of < 25 mmHg, and cerebral perfusion pressure of 50 – 80 mmHg
    - 30° elevation of the head of the bed
    - Factor VII or FFP to get INR of < 1.8
    - Mannitol infusion
    - Hypothermia or indomethacin
    - Cultures
    - Antifungal coverage
    - Vasopressors (norepinephrine)
    - To maintain cerebral perfusion pressure of > 50 mmHg, enteral nutrition

    o Psychological assessment of overdose

    o Treat complications if ALF present

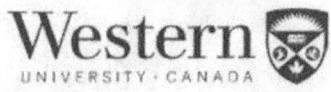

Abbreviations: ALF, acute liver failure; ICP, intracerebral pressure; MOFS, multiple organ failure syndrome

Adapted from: Chun, L.J., *et al. J Clin Gastroenterol* 2009; 43(4):342-9.

Acute Hepatitis

- o Hepatic inflammation with cell death + degeneration
- o Upwards of 50% of reported adverse reactions
- o 2 main theories for all idiosyncratic disorders
  - Metabolic idiosyncrasy
    - Susceptibility of rare individuals to a dose that is safe in majority
    - Acquired or inherited differences in metabolism or excretion
  - Immunoallergy
    - Immunological reaction due to drug causes autoimmune syndrome

Types of drug–induced acute hepatitis: immuno–allergic reaction versus metabolic idiosyncrasy

Characteristic	Immuno–allergic reaction	Metabolic idiosyncrasy
o Frequency	< 1 case per 10,000 patients exposed	1 – 50 cases per 10,000 patients exposed
o Gender predilection	Women often ≥ 2:1	Variable, slightly more common in women
o Latent period to onset	Fairly constant, 2 – 10 weeks	More variable, 2 – 24 weeks, occasionally longer than 1 year
o Relationship to dose	None	Usually none (occasional exceptions)

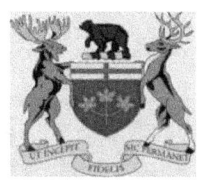

Characteristic	Immuno – allergic reaction	Metabolic idiosyncrasy
o Interaction with other agents	None	Alcohol, occasionally other drugs (i.e. isoniazid with rifampin)
o Course after stopping drugs	Prompt improvement (rare exception, i.e. minocycline)	Variable, occasionally slow improvement or deterioration (i.e. troglitazone)
o Positive rechallenge	Always; often fever within 3 days	Usual (in 2/3 of cases), abnormal liver biochemical test levels in 2 – 21 days
o Fever	Usual; often initial symptoms, part of prodrome	Infrequent, less prominent
o Extrahepatic features (rash, lymph-adenopathy)	Common	Rare
o Eosinophilia		
– Blood	33 – 67% of cases	< 10% of cases
– Tissue	Usual, pronounced	Common but mild
o Autoantibodies	Often present	Rarely present
o Examples	Nitrofurantoin, phenytoin, methyldopa, sulfonamides	Isoniazid, pyrazinamide, ketoconazole, dantrolene, troglitazone

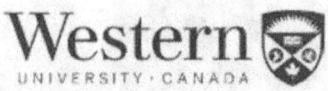

Granulomatous Hepatitis

➢ Definition

- o Drugs account for 2 – 29% of cases

➢ Differentials

- o Sarcoid
- o PBC
- o TB
- o Q fever
- o Malignancy

➢ Clinical

- o Symptoms include fever and systemic complaints within 6 months of treatment

➢ Laboratory

- o Liver biochemistry is mixed due to infiltrative nature

➢ Causative agents

- o Allopurinol
- o Carbamazepine
- o Hydralazine
- o Quinine

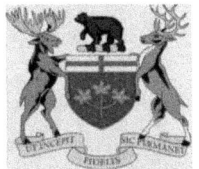

Chronic Hepatitis

- ➤ Definition
  - o Hepatitis that continues for more than 6 months

- ➤ Pathology
  - o Histology includes periportal inflammation, bridging necrosis and fibrosis

- ➤ Causes
  - o Drugs are an extremely uncommon cause (many cases have turned out to be viral in review)

- ➤ Types
  - o Chronic toxicity
    - Late realization of DILI
  - o Autoimmune
    - May respond to steroids

- ➤ Treatment
  - o Withdrawal of offending medication
  - o No approved "antidote"
  - o Treat the symptoms, i.e. pruritus
  - o No major studies conducted with the following:
    - Corticosteroids
    - Ursodeoxycholic acid (UDCA)
    - N–acetylcysteine

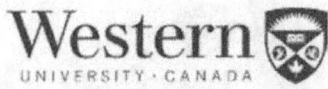

Acute Cholestasis

➢ Causes

- o OCPs are cause
  - – Cholestasis of pregnancy is RF
- o Anabolic steroids

➢ Pathology

- o Bile duct injury
- o Bile retained in canaliculi, Kupffer cells and hepatocytes
- o Minimal inflammation

Steatohepatitis

➢ Causes

- o Amiodarone
  - – Steatohepatitis is the most common liver injury
  - – Ongoing injury despite discontinuation due to stores
  - – Lag time of 1 year until the disease is present
- o Tamoxifen
  - – One of the many possible presentations
  - – Plays synergistic role with traditional risk factors

Vascular Toxicity

➢ Syndromes

- o Sinusoidal obstruction syndrome (SOS)
- o Non–cirrhotic portal hypertension (NC–PHT)
- o Nodular regenerative hyperplasia (NRH)
- o Peliosis hepatis (dilation and destruction of sinusoids)

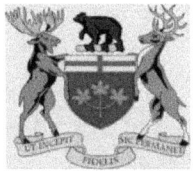

N–acetylcysteine

- o Non–tylenol ALF (INR > 1.5 and encephalopathy within 24 weeks duration) randomized to NAC or placebo

- o No difference in transplant–free survival at 3 months

- o Patients with encephalopathy grade I or II have higher transplant–free survival with NAC 52% *vs* 30%

- o DILI patients were a subgroup of this study (N = 42)
  - Transplant–free survival was 58% *vs* 27%

- o May behave differently in children

- o Those with CLD may be more susceptible to DILI
  - ↑ risk in methotrexate
  - Tamoxifen

- o Statins should not be avoided

- o Main issue is to distinguish DILI from flares of the underlying disease

Lee, W.M., *et al. Gastroenterology* 2009, 137(3): 856-64.

Suggested Reading

Chalasani, N.P., *et al.* ACG clinical guideline: The diagnosis and management of idiosyncratic drug-induced liver injury. *Am J Gastroenterol* 2014; 109(7):950-66.

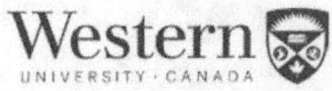

HBV Reactivation during Immunosuppression

Mohammed Aljawad

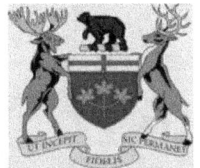

HBV Reactivation

- ➢ Definition
  - o Loss of HBV immune control in patient with inactive or "resolved" HBV infection
  - o Abrupt reappearance or increase in viral replication with liver damage occurring during and/or following immune reconstitution

- ➢ Clinically
  - o Range from subclinical to severe or fatal hepatitis
  - o Rise in HBV DNA ± return of HBeAg
  - o ALT increase (may be mild or very dramatic)
  - o May progress to liver failure and death despite antiviral therapy

Hoofnagle, J.H. *Hepatology*. 2009; 49(5 suppl):S156-S165.

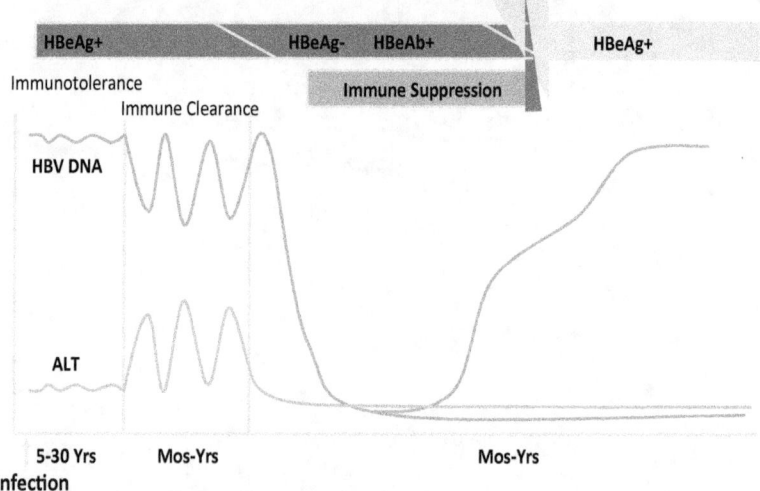

Printed with permission: Yim, H.J., *et al. Hepatology*. 2006; 43:S173-S181.

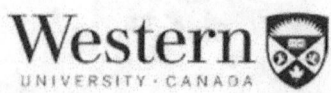

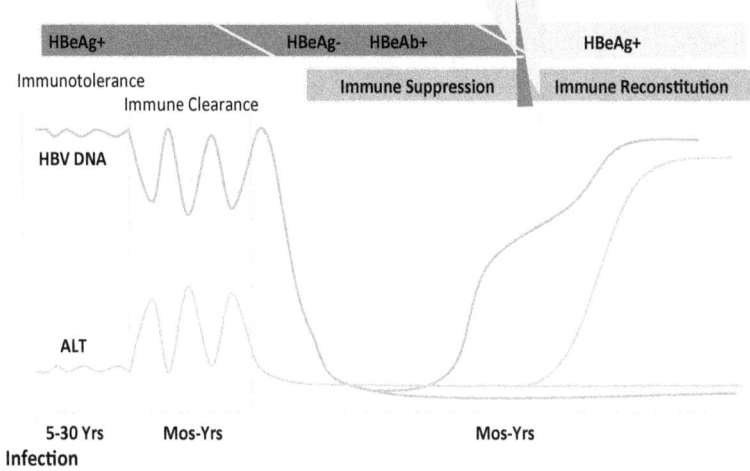

Printed with permission: Yim, H.J., *et al. Hepatology*. 2006; 43:S173-S181.

Different Causes and Forms of HBV Reactivation

- o Spontaneous
- o Progressive immunodeficiency (HIV infection)
- o Sudden withdrawal of antiviral therapy
- o Cancer chemotherapy
- o Immunosuppressive for autoimmune or allergic conditions
- o Solid organ transplantation (kidney, heart, lung)
- o Liver transplantation (reactivation in graft)
- o Bone marrow transplantation

Printed with permission: Hoofnagle, J.H. *Hepatology*. 2009; 49(5 suppl):S156-S165.

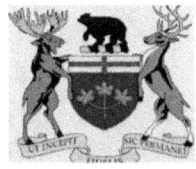

Three Phases of HBV Reactivation

Phases	Features	Diagnostic markers	Comments
1	Increase in viral replication	HBV DNA HBeAg HBsAg	Rise of > 1 log IU/mL In HBeAg negative Reverse seroconversion
2	Appearance of disease activity	ALT Symptoms Jaundice	Rise of > 3x baseline Indicative of more severe injury
3	Recovery	HBV DNA ALT HBsAg	Fall to baseline values Fall to baseline values May be cleared late

Printed with permission: Hoofnagle, J.H. *Hepatology.* 2009; 49(5 suppl):S156-S165.

> Risk of Reactivation
>   o HBV status
>   – HBsAg carrier: HBsAg(+)/HBcAb(+)
>   – Resolved infection (occult): HbsAg(–)/HbcAb(+)
>   – HBV DNA level
>   – HBeAg
>   – HBs Ab
>
>   o Type of immunosuppression

- Azathioprine
  o No reports of HBV reactivation with imuran monotherapy
  o Low risk

- Methotrexate
  o Only small number of case reports
  o Low risk

- Corticosteroids
  o Investigated in the past as any of the following:
    – Anti–inflammatory for chronic hepatitis
    – Priming agent prior to starting antiviral therapy

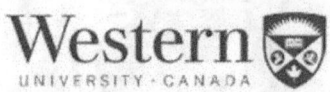

o Cummulative data
  – High risk of reactivation
  – Worsened histopathology

o Steroids increase the risk of HBV reactivation
  – 50 patients with NHL and HBsAg positive were randomized to epirubicin, cyclophosphamide and etoposide (ACE) ± prednisolone (P)
  – Prednisolone increased the risk and severity of HBV reactivation but tend toward improved NHL outcome

- Anti–TNF drugs
  o Systematic analysis of cases

	HBsAg+	HbcAb+
– No of patients (257)	89	168
– Reactivation	35 (39%)	9 (5%)
– Outcome	5 Acute liver failure	1 Death
	1 Death	

- Chemotherapy

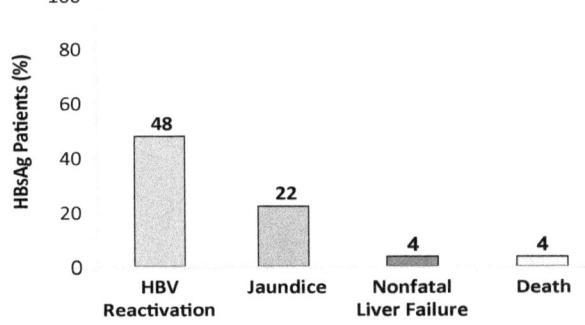

Adapted from: Lok, A.S., *et al. Gastroenterology* 1991; 100:182-8.

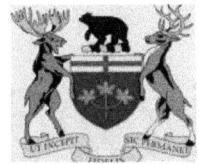

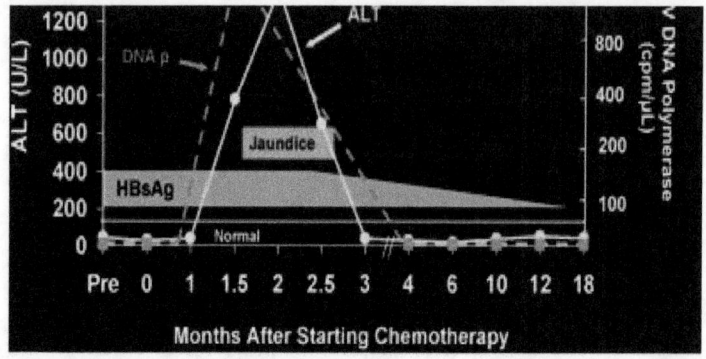

Printed with permission: Hoofnagle, J.H. *Hepatology.* 2009; 49(5 suppl):S156-S165.

- o Anti–CD20 Rituximab
    - – Complete depletion of B–cells
    - – Profound effects on antibody production
    - – Loss of HBsAb
    - – Reactivation can occur 12 months after discontinuation
- o HBV Reactivation With Rituximab in HBsAg Individuals
    - – Patients with diffuse large B–cell lymphoma
        - ▪ HBsAg-/HBc Ab+

Rituximab in HBcAb+

Studies	Estimate	(95% CI)	Reactivation rate
Yeo, 2009	0.238	(0.11, 0.512)	5/21
Matsue, 2010	0.089	(0.039, 0.206)	5/56
Koo, 2011	0.032	(0.008, 0.126)	2/62
Cheung, 2011	0.250	(0.046, 1.365)	¼
Hsu, 2013	0.189	(0.134, 0.265)	27/143
Huang, 2013	0.179	(0.092, 0.351)	7/39
Overall (I^2 = 46%, P = 0.097)	0.169	(0.131, 0.219)	47/325

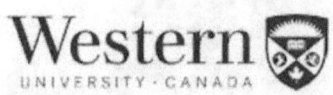

Reactivation rate 17%

Abbreviations: CI, confidence interval

- o Protective role for HBsAb
  - – 29 patients with Lymphoma given R–CHOP

HBsAb	< 100	> 100
Number	19	10
Loss of Ab	8	0
Reactivation	1	0

Pei, S.N., *et al. Ann Hematol* 2012; 91:1007–1012.

- – Retrospective study
  - ▪ 150 patients with HBcAb treated with Rituximab
- – Reactivation
  - ▪ HBs Ab+ : 0 of 104
  - ▪ HBs Ab- : 4 of 46

- ➢ Screening
  - o All patients undergoing chemotherapy or immunosuppressive therapy
  - o HBsAg should be tested in all individuals, with follow–up HBV DNA in HBsAg–positive patients
  - o Role of anti–HBc testing is less clear; recommendations from various societies are mixed
    - – EASL: HBsAg and anti–HBc
    - – AASLD: HBsAg and anti–HBc
    - – CASL: HBsAg
    - – ASCO: consider HBsAg alone
  - o How are we doing
    - – Self–reported or chart review of actual screening
  - o Few oncologists routinely screen all patients initiating chemotherapy for HBV

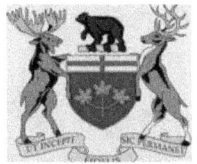

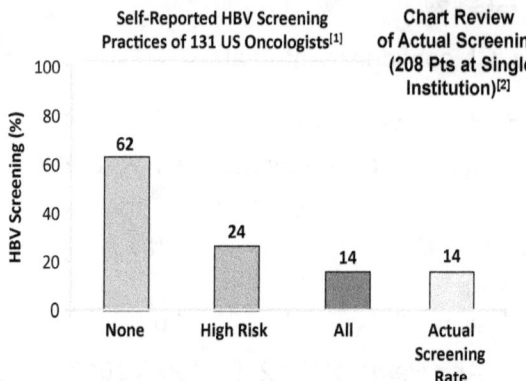

Adapted from: Khokhar, O.S., *et al.* Chemotherapy. 2009; 55:69-75.; Lee, R., *et al. Curr Oncol.* 2010; 17:32-8.

Speciality	Screening
– Oncologists	20 – 40 %
– Dermatologists	40 %
– Rheumatologists	70 %
– Gastroenterologists	unknown

- ○ Preemptive *vs* On–Demand
  - HBsAg–positive patients with lymphoma treated with high–dose chemotherapy randomized to "preemptive" *vs* "on–demand" lamivudine

- ○ 36 wk survival free from hepatitis due to HBV reactivation
  - Preemptive LAM (~ 100%)
  - On–demand LAM (if HBV DNA increased) (~ 28%)

Lau, G.K., *et al. Gastroenterology.* 2003; 125:1742-9.

- ○ HBsAg–positive patients with NHL treated with CHOP were randomized to "preemptive" *vs* "on–demand" lamivudine

- ○ Preemptive antivirals decrease the HBV reactivation from 48 – 8%

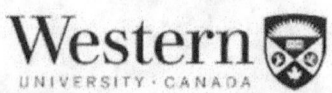

AASLD/EASL Guidelines 2008

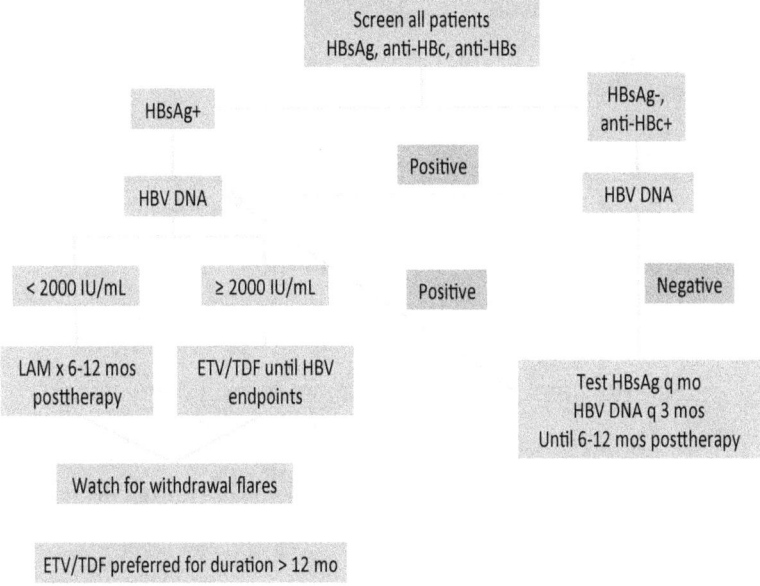

- o In HBcAb+ patients, some experts recommend prophylaxis with lamivudine in patients who receive rituximab
  - − If they are anti–HBs negative and/or
  - − If close monitoring of HBV DNA is not guaranteed
- o Prophylaxis is also recommended in patients receiving bone marrow or stem cell transplantation
- o The optimal duration of prophylaxis for these indications is not known

Hsu, C., *et al. Hepatology.* 2008; 47:844-53.

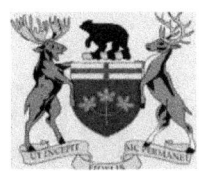

AGA 2015 Guidelines

➢ Risk of reactivation

- High risk
  - Risk of reactivation > 10 %

HBV Status	Immunosuppressive therapy
– HBsAg Carrier	B–cell depleting agent
– HBcAb	Rituximab
– HBsAg Carrier	Anthracycline derivatives doxorubicin, epirubicin
– HBsAg Carrier	Moderate to high dose steroid for more than 4 weeks

AGA recommends antiviral prophylaxis *vs* no prophylaxis

- Moderate risk
  - Risk of reactivation > 1 – 10 %

– HBsAg Carrier – HBcAb	Anti–TNF
– HBsAg Carrier – HBcAb	Cytokine or integrin inhibitors
– HBsAg Carrier – HBcAb	Tyrosine kinase inhibitors
– HBsAg Carrier	Low dose (<10 mg prednisone) ≥ 14 weeks
– HBcAb	Moderate to high dose steroid for more than 4 weeks
– HBsAg Carrier – HBcAb	Anthracycline derivatives doxorubicin, epirubicin

AGA recommends antiviral prophylaxis rather than monitoring

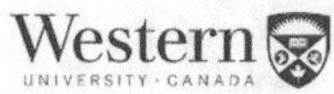

- Low Risk
  - Risk of reactivation < 1 %

– HBsAg Carrier	Traditional immunosuppressive agents
– HBcAb	
	Azathioprine, methotrexate
– HBsAg Carrier	Intra–articular corticosteroids
– HBcAb	
– HBsAg Carrier	Any dose of oral corticosteroids daily for ≤ 1 week
– HBcAb	
– HBcAb	Low dose (< 10 mg prednisone) for ≥ 4 weeks

AGA recommends against routinely using antiviral prophylaxis

"The pain, you feel today, is the strength you feel tomorrow. For every challenge encountered, there is opportunity for growth."

Unknown

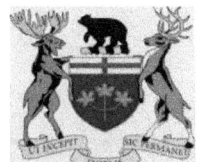

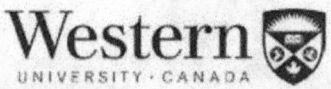

Cirrhotic *Versus* Non–Cirrhotic Portal Hypertension

Almotasem Rammal

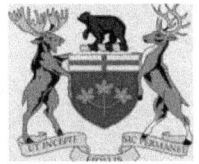

Portal Hypertension

➢ Definition

  ○ A clinical syndrome defined by a portal venous pressure gradient between the portal vein (PV) and the inferior vena cava exceeding 5 mmHg

➢ Types

  ○ Pre–hepatic

FHVP	N
RAP	N
WHVP	N
HVPG	N
PVP	↑
ISP	↑

  ○ Hepatic

FHVP	N
RAP	N
WHVP	↑
HVPG	N/↑
PVP	↑
ISP	↑

  ○ Post–hepatic

FHVP	↑
RAP	N/↑
WHVP	↑
HVPG	N/↑
PVP	↑
ISP	↑

  ○ Cirrhotic portal hypertension (CPH)
    – ↑ hepatic venous pressure gradient (HVPG) predominantly due to raised sinusoidal resistance

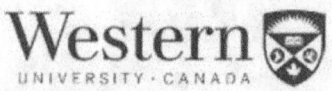

- o Non–cirrhotic portal hypertension (NCPH)
  - − HVPG is normal or only mildly ↑
  - − HPV < PV pressure
- o NCPH are most of the time is vascular in nature
- o In NCPH, liver functions are mostly normal

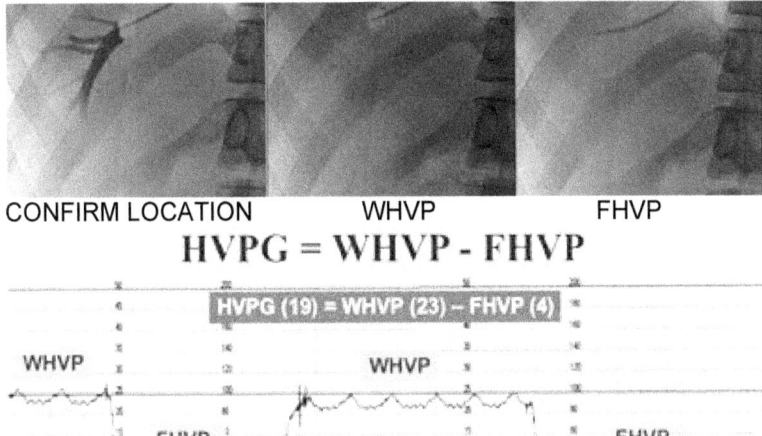

CONFIRM LOCATION   WHVP   FHVP

$$HVPG = WHVP - FHVP$$

Abbreviations: FHVP, free hepatic venous pressure; HVPG, hepatic venous pressure gradient; ISP, intrasplenic pressure; PVP, portal venous pressure; RAP, right atrial pressure; WHVP, wedged hepatic venous pressure

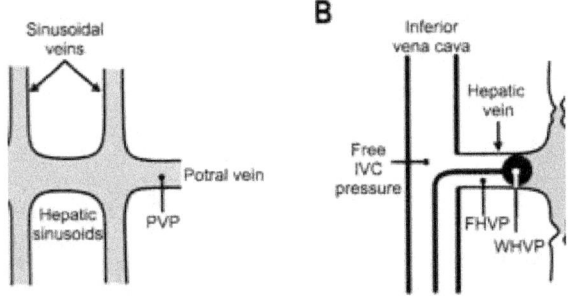

Abbreviations: FHVP, free hepatic venous pressure; IVC, inferior vena cava; PVP, portal vein pressure; WHVP, wedged hepatic venous pressure

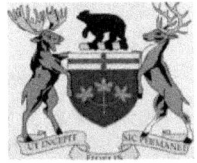

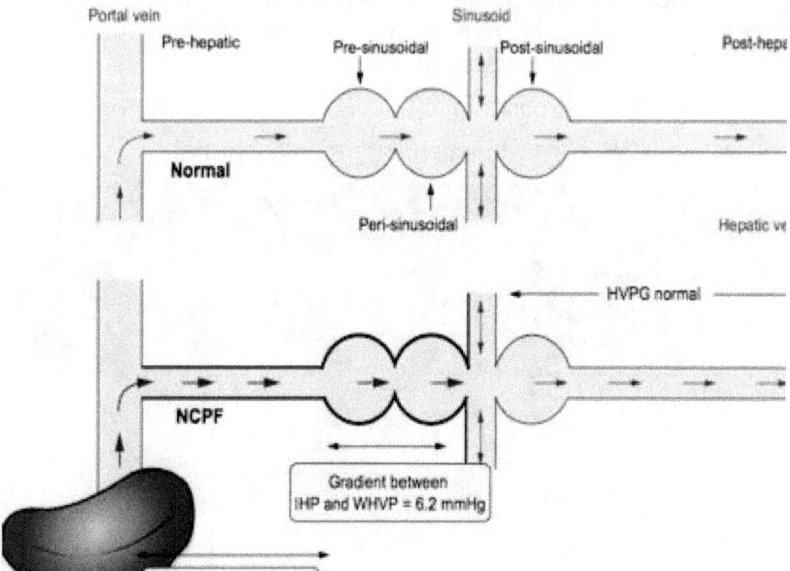

Adapted from: Khanna, R. and Sarin, S.K. *J Hepatol* 2014; 60(2):421-41.

➢ Laboratory

	Pre–hepatic	Hepatic	Post–hepatic
FHVP	N	N	↑
RAP	N	N	N/↑
WHVP	N	↑	↑
HVPG	N	N/↑	N/↑
PVP	↑	↑	↑
ISP	↑	↑	↑

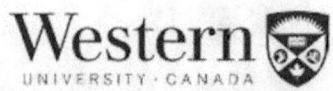

➤ **Endoscopic findings**

   o In NCPG, esophageal or gastric or anorectal varices in NCPH are characterized by:

      – Larger than in cirrhotic portal hypertension

      – Less common portal hypertensive gastropathy (PHG)

➤ **Causes and associations**

Pre–hepatic

o FHVP normal, RAP normal, WHVP normal, HVPG normal, PVP high, ISP high

o Extrahepatic portal vein obstruction (EHPVO)

o Portal vein thrombosis

o Splenic thrombosis

o Splanchnic arteriovenous fistula

o Massive splenomegaly
    – Infiltrative diseases – lymphoma, myeloproliferative disorders
    – Storage diseases – Gaucher disease

Hepatic*

FHVP normal, RAP normal, WHVP high, HVPG normal or high, PVP high, ISP high*

Pre–sinusoidal	Sinusoidal	Post–sinusoidal
o Developmental abnormalities – Acute polycystic disease – Hereditary hemorrhagic disease – Arteriovenous fistulae – Congenital hepatic fibrosis o Biliary disease – Primary biliary cirrhosis – Sclerosing cholangitis – Autoimmune cholangitis – Toxin: vinyl chloride o Neoplastic occlusion of portal vein – Lymphoma – Epithelioid hemangioendothelioma – Epithelial malignancies – Chronic lymphocytic leukemia	o Sinusoidal fibrosis – Alcoholic hepatitis – Drug (methotrexate, amiodarone) – Toxins (vinyl chloride, copper) – Metabolic (NASH, Gaucher's disease) – Inflammatory (viral hepatitis, Q fever, healed cytomegalovirus, secondary syphilis) o Sinusoidal collapse – Acute necro–inflammatory disease o Sinusoidal defenestration – Alcoholic liver disease (early phase)	o Veno–occlusive disease – Hepatic irradiation – Toxins: pyrrolizidine alkaloids – Drugs: gemtuzumab ozogamicin, actinomycin D, dacarbazine, cytosine, arabinoside, mithramycin, 6–thioguanine, azathioprine, cyclophosphamide o Phlebosclerosis of hepatic veins – Alcoholic liver disease – Chronic radiation injury – Hypervitaminosis A – E–fenol injury

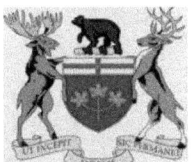

Pre–sinusoidal	Sinusoidal	Post–sinusoidal

o Granulomatous lesions
  – Schistosomiasis
  – Mineral oil granuloma
  – Sarcoidosis
 	
o Hepatoportal sclerosis
 	
o Pliosis hepatis
 	
o Partial nodular transformation
 	
o Non–cirrhotic portal fibrosis (NCPF)
 	
o Idiopathic portal hypertension
	o Sinusoidal infiltration
	  – Mastocytosis
	  – Agnogenic myeloid metaplasia
	  – Gaucher's disease
	  – Amyloidosis
	
	o Sinusoidal compression
	  – By enlarged Kupffer cells (Gaucher's disease, visceral leishmaniasis)
	  – By enlarged fat–laden hepatocytes (alcoholic hepatitis, AFLP)
		o Primary vascular malignancies
		  – Epithelioid hemangioendothelioma
		  – Angiosarcoma
		
		o Granulomatous phlebitis
		  – Sarcoidosis
		  – *Mycobacterium* species
		  – Lipogranulomas
		  – Mineral oil granuloma
		
		o Hepatic vein outflow tract obstruction (HVOTO, Budd–Chiari syndrome) – idiopathic prothrombotic states

Post–hepatic

o FHVP high, RAP normal or high, WHVP high, HVPG normal or high, PVP high, ISP high**

o Inferior vena caval obstruction: webs, thrombosis, tumor, enlarged caudate lobe

o Constrictive regurgitation

o Severe right–sided heart failure

o Restrictive cardiomyopathy

*HVPG is not feasible in HVOTO with occlusion of all 3 hepatic veins or in the supra– and intra–hepatic inferior vena caval obstruction

**Inferior vena cava pressure should also be taken both above and below the opening of the hepatic veins

Abbreviations: AFLP, acute fatty liver of pregnancy; FHVP, free hepatic venous pressure; HVPG, hepatic venous pressure gradient (difference between FHVP and WHVP); ISP, intrasplenic pressure; NASH, non–alcoholic steatohepatitis; PVP, portal vein pressure; RAP, right atrial pressure; WHVP, wedged hepatic venous pressure

Adapted from: Khanna, R. and Sarin, S.K. *J Hepatol* 2014; 60(2):421-41.

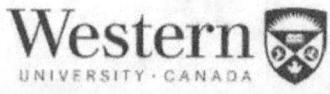

➢ Physiology

- o After a meal, portal blood flow ↑ with no ↑ in portal pressure because hepatic sinusoids have:
  - – High
    - Compliance
    - Accommodation
  - – Low
    - Resistance

- o Blood supply to the liver are as follows:
  - – 70% portal vein (PV, blood from the mesenteric circulation)
  - – 30% hepatic artery (HA, blood from celiac artery)

- o When blood flow ↑ in the PV, it ↓ in the AA, and vice versa, through an autoregulatory mechanism of the dual blood supply (portal venous inflow) to the liver
  - – 3 distinct vascular beds:
    - Intrahepatic
    - Splanchnic
    - Systemic

➢ Pathophysiology

- • Explain the pathogenesis of portal hypertension hyperdynamic circulation – systemic and splanchnic vasodilation.

- o Basic factors
  - – ↑ systemic sympathetic activity
  - – ↑ resistance
  - – ↑ flow in a hyperdynamic circulatory state
  - – ↑ collaterals (↑ angiogenesis)
  - – ↓ fenestration
  - – Ohm's law
    $$\Delta P = F \times R$$
    F, flow; ΔP, change in pressure; R, resistance
  - – ↑ portal flow and resistance

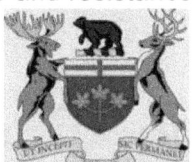

- Mechanical factors
- Regenerative nodules
- Fibrotic bands
- Defenestration and capillarization of sinusoids
- Swelling of hepatocytes and Kupffer cells
- Vascular factors
- Intrahepatic vasoconstriction and ↓ response to vasodilations

o Hepatic vasoconstriction (splanchnic vascular bed → ↑ increased intrahepatic resistance
  - Hepatic vasoconstriction
  - Law of poiseuille $R = 8 \eta L / \P r^4$
  - Resistance (R) is affected by the length and radius (r) of the vessel and by the viscosity of the blood
  - Early manisfestations:
    - ↑ nitric oxide (NO)
    - ↑ sheer stress on sinusoids
    - ↑ eNOS → NO (nitric oxide) → intrahepatic vasodilation
    - ↑ ET–1 (endothelin–1) → binds to:
      - ET–A receptors on HSC → ↑ HSC contraction → intrahepatic vasoconstriction
      - Binds to ET–B receptors on endothelial cells → activates eNOS → vasodilation
    - In cirrhosis, there may be ↑ NO production
    - In splanchnic endothelial cells from ↑ sheer stress, ↑ cytokines and ↑ phosphorylation of eNOS leading to vasodilation in splanchnic and systemic vascular beds (note below that there is ↓ intrahepatic NO, ↓ intrahepatic vasodilation and ↑ intrahepatic vasoconstriction)

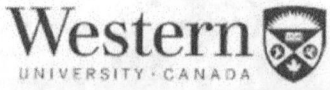

- Late (cirrhosis)
  - ↓ production of NO
  - ↓ activation of eNOS protein in endothelial cells
  - ↑ caveolin–1 (an eNOS inhibiting protein)
  - ↓ AKT (protein kinase B)
  - Phosphorylation of eNOS
  - ↑ GRK (G protein–coupled receptor kinase, which inhibits eNOS)
  - ↑ VEGF (vascular endothelial growth factor) from shear stress may ↑ eNOS (VEGF is a NO stimulatory growth factor)

- Give the components of each of the vasodilating and vasoconstricting systems involved in the **disturbed hemodynamics** in cirrhosis.

➢ Vasodilator systems

- Adenosine
- Adrenomedullin
- Arterial natriuretic peptide (ANP)
- Bradykinin
- Brain natriuretic peptide (BNP)
- Calcitonin gene–related peptide (CGRP)
- Carbon monoxide (CO)
- Endocannabinoids
- Endothelin–3 (ET–3)
- Endotoxin
- Enkephalins
- Glucagon
- Histamine
- Hydrogen sulphide
- Interleukins
- Natriuretic peptide of type C (CNP)
- Nitric oxide (NO)
- Prostacyclin (PGI$_2$)
- Substance P
- Tumor necrosis factor–α (TNF–α)
- Vasoactive intestinal polypeptide (VIP)

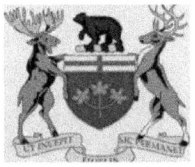

➤ Vasoconstrictor systems
   o Adrenaline and noradrenaline
   o Angiotensin II
   o Endothelin–1 (ET–1)
   o Neuropeptide Y
   o Renin–angiotensin–aldosterone system (RAAS)
   o Sympathetic nervous system (SNS)
   o Vasopressin (anti–diuretic hormone [ADH])

Printed with permission: Møller, S. and Henriksen, J.H. *Gut* 2008; 58: page 271.

   o **Vasodilation in splanchnic and systemic** (peripheral) vascular beds lead to the following:
      – ↑ cardiac output
      – ↓ mean arterial pressure
      – ↑ systemic blood flow into the splanchnic circulation
      – Overall effect is ↓ intrahepatic NO and ↓ intrahepatic vasodilation (effects on endothelial cells, as well, as possibly on HSCs)
      – ↓ intrahepatic vasodilation results in ↑ intrahepatic vasoconstriction
      – ↑ intrahepatic vasoconstriction leads to ↑↑ intrahepatic resistance (law of Poiseuille)

• Giving nitric oxide (NO) in cirrhotics will restore the intrahepatic vasodilation arising from the endothelial cells, but the HSC in cirrhosis contribute to the vasoconstriction and are less responsive to NO. Replacement in cirrhosis, as a benefit of restoring ↓ NO levels, does not fully restore the vessel diameter to normal.

   o In cirrhosis, there is ↑ intestinal endotoxin (LPS) → ↑ TGF–β, ↑ ET–1, with binding to ET–A receptors on HSC and intrahepatic vasoconstriction

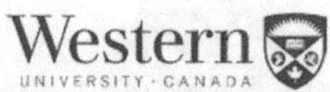

- o ↑ sympathetic activity (norepinephrine)
  - Will also act as an intrahepatic vasoconstrictor
  - Angiotension
  - Leukotrienes
  - Thromboxane
- o Hyperdynamic circulation

- Explain the pathophysiological components producing the hyperdynamic circulation and cardiovascular dysfunction in patients with cirrhosis.
  - o Peripheral and splanchnic arterial vasodilatation
    - Baroreceptor–induced increase in heart rate
  - o Autonomic dysfunction
    - Increased sympathetic nervous activity
    - Vagal impairment
  - o Alterations in cardiac preload
    - Increased portosystemic shunting
    - Increased blood volume
    - Effects of posture
    - Decreased blood viscosity
  - o Alterations in oxygen exchange
    - Anemia
    - Hypoxemia
    - Hepatopulmonary syndrome
    - Portopulmonary hypertension

Printed with permission: Møller, S. and Henriksen, J.H. *Gut* 2008; 58:271.

- o Collateral Circulation
  - As the portal pressure increases
    - There is ↑ flow of blood into the portal vein → systemic collateral circulation increase
    - Direction of blood flow reverses

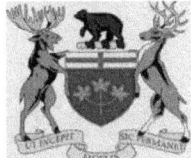

- Blood flows abnormally from the portal circulation into the venous component of the systemic system

- In portal hypertension (PHT) and hepatic cirrhosis, define "hepatofugal" blood flow.

  o When the HVPG (hepatic venous portal gradient) is > 12 mmHg, blood flows backwards up into the esophageal vein, and from there, into the portal vein

- Give the circumstance when splenectomy is not curative for SVT.

  o An SVT combined with portal vein thrombosis (PVT) canot be cured by splenectomy.

- Give the sites of communication of the portal to the systemic circulation develop in portal hypertension. Name the involved and connected blood vessels in this abnormal flow.

Sites	Vessel(s)
o Rectum	Inferior mesenteric vein → pudendal vein
o Umbilicus	Umbilical vein → left portal vein
o Retroperitoneum (in women)	Ovarian vessels → iliac veins
o Gastroespohageal area	Hepatic venous pressure gradient - > 10 mmHg for collaterals to develop - > 12 mmHg for esophageal varices to bleed - > 16 mmHg for gastric varices to bleed Most common site of bleeding, palisade zone, do not drain to periesophageal veins, and from there to the azygous system

Printed with permission: Møller, S. and Henriksen, J.H. *Gut* 2008; 58:271.

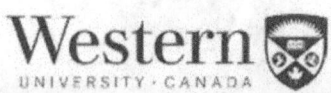

➢ Causes and associations

- **Classify** the causes of portal hypertension based on the site of increased resistance to portal blood flow.
  - ○ Prehepatic
  - ○ Intrahepatic
    - – Presinusoidal
    - – Sinusoidal
    - – Post–sinusoidal
  - ○ Post–hepatic

- Give the anatomical site with increased resistance when liver disease is associated with ↑ portal pressure (PP) and HVPG is normal.
  - ○ There will be ↑ PP but normal HVG when the site of increased resistance is presinusoidal.

- Give the causes of liver disease in which there may be **portal hypertension without cirrhosis**, due to a presinusoidal component of the intrahepatic disease.
  - ○ Alcoholic liver disease (ALD) presinusoidal perivenular lesions
  - ○ Autoimmune hepatitis (AIH)
  - ○ Primary biliary cirrhosis PBC)
  - ○ Hereditary hemochromatosis HH)
  - ○ Schistosomiasis (*S. mansoni, S. japonicum*)
    - – Presinusoidal granulomas
    - – Inflammation
    - – Periportal fibrosis
  - ○ Sarcoidosis (early disease; later the site of ↑ intrahepatic resistance is postsinusoidal)
  - ○ 1° or 2° liver malignancy

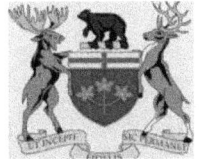

➢ Causes of non–cirrhotic portal hypertension

- Pre–hepatic
  - Extrahepatic portal vein obstruction (EHPVO)
    - Portal vein thrombosis
    - Splenic vein thrombosis
  - Massive splenomegaly
  - Infiltrative diseases, i.e. Lymphoma
    - Myeloproliferative disorders

- Post–hepatic
  - Inferior vena caval (IVC) obstruction, thrombosis, tumor
  - Constrictive pericarditis
  - Tricuspid regurgitation
  - Severe right–sided heart failure
  - Restrictive cardiomyopathy

- Presinusoidal
  - Non–cirrhotic portal fibrosis (NCPF) and idiopathic portal hypertension (IPH)
  - Hepatoportal sclerosis
  - Congenital hepatic fibrosis
  - Vinyl chloride, azathioprine hepatotoxicity
  - Schistosomal portal hypertension

- Sinusoidal
  - Alcoholic hepatitis
  - Hypervitaminosis A
  - Incomplete septal fibrosis
  - Nodular regenerative hyperplasia
  - Methotrexate hepatotoxicity

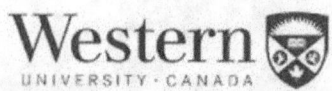

- Post–sinusoidal:
  - Veno–occlusive disease
  - Hepatic vein thrombosis (BCS)

Portal Vein Thrombosis (PVT)

- ➤ Pathogenesis
  - Obstruction of portal vessels and sinusoids
  - Vessel wall injury
  - ↓ blood flow
  - Venous stasis

- ➤ Types of disorders
  - Hepato–portal sclerosis
  - Incomplete fibrotic septa
  - Nodular regenerative hyperplasia
  - Perisinosoidal fibrosis
  - Sinusoidal obstruction syndrome

- ➤ Causes and associations
- Early
  - Infections
    - Acute appendicitis
    - Cholangitis
    - Schistosomiasis
  - Immune
    - Systemic lupus erythematosis (SLE)
  - Infiltration
    - Myeloproliferative disorder (MPD)
    - Infiltration

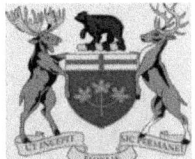

- o Iatrogenic
  - – Drugs, toxins
- o Thrombophilia
  - – Drugs, toxins
- Later
  - o Cavernous transformation of portal vein (formation of multiple periportal venous channels)
  - o Portal vein thrombi extension into the splanchnic circulation
  - o Hypercoagulable states
    - – Anti–phospholipid syndrome
    - – Anti–thrombin deficiency
    - – Factor V Leiden mutation
    - – Methylenetetrahydrofolate reductase mutation TT677
    - – Myeloproliferative disorders
    - – Nephrotic syndrome
    - – Oral contraceptives
    - – Paroxysmal nocturnal hemoglobinuria
    - – Polycythemia rubra vera
    - – Pregnancy
    - – Prothrombin mutation G20210A
    - – Protein C deficiency
    - – Protein S deficiency
    - – Sickle cell disease
  - o Impaired portal vein flow
    - – Budd–Chiari syndrome
    - – Cirrhosis
    - – Nodular regenerative hyperplasia
    - – Sinusoidal obstruction syndrome
  - o Inflammatory diseases
    - – Umbilical vein (infants)
    - – Behçet syndrome

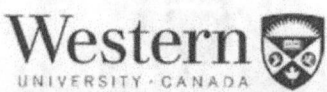

- – Inflammatory bowel disease
- – Pancreatitis

- o Infections
  - – Appendicitis
  - – Cholangitis
  - – Cholecystitis
  - – Diverticulitis
  - – Liver abscess

- o Intra–abdominal cancer
  - – Pancreas
  - – Cholangiocarcinoma
  - – HCC
  - – Bladder cancer

- o Intra–abdominal procedures
  - – Alcohol injection
  - – Abdominal surgery
  - – Colectomy
  - – Fundoplication
  - – Gastric banding
  - – Hepatic chemoembolization
  - – Hepatobiliary surgery
  - – Islet cell injection
  - – Liver transplantation
  - – Peritoneal dialysis
  - – Radiofrequency ablation of hepatic tumor(s)
  - – Sclerotherapy of esophageal varices
  - – Splenectomy
  - – TIPS procedure
  - – Umbilical vein catheterization

Adapted from: Valla, D. C. *Sleisenger & Fordtran's Gastrointestinal and Liver Disease: Pathophysiology/ Diagnosis/Management.* 10th Ed. 2016: page 11397.

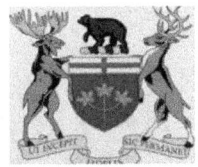

Clinical Alert!

- o "…..long term anti–coagulation does not increase the risk or severity of variceal bleeding and prevents further portal and mesenteric venous thrombotic complications" (Feldman, M., *et al. Sleisenger and Fordtran's Gastrointestinal and Liver Disease.* 9th Edition. Saunders/Elsevier, Philadelphia, 2010, page 1379).

➤ Clinical
  - o Bowel ischemia and mesenteric infarction

- Give the **clinical features and treatment** for hepatic artery stenosis and hepatic artery thrombosis, as well as portal vein stenosis or thrombosis.

Time of occurrence	Leading symptoms	Treatment
• Hepatic artery stenosis	– Slight increase in LFTs – Mild or late biliary complications	▪ Reoperation, with resection of the anastomosis and end–to–end reconstruction
o Early	– Acute liver failure – Fulminant increase in LFTs – Hemodynamic instability – Ascites – Variceal bleeding	▪ Urgent thrombectomy ▪ Urgent retransplantation
o Late	– Slight increase in LFTs – Portal hypertension – Ascites – Variceal bleeding	▪ Endoscopic treatment Rt–PA lysis therapy ▪ Elective retransplantation

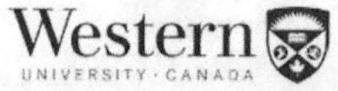

Time of occurrence	Leading symptoms	Treatment

- Hepatic artery thrombosis

o Early	– Fulminant increase in LFTs – Acute liver failure – Hemodynamic instability	▪ Urgent acute thrombectomy or ▪ Urgent retransplantation
o Late	– Biliary complications – Strictures – Intrahepatic abscesses – Cholangitis and sepsis	▪ Management of biliary complications using ERC, PTC Rt–PA lysis therapy ▪ Elective retransplantation

- Portal vein stenosis | – Slight increase in LFTs, Portal hypertension, Ascites | ▪ Resection and end–to–end reconstruction

• Portal vein stenosis	– Slight increase in LFTs, Portal hypertension, Ascites	▪ Resection and end–to–end reconstruction

Printed with permission: Mueller, A.R., *et al. Best Practice & Research Clinical Gastroenterology* 2004; 18(5): page 884.

➢ Treatment
- o Acute stage of portal vein thrombosis
  - Anticoagulant therapy is essential to achieve recanalization
  - There is no consensus as to the need for anticoagulation in chronic portal vein thrombosis
- o In a cohort study of anticoagulated and non–anticoagulated patients, anticoagulation is characterized by:
  - No ↑ risk or severity of bleeding
  - ↓ prevalence of splanchnic infarction

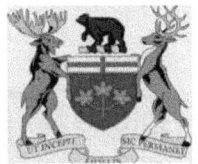

Cavernoma Cholangiopathy

- o Symptoms of bile duct obstruction
- o Recruitment of the peribiliary venous plexuses to serve as portal collaterals is believed to be responsible for common bile duct compression and upstream biliary dilatation
- o Conservative treatment with ursodeoxycholic acid is an option
- o Endoscopic treatment with ERCP

Budd–Chiari Syndrome

- ➢ Definition: obstruction of the hepatic venous outflow from the right atrium to the small hepatic venules

- ➢ Causes and associations
  - o Primary
    - – Characterized by obstruction of hepatic venous outflow in the absence of any of the following:
      - ▪ Right–sided heart failure
      - ▪ Constrictive pericarditis
  - o Secondary
    - – Neoplastic invasion or compression

- • Give the causes of Budd–Chiari Syndrome (BCS).
  - o Hypercoagulable states
    - – Inherited
      - ▪ Factor V Leiden mutation
      - ▪ Prothrombin mutation
      - ▪ Antithrombin deficiency
      - ▪ Protein C deficiency
      - ▪ Protein S deficiency
      - ▪ Antiphospholipid syndrome

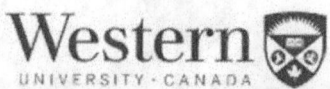

- Acquired
    - Myeloproliferative disorders
    - Cancer
    - Pregnancy
    - Oral contraceptive use
    - Paroxysmal nocturnal hemoglobinuria (PNH)
    - Polycythemia rubra vera (PRV)

o Tumor invasion
- Hepatocellular carcinoma
- Renal cell carcinoma
- Adrenal carcinoma

o Miscellaneous
- Aspergillosis
- Behçet syndrome
- Inferior vena cava webs
- Trauma
- Inflammatory bowel disease
- Dacarbazine therapy

o Idiopathic

o Most common causes
- Africa, Asia
    - MOIVC (membranous obstruction of the inferior vena cava)
- NA/Europe
    - Thrombosis of hepatic veins from thrombogenic states, i.e. myeloproliferative disorders (JAK2 mutations of the gene coding for tyrosine kinase Janus kinase 2)

➤ Clinical
o Presentations
- Asymptomatic illness
- A fulminant form
- Chronic disease

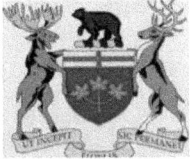

- o The main clinical picture are the following:
    - – Abdominal pain
    - – Ascites
    - – Hepatosplenomegaly
    - – Signs of portal hypertension
- o Hepatocellular carcinoma (HCC) is not uncommon

➢ Diagnostic imaging

- o Doppler ultrasound
- o MRI (contrast–enhanced); multiphasic CT
- o Liver biopsy (zone 3 congestion)

CLINICAL CHALLENGE

A young woman presents with a rapid onset of abdominal pain, hepatomegaly and ascites. MRI demonstrates an enlarged caudate lobe.

- • Give the clinical diagnosis and explain the changes on diagnostic imaging.
    - o Budd–Chiari syndrome (BCS) is caused by obstruction of the blood flow in the hepatic vein which flow away from the liver.
    - o The damage occurs mostly in zones 3 and 2 because of the total ↓ in the HV, and because the caudate lobe has additional blood flow through the accessory hepatic veins, the caudate lobe may hypertrophy.
    - o If a venogram was peformed, it might show a "spider web" appearance suggestive of BCS (BCS → ↓ HV flow → ↑ accessary HV flow → spider appearance on venography).
    - o Curiosity: a very large caudate lobe may compress the IVC (inferior vena cava) and further ↓ HV outflow.

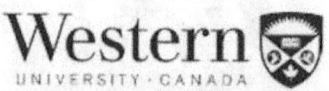

- Give the acute and chronic **pathological changes** of Budd–Chiari syndrome.

  - o Acute centrilobular, portal sinusoids
    - – Congestion
    - – Sinusoidal distention
    - – Hemorrhage
    - – Necrosis
    - – Little inflammation
    - – Wide subendothelium

  - o Chronic
    - – Patchy, asymmetrical involvement
    - – Perivenular sclerosis
    - – Hepatocellular necrosis
    - – Regenerative nodules
    - – Cirrhosis

Abbreviations: HV, hepatic vein; IVC, inferior vena cava; PV, portal vein

Adapted from: Stevens, W.E. *Sleisenger & Fordtran's Gastrointestinal and Liver Disease: Pathophysiology/ Diagnosis/Management* 2006: page 1756.; and Printed with permission: Kamath, P.S. *Clinic Gastroenterology and Hepatology Board Review* 2008: page 343; and 2010, page 1372.

  - o Note: the "uncorrected" MELD score does not take into account the refractory ascites which is common in BCS

➢ Treatment
  - o Anticoagulation is recommended in all patients
  - o Percutaneous transluminal angioplasty is indicated whenever short–length stenosis of the hepatic veins or inferior vena cava is present

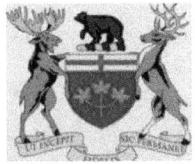

- o Failure of the above strategies is an indication for transjugular intrahepatic portosystemic shunting (TIPS)
- o Liver transplantation. Retrospective analyses of European [18] and US [19] case–series have reported 5–year survival rates of 80% in transplanted patients
- o Acute
  - – Supportive care, including the following:
    - Large volume paracentesis of ascites
    - Treating the underlying condition
  - – Anticoagulation
  - – Thrombolysis
  - – Angioplasty (obstruction of IVC plus HV → form portocaval shunt)
  - – Stent placement
  - – TIPS ("bridge" for liver transplantation)
- o Fulminant
  - – Hepatic failure (↑ MELD score)
  - – Liver transplantation (LT)
- o Chronic
  - – If the acute care as per above fails, and there is decompensated cirrhosis, then do the following:
    - TIPS
    - Portosystemic shunt surgery (PSS)
      - – PV becomes the hepatic outflow tract
      - – No IVC stenosis
      - – IVC pressure < 20 mmHg
      - – Embolectomy (selected cases)
      - – Liver transplant

- Give features present in patient with Budd–Chiari syndrome that should be considered before LT.

  - o Associated hepatic malignancy
  - o Other contraindications for LT

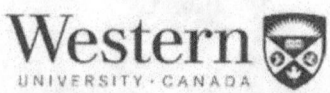

- Give the **treatment** options and indications of the different modalities for patients with Budd–Chiari Syndrome (BCS), advantages and disadvantages.

Treatment	Indication	Advantages	Disadvantages
o Thrombolytic therapy	– Acute thrombosis	▪ Reverses hepatic necrosis	Risk of bleeding Limited success
o Angioplasty with and without stenting	– IVC webs – IVC stenosis – Focal hepatic vein stenosis	▪ No long term sequelae ▪ Averts need for surgery	High rate of restenosis or shunt occlusion
o TIPS	– Possible bridge to liver transplantation in fulminant BCS – Acute BCS (HE)	▪ Low mortality ▪ Useful even with compression of IVC by caudate lobe	High rate of shunt stenosis Extended stents may interfere with liver transplantation
o Surgical shunt	– Subacute BCS if portacaval pressure gradient <10 mmHg or occluded IVC	▪ Definitive procedure for many patients ▪ Low rate of shunt dysfunction with portacaval shunt	Risk of procedure-related death Limited applicability
o Liver transplant-ation	– Subacute BCS – Portacaval pressure gradient >10 mmHg – Fulminant BCS – Presence of cirrhosis – Failure of porto-systemic shunt	▪ Reverses liver disease ▪ May reverse underlying thrombophilia	Risk of procedure-related death Need for long term immunosuppression

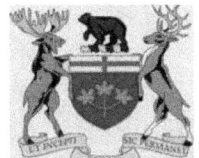

Abbreviations: HE, hepatic encephalopathy; IVC, inferior vena cava; TIPS, transjugular intrahepatic portosystemic shunt

Printed with permission: Kamath, P.S. *Mayo Clinic Gastroenterology and Hepatology Board Review* 2008: page 344.

Sinusoidal Obstruction Syndrome (SOS; aka Veno–Occlusive Disease)

➢ Definition

- o A non–thrombotic obstruction of the liver sinusoids that may extend to the central vein causing post–sinusoidal portal hypertension
- o Triggered by injury to the endothelial cells
- o Ingestion of plants containing pyrrolizidine alkaloid
- o Myeloablative conditioning prior to bone marrow or hematopoietic stem cell transplantation
- o Use of oxaliplatin as chemotherapy for colorectal liver metastasis

➢ Causes and associations

- o Common associations
  - – Bone marrow transplantation (BMT) occurs
    - ▪ Within 2 weeks after BMT
    - ▪ In 50% of BMT
    - ▪ 70% mortality rate
  - – Chemotherapy
  - – Azathioprine
- o Hepatic irradiation
- o Older age
- o HCV infection

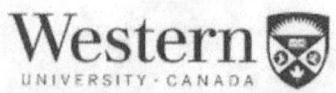

- o Hereditary hemochromatosis (HH)
- o Pre–existing chronic liver diseases
- o Recent bacterial and viral infections

➢ Clinical
- o Resembles BCS
- o Painful hepatomegaly
- o Develops within 10 – 20 days after BMT
- o Symptoms
  - – ↑ weight
- o Ascites, right upper quadrant pain, hepatomegaly and jaundice
- o Clinical diagnosis is sometimes challenging and imaging findings are nonspecific
- o Liver biopsy is required
- o Portal hypertension is due to disorders that should be treated in accordance with its manifestations

- Give the timing and method of diagnosis of 5 liver and biliary diseases following **stem cell** transplantation.

Diseases	Timing	Diagnosis
o Sinusoidal obstruction syndrome	Onset before day 20	– Typical clinical features plus exclusion of other causes of jaundice and weight gain – Imaging (doppler ultrasound or CT) – Transvenous measurement of wedged hepatic venous pressure gradient and liver biopsy – Note for atypical presentations (acute hepatitis, anasarca)

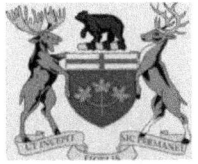

Diseases	Timing	Diagnosis
○ Cholestasis and infection (cholangitis lenta)	Following sepsis or neutropenic fever (usually before day 30)	– Exclude other causes of cholestasis – Inferential diagnosis in a patient with cholestatic jaundice
○ Acute graft–versus host disease	Day 15 – 50	– Confirm GVHD in skin, gut – Exclude other causes of cholestasis – Liver biopsy
○ Acute viral hepatitis	HSV, day 20 – 50 Adenovirus, day 30 – 80 VZV, day 80 – 250 HBV and HCV, during immune reconstitution	– Pre–transplant blood test (antigen, antibodies, PCR results) – Isolation of virus from other sites (stool and urine for adenovirus) – PCR of serum for specific viruses
○ Fungal abscess	Day 10 – 60	– Liver biopsy histology/PCR/immunostains – Hepatic pain, fever
○ Bacterial infection	Day 10 – 80	– Liver imaging (MRI > CT) – Serum fungal antigen(s) – Hepatic pain, fever – Liver imaging – Liver biopsy, culture
○ Drug–liver injury	Day 0 – 100	– Clinical evidence linking elevations of serum ALT or alkaline phosphatase to drugs known to cause liver injury

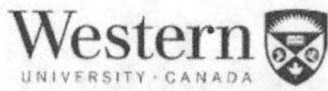

Diseases	Timing	Diagnosis
o Ischemic liver disease	Day 0 – 30 Day 15 – 60	– Clinical evidence linking shock to subsequent rises in serum ALT
o Biliary obstruction	Day 10 – 50	– History, examination – Biliary ultrasound
o Idiopathic hyper–ammonemia	After day 80	– ERCP > magnetic resonance cholangiography – Unexplained confusion, coma – Blood ammonia
o Chronic hepatitis C	Pre-transplant Long term follow–up after transplant	– HCV RNA in serum – Elevation of serum ALT after immune reconstitution
o Iron overload	After day 80	– Transferrin saturation – Marrow iron qualification – Liver iron quantification (Ferrisca MRI, liver biopsy quantification)
o Chronic GVHD	Years after transplant	– Prior acute GVHD history – Chronic GVHD in other organs – Consistent elevations of serum ALT, alkaline phosphatase – Noted hepatitis presentation
o Nodular regenerative hyperplasia (NRH)		– Liver biopsy (reticulin stain) – Signs of portal hypertension but preserved liver function – Laparoscopic appearance of the liver

Printed with permission: McDonald, G.B. and Frieze, D. *Gut* 2008; 57:987-1003, Table 3 page 995.

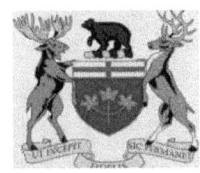

- ➤ Laboratory
  - ○ Conjugated hyperbilirubinemia > 2 mg/dL
  - ○ Thrombocytopenia

- ➤ Diagnostic imaging
- • Give the non–specific changes seen on diagnostic imaging (abdominal ultrasound, CT or MRI) suggesting the diagnosis of SOS (Sinusoidal Obstruction Syndrome).
  - ○ Liver, spleen
    - – Hepatosplenomegaly
  - ○ Portal vein (PV)
    - – Dilated
    - – Flow in PV is slow or reversed
  - ○ Umbilical vein
    - – Recanalization
  - ○ Gallbladder has thick walls

- ➤ Differential
  - ○ SOS develops after BMT on days 10 – 20
  - ○ Distinguish from GVHD (graft–versus–host disease) which develops after day 15
  - ○ Sepsis and drug toxicity do not usually cause painful hepatomegaly or ascites, as does SOS

- ➤ Predictors of severity
  - ○ Jaundice
  - ○ Ascites
  - ○ HVPG (hepatic venous pressure gradient) > 20 mmHg
  - ○ Multiorgan failure
  - ○ Mortality rate is ~ 25% from multiorgan failure and from non–liver failure

Note: be prepared for questions such as: without performing a liver biopsy, distinguish between SOS and GVHD of the liver (easy – see above)

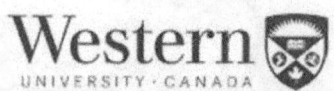

Schistosomal portal hypertension

➢ Demography

- o Schistosomiasis, a parasitic disease is endemic in over 70 countries worldwide

- o *Schistosoma mansoni.* In Brazil alone, roughly 3 – 4 million patients are believed to be infected with *S. mansoni* many of whom have hepatosplenic schistosomiasis

➢ Clinical
- o Common
  - Esophageal varices
- o Uncommon
  - Ascites and hepatic encephalopathy are uncommon
- o Migration of ova and dead parasites to the liver → formation of hepatic granulomas and periportal fibrosis → presinusoidal obstruction of portal blood flow, massive splenomegaly → development of portosystemic collaterals and gastroesophageal varices

➢ Management of upper gastrointestinal bleeding (UGIB) in patients with non–cirrhotic portal hypertension
- o Acute UGIB – Permissive hypotension has systolic blood pressure of 90 – 100 mmHg
  - Hemoglobin < 10 g/dL
  - Vasoconstrictors: terlipressin, somatostatin, octreotide
  - Endoscopic management (preferably band ligation of esophageal varices)

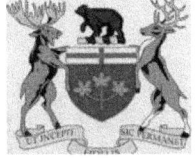

- o Rebleeding prophylaxis
  - Pharmacological treatment with beta–blockers (propranolol is controversial in schistosomiasis due to pulmonary hypertension)
  - Endoscopic management: preferably band ligation over sclerotherapy
  - Surgical management: shunt procedures versus deconnection surgeries (as esophagogastric devascularization with splenectomy in schistosomiasis)

Esophagogastric Devascularization with Splenectomy (EGDS)

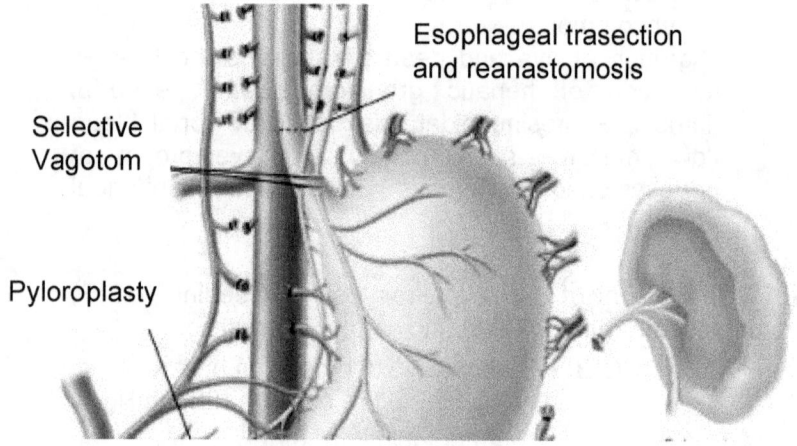

Esophageal trasection and reanastomosis

Selective Vagotom

Pyloroplasty

ACS SURGERY 2004 WebMD Inc

Sarcoidosis

- o Presinusoidal portal hypertension secondary to portal non–caseating granulomas with liver sarcoidosis

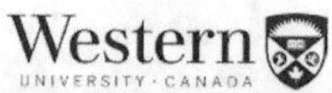

Obliterative Portal Venopathy

- o Fibrosis and stenosis or occlusion of small portal vein branches
- o Chemical agents (i.e. vinyl chloride)
  - – Drugs (i.e. azathioprine)
- o Immune–mediated conditions (i.e. thyroiditis, lupus, autoimmune hepatitis or sarcoidosis)
- o In HIV–positive patients, the vascular injury of obliterative portal venopathy has been associated with the use of anti–retrovirals, i.e. didanosine and stavudine

Non–Cirrhotic Portal Fibrosis (NCPF; Idiopathic PHT [IPH] or Hepatoportal Sclerosis)

- ➢ Definition
  - o A disorder of unknown etiology, clinically characterized by features of PHT that is of moderate to massive splenomegaly, with or without hypersplenism, preserved liver functions and patent hepatic and portal veins

o Japanese criteria for IPH	Additional points
– Clinical disorder of unknown etiology	– Normal to near–normal liver function tests
	– Varices demonstrable by endoscopy or radiography
– Splenomegaly, anemia and portal hypertension	– Decrease of one or more of the formed blood elements
	– Liver scan shows not typical of cirrhosis
– Absence of cirrhosis, blood disease, parasites in the hepatobiliary system and occlusion of the hepatic and portal veins	– Patent hepatic veins with normal to slightly elevated WHVP
	– Grossly non–cirrhotic liver surface
	– Hepatic histology is not indicative of cirrhosis
	– Patent extrahepatic portal vein with frequent collateral vessels
	– Elevated portal pressure
	* Not all these investigations are required for the diagnosis

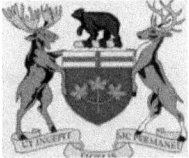

- ➢ Demography
  - o NCPF accounts for approximately 10 – 30% of all cases of variceal bleeding in several parts of the world including India
  - o More common in young males in the 3rd to 4th decades belonging to low socioeconomic groups

- ➢ Pathlogy
  - o Idiopathic Portal Hypertension (IPH) and Hepatoportal Sclerosis (HPS) are associated with ↑ PP (portal pressure) and no obstruction of the extrahepatic portion of the PV (portal vein)

- • Give the distinctive hepatic histopathological features of IPH *vs* HPS seen on liver biopsy.

  - o IPH
    - – Normal
  - o HPS
    - – Intrahepatic portal veins show the following:
      - ▪ Subendothelial thickening
      - ▪ Thrombosis
      - ▪ Recanalization

- ➢ Pathogenesis
  - o Endotoxin mediated injury
    - – With or without induced autoimmunity
  - o Familial clustering, association with human leukocyte antigen (HLA)–DR3

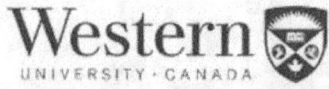

Extrahepatic Portal Venous Obstruction (EHPVO)

➤ Definition
- A childhood disorder characterized by a chronic blockage of PV blood supply leading to PHT and its sequelae in the setting of a well–preserved liver function.
- EHPVO is a major cause of PHT (54%) and upper gastrointestinal bleeding in children (68 – 84%) from the developing world.

➤ Causes and associations
- Primary myeloproliferative disorders:
  - With or without janus kinase 2 (JAK2) mutation (V617F)
- Factor V Leiden mutation (rs6025)
- Prothrombin gene mutation (G20201A)
- MTHFR gene mutation (C677T)
- Hyperchromocysteinemia
- Protein C deficiency
- Protein S deficiency
- Antithrombin III deficiency
- Antiphospholipid syndrome and anticardiolipin antibodies
- Paroxysmal nocturnal hemoglobinuria
- Local inflammatory conditions
  - Pancreatitis
  - Abdominal sepsis
  - Liver abscess
- Portal vein injury
  - Trauma (splenectomy, pancreatic surgery, colectomy)
  - Umbilical vein catheterization
  - Umbilical sepsis

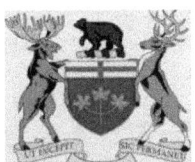

- o Pregnancy
- o Oral contraceptive
- o Post–liver transplantation
- o Idiopathic

➢ Differential

NCPF *vs* EHPVO

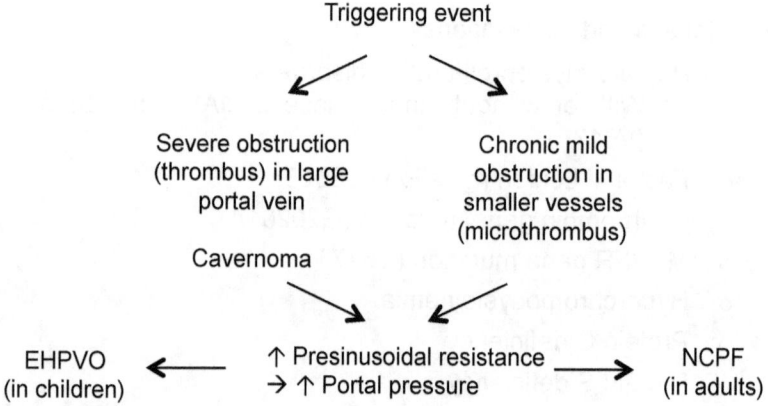

Abbreviations: EHPVO, extrahepatic portal venous obstruction; NCPF, non–cirrhotic portal fibrosis

Abbreviations: AC, anti–coagulation; EHPVO, extrahepatic portal venous obstruction; NCPF, non–cirrhotic portal fibrosis; PHTN, portal hypertension

➢ Summary
- o NCPF is one of the most comment cause of variceal bleed in Asia (India)
- o NCPF is usually secondary to vascular and pro thrombotic diseases

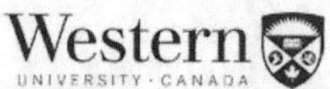

- ○ Usually has normal liver function
- ○ Management the complication of PHT is almost the same but they tend to have more variceal bleed
  - – Anti–coagulation (AC)
    - ▪ Usual treatment
- ○ Prognosis is usually good

The Stomach in Portal Hypertension

- Give the mucosal changes in the stomach associated with **portal hypertensive gastropathy**.
  - ○ Mosaic–like mucosal pattern
    - – Small, polygonal areas surrounded by a whitish–yellow depressed border (snake skin appearance) can be categorized as mild (pink mucosa) and moderate (diffuse red mucosa)
  - ○ Red point lesions
    - – Small (< 1 mm), red, flat, point–like marks
  - ○ Cherry red spots
    - – Large (> 2 mm), round, red colored, protruding lesions
  - ○ Black–brown spots
  - ○ Irregularly–shaped black and brown flat spots that do not fade upon washing (these changes might represent intramucosal hemorrhage)

*These changes are characterized endoscopically by the presence of 4 main findings, as described by the New Italian Endoscopic Club (NIEC).

Printed with permission: Macmillan Publishers Ltd: Perini, *et al. Nature Clinical Practice Gastroenterology and Hepatology* 2009; 6(3):150-8.

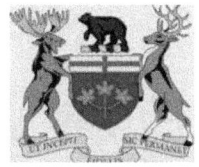

➤ Differentials

- Compare and contrast portal hypertensive gastropathy (PHG) from gastric antral vascular ectasia (GAVE).

	PHG	GAVE
o Distribution	Proximal stomach	Distal stomach
o Mosaic pattern	Present	Absent
o Red signs	Present	Present
o Biopsy		
– Thrombi	-	+++
– Spindle cell proliferation	+	++
– Fibrohyalinosis	+	+++
o Treatment	Beta–blockers TIPS	Argon laser Banding Cryotherapy Antrectomy

*Note: In portal hypertension, gastric vascular ectasia may occur at sites other than the antrum

Printed with permission: Garcia-Tsao, G. and Kamath, P.S. *2007 AGA Institute Postgraduate Course*: page 619.

TIPS – Transjugular Intrahepatic Portosystemic Shunt

- o In about 10% of TIPS, thrombosis occurs within 24 hours and the prophylactic use of anticoagulation is not established.

- o Over the long term, dysfunction of the shunt will occur in ~ half because of pseudo–intimal hyperplasia in the parenchymal tract or outflow hepatic vein, associated with the development of a coating of collagenous matrix covered by endothelial cells.

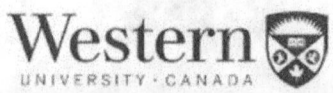

- o Doppler ultrasound may be used to establish the potency of TIPS.

- o There are numerous signs reported on Doppler ultrasound which have been used to predict the presence of dysfunction of the shunt, but these signs have low sensitivity rate (10 – 12.6%) and an acceptable specificity (88 – 100%).

- o Patency of TIPS is best demonstrated with re–catheterization of TIPS.

- o Overall, TIPS causes
  - ↓ rebleeding from any of the following:
    - Esophageal varices (EV)
    - Gastric varices (GV)
    - ECTV (ectopic varices)
  - ↑ HE (hepatic encephalopathy)
  - No change in overall survival

- o Proven benefit of TIPS
  - No primary prophylaxis of bleeding from EV or GV
  - Prevent rebleeding from the following:
    - EV, GV, ECTV - Yes
    - PHG failing BB - Yes
    - GAVE - No
  - Refractory cirrhotic ascites, intolerant to LVP - Yes
  - Hepatic hydrothorax, resistant to ↓ Na^+ and diuretics - Yes
  - Budd–Chiari syndrome, moderate disease, failed anticoagulation - Yes (controversial)
  - HRS

Abbreviations: BB, beta blocker; ECTV, ectopic varices; EV, esophageal varices; GAVE, gastric antral vascular hyperplasia; GV, gastric varices; HRS, heptorenal syndrome; LVP, large volume paracentesis; PHG, portal hypertensive gastropathy

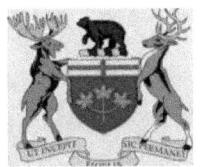

- Give the **relative contraindications** of TIPS.

  o Liver failure
    - Hepatic encephalopathy
    - Jaundice (serum bilirubin > 5 mg/dL)
    - Coagulopathy (INR > 2)
  o Progressive renal failure
  o Presence of associated acute infection
  o Severe cardiopulmonary disease
  o MELD > 18
  o R–HF

Abbreviations: HE, hepatic encephalopathy; R–HF, right heart failure; TIPS, transjugular intrahepatic portosystemic shunts

- Give the **complications** of TIPS (transjugular intrahepatic portosystemic shunt) procedure.

  o Technical complications
    - Neck puncture
    - Indequate access to hepatic vein
    - Creation of parenchymal tract to portal vein
    - May make later liver transplantation more difficult
  o Vessels
    - Puncture of pulmonary artery (PA), pulmonary vein (PV), liver capsule
    - Ischemia (hepatic artery thrombosis)
  o Stent
    - Inadequate deployment of stent across the parenchymal tract
    - Stent–related complications: thrombosis, stenosis
    - Stent migration into the portal vein or inferior vena cava

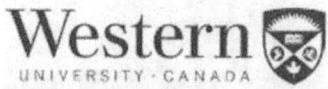

- o Liver
  - – Hepatic encephalopathy (HE) (new, worse, or chronic)
  - – Intraperitoneal bleeding
  - – Hepatic infarction
  - – Hepatic rupture
  - – Fulminant hepatic failure (acute liver failure [ALF])
- o CPS
  - – Pulmonary hypertension and right heart failure
- o Unique
  - – Unique complications of TIPS: hemolytic anemia, infectious endotipsitis
- o Systemic
  - – Sepsis
  - – Multiple organ failure syndrome
  - – Long term presence of foreign body

Abbreviation: CPS: cardiopulmonary systems

Adapted from: Sanyal, A.J. *2006 AGA Institute Postgraduate Course:* page 195.

Practical Tips for Liver Biopsy (LBx)

Peri–LBx management	Days to stop before LBx	Days to restart after LBx
o Drugs		
– Antiplatelet drugs	10	2 – 3
– Anticoagulants	5	1
– Heparin	1	
o Restrictions		
– Food	No	
– Exercise	No	
– Sedation	No	
– Heavy lifting	Probably a good idea	

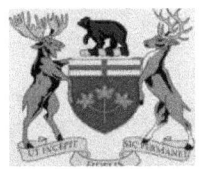

- o Post–biopsy
  - – Monitoring vital signs   Yes
  - – Observation time   4 hours
- o Hemostasis
  - – "…..the time to spontaneous cessation of surface bleeding (from the liver after biopsy with a 1.8 mm diameter Menghini needle) did not correlate with abnormalities in the PT, platelet count or whole blood clot time".
  - – In patients with hemophilia, correct the bleeding diathesis before LBx
  - – Inpatients on hemodialysis or with chronic renal failure
    - ▪ DDAVP (desmopressin) 0.3 mg/kg BW may be given pre–LBx
    - ▪ Patients on chronic hemodialysis should be dialyzed before LBx

Hereditary Hemorrhagic Telangiectasia (HHT) **and Osler-Weber–Rendu Disease** (OWRD)

- o HHT and OWRD may be associated with portal hypertension and bleeding esophageal varices as the result of the development of shunts between the hepatic artery (HA), hepatic vein (HV) and portal vein (PV).

- • Give the diagnostic criteria for HHT and OWRD.

The diagnostic criteria for HHT and OWRD include:
- o Positive family history
- o Epistaxis
- o Telangiectasias
- o AV fistulae (lung, liver)

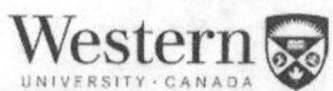

Intrahepatic Shunts

- Give the different clinical presentations arising from shunting between HA (hepatic artery), HV (hepatic vein) and PV (portal vein) in HHT (hereditary hemorrhagic telangiectasia).

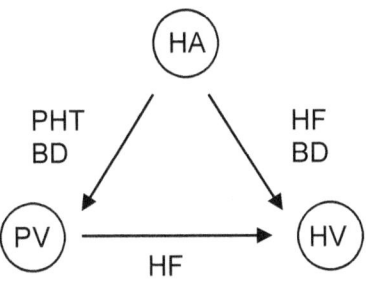

Abbreviations: BD, biliary disease; HF, heart failure; PHT, portal hypertension

- o High–output heart failure (HF) (hepatic artery [HA] and/or portal vein [PV] to hepatic vein [HV] shunt)
  - – Shortness of breath on exertion
  - – Orthopnea
  - – Ascites
  - – Edema
- o Portal hypertension (PHT) (hepatic artery [HA] to portal vein [PV] shunt)
  - – Esophageal varices
  - – Nodular regenerative hyperplasia
- o Biliary disease [BD] (hepatic artery [HA] to hepatic vein [HV] and/or portal vein [PV] shunt)
  - – Severe cholestasis
  - – Recurrent cholangitis
- o Hepatic disintegration

Abbreviation: BD, biliary disease; HA, hepatic artery; HV, hepatic vein; PHT, portal hypertension; PV, portal vein

Adapted from: Sabbà, C. and Pompili, M. *Aliment Pharmacol Ther* 2008; 28(5):523-33.

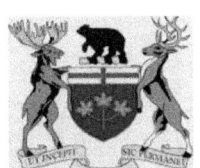

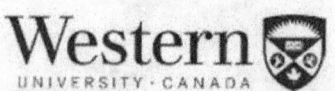

Hepatitis B in Pregnancy

Bandar Al-Judaibi

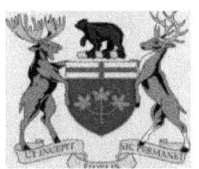

Chronic Hepatitis B (CHB) virus (HBV) – disease burden

➤ Demography

- o Chronic hepatitis B (CHB) affects 350 million individuals worldwide

- o Estimated prevalence of HBV carriers in Canada is approximately 2%

- o Rate of cirrhosis or chronic liver failure is 20 – 25% and rate of HCC is ~ 5%

Shaikh, T., *et al. Can J Infect Dis* 2011; 12:351.; Lai, C.L., *et al.* Lancet 2003; 362:2089-94.; McMahon, B.J. *Clin Liver Dis* 2010; 14:381-96.

➤ Modes of transmission

- o Over 50% of CHB infections are acquired by vertical transmission (VT) from their mothers

- o > 90% of VT infections become chronic due to induction of an immune–tolerance

- o Management of CHB during pregnancy and strategies to prevent VT would reduce the new HBV infection as well as the morbidity and mortality

Jonas, M.M. *Liver Int.* 2009; 29 Suppl 1:133-9.

➤ Prevention of CHB

- o Vaccination
  - – Universal neonatal vaccination recommended by AASLD and CASL
  - – Most provinces still vaccinate during adolescence!
  - – Incidence of HBV infection has fallen to 82% since the implementation of universal vaccination at birth in the early 1990s (USA)

Alter, M.J. *Hepatol* 2003; 39(Suppl 1):S64-9.; Coffin, C.S., *et al. Can J Gastroenterol* 2012; 26(12):917-38.

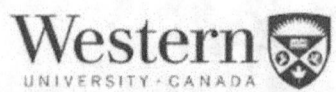

- o Prenatal screening
  - – Universal prenatal screening for HBV identifies HBsAg–positive women before they give birth
  - – Newborns receive the appropriate post–exposure prophylaxis to reduce VT
  - – Infected mothers should receive the appropriate medical care during and after pregnancy
  - – HBsAg–negative mothers can be vaccinated

Degli-Esposti, S. and Shah, D. *Gastroenterol Clin N Am* 40 (2011) 355-72.

Effect of CHB on Pregnancy

- o CHB does not significantly influence fertility unless the patient has cirrhosis or liver failure
- o CHB during pregnancy does not increase the maternal or fetal morbidity and mortality
- o HBsAg–positive mothers have ↑ risk of the following:
  - – Gestational diabetes mellitus
  - – Antepartum hemorrhage
  - – Threatened preterm labor
- o Usually, no worsening of chronic liver disease during pregnancy
- o Hormonal changes can lead to elevations of HBV DNA and fluctuations in liver function tests
- o Antepartum CHB flares and liver failure have been rarely reported
- o Postpartum hepatitis flares leading to hepatic decompensation

Tan, J., *et al. Liver Transpl* 2008; 14: 1081-91.; Wong, S., *et al. Am J Perinatol* 1999; 16:485-8.; Tse, K.Y., *et al. J Hepatol* 2005; 43:771-5.; Ter Borg, M.J., *et al. J Viral Hepat* 2008; 15:37-41.; Nguyen, G., *et al. Aliment Pharmacol Ther* 2009; 29:755-64.

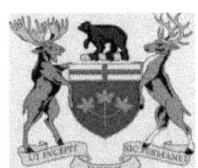

Transmission of HBV

❖ Vertical transmission

- o Risk of VT of HBV infection
  - HBeAg–positive mother: 70 – 90% risk
  - HBeAg–negative mother: 10 – 40% risk

- o Viral factors
  - HBV DNA is the most important risk factor for VT

- o Maternal factors
  - Prolonged uterine contractions and preterm labor may result in transplacental leakage → maternal–fetal microtransfusions
  - Mothers with prior infant who failed from immunoprophylaxis have a higher risk of VT in subsequent pregnancies

- o Intrauterine transmission
  - Not the predominant mode of transmission
  - HBsAg is common in cord blood but does not predict a chronic infection
  - Important source of immunoprophylaxis failure***

- o Transmission during delivery
  - Most frequent route of VT
  - Mechanisms of VT may include:
    - Micro-transfusion of mother's blood to the fetus during contractions
    - Infection after the rupture of membranes
    - Direct contact of the infant's mucosal membrane with the infected secretions or blood from the maternal genital tract

Xu, D.Z., et al. J Med Virol 2002; 67:20-6.; Wong, V.C., et al. Br J Obstet Gynaecol 1980; 87:958-65.; Keeffe, E.B., et al. Clin Gastroenterol Hepatol 2008; 6:1315; Lin, H.H., et al. J Pediatr 1987; 111(6 Pt 1):877-81.; Kumar, A. Indian J Gastroenterol 2012; 31:43-54.

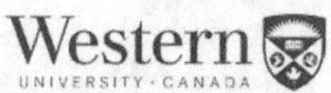

➢ Strategies to prevent VT

❖ Antepartum
- o Hepatitis B immunoglobulin (HBIg) injection
- o Previous studies: HBIg given at antepartum stage could induce > 2 log decline in maternal HBV DNA with a modest reduction in VT
- o However, a recent large controlled study showed that antepartum HBIg is not effective in preventing VT
- o Therefore, this strategy is not currently recommended

❖ Postpartum immunoprophylaxis
- o Most guidelines recommend infants born to HBsAg–positive mothers to receive both HBIg and HBV vaccine within 12 hours of birth
- o This should be followed by at least 2 more doses of HBV vaccine within the first 6 months of life
- o Combining HBIg and at least 3 doses of HBV vaccine is more effective in reducing VT than HBIg or the HBV vaccine alone
- o After the vaccine protocol is completed HBsAg and anti–HBs should be tested at 9 months of age
- o HBsAg–negative infants with anti–HBs levels > 10 U/ml are protected and no further medical management is required
- o This strategy reduces VT by 90 – 95%

Zhu, Q., et al. Clin Med J (Engl) 2003; 116:685-7.; Yuan, J., et al. J Viral Hepat 2006; 13:597-604.

❖ Horizontal transmission (HT)
- o Postpartum transmission
  - – 34% of infants born to HBeAg+ mothers who are not infected at birth acquire HBV in the next 6 months
  - – Transmission in postpartum period is likely the result of close contact between the mother and baby
  - – Several studies have shown that breastfeeding carried no additional risk of HBV transmission

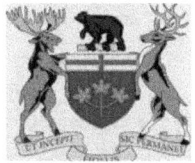

❖ Summary of two studies evaluating maternal antiviral therapy to prevent mother–to–infant transmission of hepatitis B virus (HBV)

Parameter	Xu, *et al.*, 2009	Han, *et al.*, 2011
○ Intervention	Lamivudine 100 mg 1x daily *vs* placebo	Telbivudine 600 mg 1x daily *vs* untreated controls
○ Timing of treatment	Weeks 32 gestation to week 4 postpartum	Week 20 – 32 gestation to week 4 postpartum
○ Design	RCT, double blind	Non–randomized, open–label
○ Maternal HBV criteria	DNA > 10^9 virus copies/mL (one subject was HBeAg-)	HBV DNA > 10^7 virus copies/mL and HBeAg+
○ Number	56 lamivudine, 59 placebo	135 telbivudine, 94 controls
○ Caesarean section rate	Approximately 50% in both groups	56% telbivudine 47% placebo
○ HBV DNA, $\log_{10}$ copies/mL	Lamivudine 2.2 x 10^9 Placebo 2.7 x 10^9	Telbivudine 8.10 Control 7.98
○ HBV DNA at delivery, $\log_{10}$ copies/mL	Lamivudine 5.1 x 10^9 Placebo 2.2 x 10^9	Telbivudine 2.4 Control 7.82
○ HBsAg+ infants	18% lamivudine, 39% placebo ($P = 0.014$)	0% telbivudine, 8% control ($P = 0.002$)
○ Antiviral resistance	Not tested	Not reported

- Negative; + Positive; RCT, randomized controlled trial

Adapted from: Xu, W.M., *et al. J Viral Hepat* 2009; 16:94-103.; Petersen, J. *J Hepatol* 2011;55:1215-21.

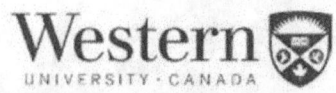

❖ Summary of Nanjing single–center experience of mother–to–infant transmission of hepatitis B virus (HBV) *vs* HBV prophylaxis failure rate

Maternal HBV DNA level at deilivery*	Infection rate, n/n (%)
< 6 $\log_{10}$ copies/mL	0/0 (0)
6–6.99 $\log_{10}$ copies/mL (2 x 5–6 $\log_{10}$ IU/mL	9/298 (3.2)
7–7.99 $\log_{10}$ copies/mL (2 x 6–7 $\log_{10}$ IU/mL	29/531 (5.46)
> 8 $\log_{10}$ copies/mL (2 x 7–8 $\log_{10}$ IU/mL	23/239 (9.62)

*1 IU/mL = approximately five virus genome copies (or virus genome equivalents)/mL.

○ High HBV DNA level increases the risk of immunoprophylaxis failure

Pan, C., *et al. Hepatology* 2011; 54(Suppl 4):878A.

➢ Oral antiviral drugs for the treatment of hepatitis B virus infection and their use in pregnancy

○ FDA pregnancy category
  – B
    ▪ Telbivudine
  – C
    ▪ Adefovir
    ▪ Entecavir
    ▪ Lamivudine

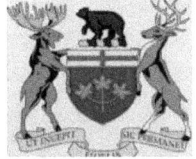

Antiretroviral pregnancy registry data
➢ Safety of antiviral therapy in pregnancy

With an exposure to	Defects/liver births	Birth defects/live births
Lamivudine	122/3966 (3.1%)	178/6427 (2.8%)
Tenofovir	27/1219 (2.2%)	15/714 (2.1%)
Telivudine	0/8	0/9
Adefovir dipivoxil	0/43	0/0
Entecavir	1/30	0/2
Any NRTI	165/5582 (3.0%)	216/7772 (2.5%)
Any NtRTI	27/1262 (2.1%)	15/712 (2.1%)

Printed with permission: Piratvisuth, T. *Liver Int* 2013; 33 Suppl 1:188-94.

C–section *vs* vaginal delivery

o Chinese studies VT risk with vaginal delivery, vacuum extraction or forceps or C–section
- 301 infants of HBsAg–positive mothers
- All received HBIg and HBV vaccine at birth
- No difference in rates of HBsAg+ at birth between the 3 groups: 8.1, 7.7 and 9.7%, respectively

o Rates of chronic infection were not significantly different between the groups during follow–up

o Meta–analysis of 4 RCTs (789 mothers) showed elective C–section reduced VT *vs* vaginal delivery
- VT rates: 10.5% for C–section *vs* 28% for vaginal delivery

o Elective C–section may play a role in reducing VT in highly viremic HBeAg–positive mothers BUT.....
- Studies included had methodological flaws
- Is this effect independent of use of antivirals?
- Most obstetric guidelines do not endorse routine use of C–section to prevent VT

Yang, J., *et al. Virol J* 2008; 5:100.

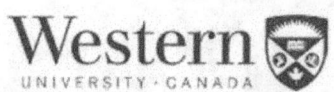

Breastfeeding

- o With appropriate immunoprophylaxis, breastfeeding does not increase the risk of HBV transmission
  - – Hill, *et al.* found a similar infection rate in breast–fed and formula–fed infants (0% *vs* 3%)
- o Meta–analysis of 1624 infants confirmed that breastfeeding did not increase the risk of VT
- o WHO recommends breastfeeding in infants of HBsAg–positive mothers even in endemic areas where the HBV vaccination is not readily available

Hill, J.B., *et al. Obstet Gynecol* 2002; 99:1049-52.; Shi, Z., *et al. Arch Pediatr Adolesc Med* 2011; 165:837-46.

Breastfeeding and Antivirals

- o Breastfeeding is not recommended for mothers on antiviral therapy
- o Antiviral drugs should be discontinued postpartum
- o Mothers should be monitored to detect hepatitis flares after discontinuing the treatment
  - – Secondary to drug withdrawal or postpartum state
  - – Monitor with serial ALT and HBV DNA levels

Bzowej, N.H. *Curr Hepatitis Rep* 2012; 11:82-89.

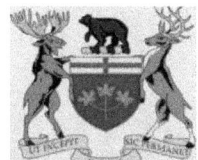

Algorithm for management of hepatitis B virus during pregnancy

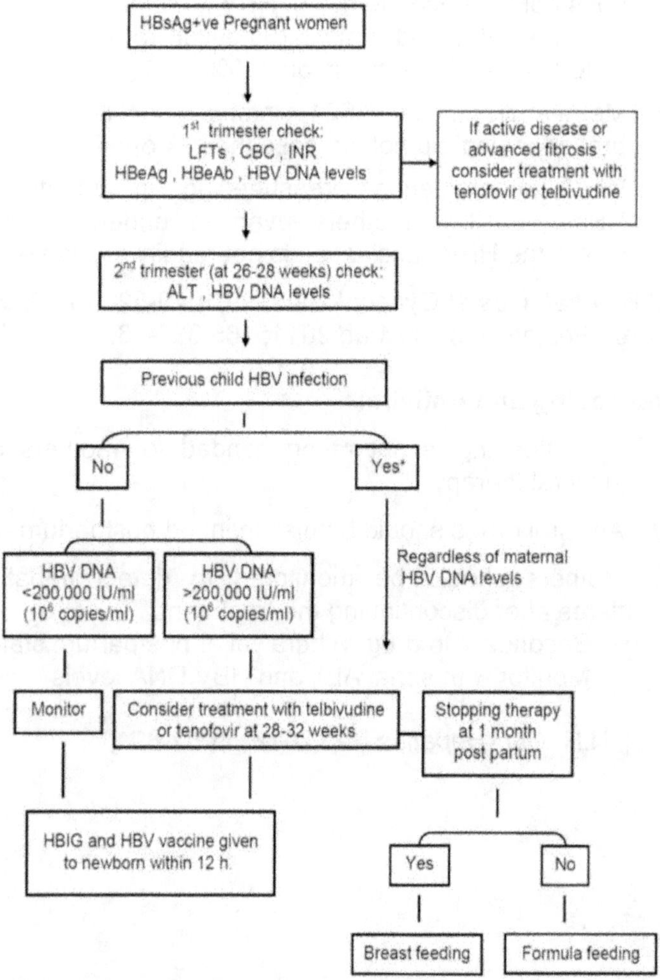

```
                    ┌─────────────────────────┐
                    │ HBsAg+ve Pregnant women │
                    └───────────┬─────────────┘
                                │
                                ▼
      ┌──────────────────────────────┐      ┌─────────────────────┐
      │ 1ˢᵗ trimester check:          │      │ If active disease or│
      │ LFTs , CBC , INR             ├─────▶│ advanced fibrosis : │
      │ HBeAg , HBeAb , HBV DNA levels│      │ consider treatment  │
      └──────────────┬───────────────┘      │ with tenofovir or   │
                     │                       │ telbivudine         │
                     ▼                       └─────────────────────┘
      ┌──────────────────────────────────┐
      │ 2ⁿᵈ trimester (at 26-28 weeks) check:│
      │ ALT , HBV DNA levels             │
      └──────────────┬───────────────────┘
                     │
                     ▼
      ┌──────────────────────────────┐
      │ Previous child HBV infection │
      └──────────────────────────────┘
```

1ˢᵗ trimester check:
LFTs , CBC , INR
HBeAg , HBeAb , HBV DNA levels

If active disease or advanced fibrosis : consider treatment with tenofovir or telbivudine

2ⁿᵈ trimester (at 26-28 weeks) check:
ALT , HBV DNA levels

Previous child HBV infection

No   Yes*

HBV DNA <200,000 IU/ml (10⁶ copies/ml)   HBV DNA >200,000 IU/ml (10⁶ copies/ml)

Regardless of maternal HBV DNA levels

Monitor   Consider treatment with telbivudine or tenofovir at 28-32 weeks   Stopping therapy at 1 month post partum

HBIG and HBV vaccine given to newborn within 12 h.

Yes   No

Breast feeding   Formula feeding

*Individual consideration after a discussion on risk and benefits with mother.

Printed with permission: Piratvisut, T. *Liver Int* 2013 Feb; 33 Suppl 1:188-94.

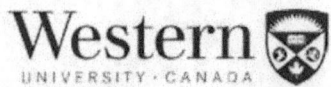

Summary of management of CHB in pregnancy

- o Initiation of antiviral therapy during the reproductive years
  - − Unknown how long do we wait to see if HBeAg+ patient will spontaneously seroconvert
  - − Consider interferon where possible due to finite nature of therapy
  - − Tenofovir probably the best oral choice (pregnancy class B, no resistance, potent)

- o Patients already on antiviral therapy: Stop, Switch or Continue Drug
  - − Organogenesis occurs between 4 – 14 weeks so stopping after that does not seem logical
  - − If you see patient early in the 1st trimester, consider risk of stopping therapy *vs* risk to fetus of continuing antiviral therapy
    - Hepatitis flare and decompensation (in those with advanced fibrosis)
    - High viral load → immunoprophylaxis failure
    - No clear cut increase in the risk of birth defects
  - − Consider switching from class C (i.e. Entecavir) to class B drug

Bzowej, N.H. *Curr Hepatitis Rep* (2012) 11:82-9.; Degli Esposti, S. and Shah, D. *Gastroenterol Clin North Am* (2011) 40:355-72.

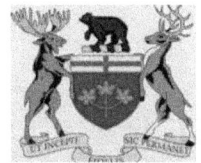

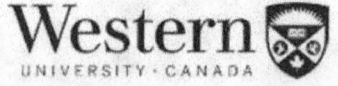

Pregnancy and Liver Disease

Amindeep Sandhu

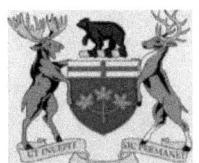

Normally.....

- o Pregnancy has many normal physiological and anatomic liver changes
- o Physical: palmar erythema, spider angiomas (increased estrogen)
- o Laboratory
  - 1st TM → Low albumin, TP
  - 2nd and 3rd TM → Elevated ALP, Decreased GGT, Billirubin
  - All TM → Marked elevations of TC, Tg concentrations
  - ALT, INR, LDH unaffected
- o Imaging unaffected

Abbreviations: ALP, alkaline phosphatse; ALT, alanine transaminase; GGT, gamma glutamyl transferase; LDH, lactate dehydrogenase; O/E, on examination; TC, total cholesterol; Tg, triglyceride; TM, trimester

Hyperemesis Gravidarum

➢ Demography
- o 1% of all pregnancies – does not affect fetal outcome
- o Week 4 – 20; First trimester

➢ Clinical
- o Severe nausea and vomiting
- o Dehydration
- o Complications
  - > 5 – 10% weight loss
  - Dehydration → ketosis and starvation ketoacidosis
  - Malnutrition – thiamine, B6, B12 deficiencies are not uncommon
  - Those related to metabolic derangements - low Na, K

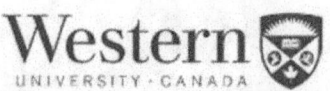

➤ Laboratory
- o ↑ transaminases (ALT > AST)
  - – Usually not greater than 2 – 300
  - – Proportional to severity of vomiting
  - – May occasionally be as high as 1000
- o Bilirubin < 4 mg/dL

➤ Pathophysiology
- o Related to rapid rise of β–HCG, estrogen, progesterone → GI distention, decreased gut motility, elevated liver enzymes
- o May be associated with *Helicobacter pylori* infection

➤ Treatment
- o Intravenous infusion of fluids
- o Anti–emetics
  - – 1st line
    - ▪ H1 antagonists, i.e. diphenhydramine
  - – 2nd line
    - ▪ Dopamine antagonists, i.e. prochlorperazine
- o Thiamine to ↓ risk of Wernicke encephalopathy (little data)
  - ▪ Resolves with fluids, NPO

Intrahepatic Cholestasis of Pregnancy

➤ Demography
- o Occurs in 2nd and 3rd trimester; resolves after birth
- o Incidence: $200/10^5$ in USA, highest in Bolivia, Chile

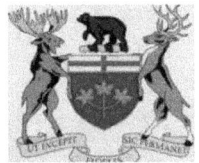

- ➤ Clinical
  - ○ Pruritis
    - – Often intolerable
    - – Palms, feet, nocturnal
  - ○ Often no abdominal pain or encephalopathy
  - ○ Excoriations from scratching
    - – Jaundice seen in < 10% (jaundice without pruritis is rare; search for other causes)

- ➤ Pathogenesis
  - ○ Unknown – estrogen is known to cause cholestasis

- ➤ Laboratory
  - ○ Total fasting bile acid concentrations (10 – 100x ULN)
  - ○ ↑ serum bile acids
    - – Cholic > chenodeoxycholic acid
  - ○ ↑ ALP 1 – 4x ULN, GGT often normal or slightly high
  - ○ ↑↑ bile acids (out of proportion to ↑ GGT)
  - ○ ↑ AST and ALT, often > 1000
  - ○ Bilirubin is modestly elevated
  - ○ INR is often normal, elevated due to Vitamin K deficiency associated with cholestasis or the use of bile acid sequestrants – not due to liver dysfunction

- ➤ Diagnostic imaging
  - ○ Abdominal ultrasound
    - – Normal parenchyma, ducts

- ➤ Diagnosis
  - ○ Pruritis + ↑ bile acid levels + ↑ AST and ALT + exclusion of other causes (viral cause is important with high enzymes)

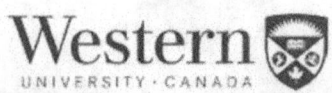

➢ Pathology
  o Liver biopsy is rarely necessary – cholestasis without inflammation

➢ Treatment
  o ↓ symptoms in mother
  o ↓ risk of maternal/fetal complications
  o Early delivery (week 32: fetal distress; 37 – 38 if not)
  o UDCA – increases bile flow, relieves pruritis = 1st line
    - Meta–analyses of 9 RCTs, 454 patients → better outcomes *vs* alternative agents (dex, cholestryamine)
    - Pruritis improvement: 61% *vs* 27%
    - Improvement of bile acid concentrations and transaminases, lower premature delivery rate
    - Dosing: 500 *bid* or 300 *tid* until delivery
  o Vitamin K repletion
  o Hydroxyzine (20 – 50 mg/d): may improve the pruritis, may aggravate the respiratory difficulties of preterm babies
  o Cholestyramine (8 – 16 g/day): decreases ileal absorption of bile salts = ↑ fecal excretion
    - Considered 2nd line, inferior to UDCA
    - Effect on pruritis is limited, can ↑ steatorrhea and ↑ vitamin K deficiency

➢ Prognosis
  o Recurrence in subsequent pregnancies
    - 60 – 70%
  o Use of OCP (Estrogen–Progestin, Progestin only) not contraindicated (does not ↑ recurrence)

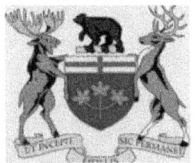

- o Fetal Risks
  - – Prematurity (40%), meconium–stained amniotic fluid, intrauterine death (0.3%), neonatal ARDS (bile acid enters the lungs)
- o Maternal
  - – Good prognosis, often a clue to any underlying disease, check for HBV/HCV post–delivery, ↑ gallstone risk

HELLP

- ➤ Definition
  - o Syndrome of MAHA, elevated liver enzymes, low platelets (thrombocytopenia)

- ➤ Demography
  - o 0.5% all pregnancies, 10 – 20% if severe preeclampsia
  - o Likely represents severe form of preeclampsia

- ➤ Risk factors
  - o Family or personal history of preeclampsia and HELLP
  - o Nulliparity is not a risk factor (as is preeclampsia)

- ➤ Criteria for the diagnosis of preeclampsia
  - o Systolic blood pressure of ≥ 140 mmHg or diastolic blood pressure of ≥ 90 mmHg on 2 occasions at least 4 hours apart after 20 weeks of gestation in a previously normotensive patient
  - o If systolic blood pressure is ≥ 160 mmHg or diastolic blood pressure is ≥ 110 mmHg, confirmation within minutes is sufficient

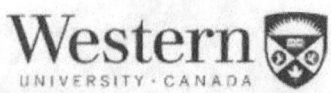

- o   Proteinuria with ≥ 0.3 g in a 24–hour urine specimen or protein (mg/dL) creatinine (mg/dL) ratio of ≥ 0.3

- o   Dipstick result is 1+, if a quantitative measurement is unavailable

- In patients with new onset hypertension without proteinuria, the new onset of any of the following is diagnostic of preeclampsia:

  - o   Platelet count: < 100,000 µL

  - o   Serum creatinine: > 1.1 mg/dL or doubling of serum creatinine in the absence of other renal disease

  - o   Liver transaminase is at least twice the normal concentrations (2x the upper limit of normal)

  - o   Pulmonary edema

  - o   Visual changes

Adapted from: American College of Obstetricians and Gynecologists; Task Force on Hypertension in Pregnancy. *Obstet Gynecol* 2013, 122:1122-31.

➢   Symptoms and signs

  - o   Usually present at 28 – 36 weeks

  - o   Abdominal pain – epigastric, RUQ

  - o   N/V, malaise, visual changes

  - o   HTN (> 140/90) and proteinuria

  - o   Jaundice and ascites may be the initial presentation

Abbreviations: HTN, hypertension; N/V, nausea/vomiting; RUQ, right upper quadrant

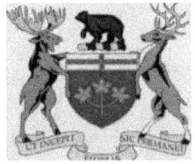

❖ Reported frequency of signs and symptoms of HELLP syndrome

Signs and symptoms	Frequency (%)
o Proteinuria	86 – 100
o Hypertension	82 – 88
o Right upper quadrant and epigastric pain	40 – 90
o Nausea, vomiting	29 – 84
o Headache	33 – 61
o Visual changes	10 – 20
o Jaundice	5

➤ Laboratory

- o ALT, AST < 500 (median is 250, higher if there is hepatic infarction)
- o Platelets < 100,000
- o LDH > 600
- o Bilirubin median 1.5 mg/dL

➤ Diagnosis

- o MAHA → elevated LDH > 600, low haptoglobin < 1, schistocytes are diagnostic
- o Platelets < 100
- o Total Bilirubin > 20.5
- o AST > 70 (reflects RBC hemolysis, hepatocellular necrosis)
- o All of these are required for the Tennessee Classification

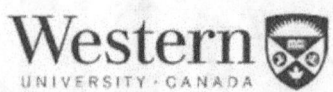

➤ Complications

- o Hepatic rupture with hematoma beneath the Glisson's capsule (hepatic preeclampsia)

- o Hematoma: contained or ruptured into the peritoneal cavity → usually if preecclampsia

- o Hematoma can cause epigastric pain and N/V
  - If contained → supportive care (IVF, pRBCs, platelet transfusion)
  - Full resolution takes months, perform follow–up imaging if with stable size and laboratory parameters are improving

- o Rupture → shock, hemoperitoneum, AST/ALT > 1000
  - Percutaneous embolization of hepatic arteries, if stable
  - Surgery is unstable and would result to worsening of pain and expansion

- o Infarction: transaminases > 1000, fever, usually associated with underlying hypercoagulability (i.e. APLAS)

➤ Outcomes

- o Mother
  - Postpartum → platelets drop within 48 hours of delivery, LDH peaks; platelets usually > 100 by day 6
  - Associated with DIC (21%), ARF (16%), pulmonary ddema (6%), liver hematoma (1%), retinal detachment (1%)
  - Recurs in future pregnancies in 3 – 27%, risk of preecclampsia in future pregnancies is 40%

- o Mortality
  - Mother   3%
  - Fetus   35 – 45%

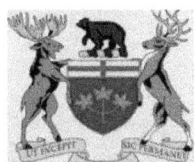

➢ Treatment
- o Treat HTN → labetolol, hydralazine, nifedipine
- o Severe HTN → symptomatic → $MgSO_4^-$
- o Delivery
  - − Immediate, regardless of weeks, if with DIC, MOD, pulmonary edema, RF, liver hemorrhage and infarction, fetal distress
  - − Immediate, if >/= 34 weeks (1 C)
  - − </= 34 weeks → steroids to enhance fetal pulmonary maturity and delivery, C/S if </= 30 weeks
- o Platelet transfusions − if with active bleeding, < 20 − 50 and during delivery
- o Dexamethasone → if platelets < 100, but used by many centers without evidence, Cochrane reviews demonstrated no efficacy; no good RCTs

Abbreviations: C/S, caeserian section; DLC, disseminated intravascular coagulopathy; HTN, hypertension; MOD, multiple organ dysfunction; RCT, randomized controlled trials; RF, respiratory failure

Acute Fatty Liver of Pregnancy

➢ Demography
- o $10/10^5$ deliveries
- o Characterized by microvesicular fatty infiltration of hepatocytes
- o First described in 1940s, almost 100% fatal at the time
- o Early detection and prompt delivery immensely improve the outcomes
- o More common: multiple gestations, underweight mom
- o Almost always in the 3rd trimester

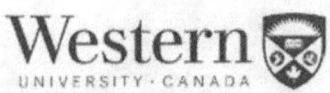

- Clinical
  - Nausea and vomiting – 75%, epigastric pain – 50%, anorexia, jaundice
  - 50% have signs of preecclampsia
  - Extrahepatic complications: infection, DIC, GIB, intra–abdominal bleeding, central DI, pancreatitis, ARF

- Laboratory
  - AST/ALT ≤ 500, may be > 1000, leukocytosis, thrombocytopenia
  - Can cause coagulopathy or ↑ INR and ↓ platelets
  - ↓ glucose, ↑ uric acid

- Pathogenesis
  - Associated with inherited defects in mitochondrial oxidation of fatty acids
  - LCHAD = Long chain 3–hydroxyacyl CoA dehydrogenase deficiency due to genetic defect
  - Accumulation of long chain metabolites produced by the fetus or placenta which is toxic to the liver
  - Pathogenesis is still poorly understood
  - Women with AFLP and their children suggested to go for molecular testing for LCHAD mutation → G1528C

- Diagnosis
  - Clinical overlap with HELLP, often cannot be differentiated
  - Liver biopsy is diagnostic → microvesicular fatty infiltration of hepatocytes, "foamy appearance"
    - Fatty parts are prominent in the central and mid–zonal parts of the lobule
    - Usually spares the rim of cells around portal tracts
    - Invasive
    - Only if the diagnosis is in doubt, as diagnosis will result to delivery of the baby

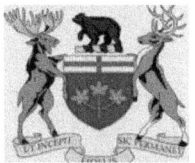

- ➤ Histopathology
  - o Microvesicular steatosis

- ➤ Treatment
  - o No specific therapy
  - o Stabilize by giving glucose infusion D10W as hypoglycemia is common and reverse coagulopathy
  - o FFP, cryoprecipitate, RBCs, platelets as necessary
  - o Immediate delivery
  - o Substantial morbidity to mother and baby without delivery
  - o May worsen few days after delivery, but improvement is seen within 7 – 10 days

American College of Gastroenterology Guidelines: Liver Disease in the Pregnant Patient

- o Use of gestational age of pregnancy is the best guide to the differential diagnosis of liver disease in pregnant woman
- o Hyperemesis gravidarum should be considered in the differential diagnosis of abnormal liver tests presenting in the first trimester
- o Cholestasis of pregnancy is common, and should be considered in the differential diagnosis of abnormal liver tests presenting initially in the second trimester. Affected pregnancies are at increased risk for prematurity and stillbirth, and early delivery should be considered when possible.

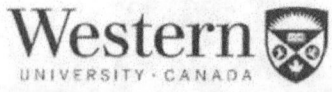

- o HELLP (hemolysis, elevated liver tests, low platelets) syndrome and acute fatty liver of pregnancy should be considered in the differential diagnosis of abnormal liver tests in the second half of pregnancy, usually seen also in the third trimester
- o Patients with acute fatty liver of pregnancy have true hepatic dysfunction, and may, or may not, have signs of preeclampsia and HELLP syndrome
- o Consider viral or drug–induced hepatitis, gallstone disease, or malignancy in the differential diagnosis of abnormal liver tests in any of the trimesters of pregnancy
- o Chronic hepatitis B or C poses a risk of transmission of the off-spring

Printed with permission: Riely, C.A. *Am J Gastroenterol* 1999, 94:1728-32.

Other Entities

Herpes Simplex Viral (HSV) Hepatitis

- o Usually 3rd trimester, HSV–1 and 2
- o Prodrome of fever and malaise for 4 – 14 days
- o RUQ pain and oral and genital lesions seen in 30%
- o Transaminases > 1000, moderately increased bilirubin, rapid progression to fulminant hepatic failure
- o CT shows multiple low density, non–enhancing areas that represent hemorrhagic necrosis
- o Maternal mortality = > 80% without treatment
- o Must start IV acyclovir early
- o Transmission to infants in 45%

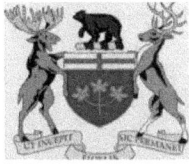

Portal Hypertension in Pregnancy

- ○ ↑ portal pressure due to ↑ plasma volume and ↑ cardiac output + ↑ vascular resistance from compression of IVC
- ○ Risk of variceal hemorrhage is greatest in the 2nd trimester and during labor (75% if associated with pre–existing varices)
- ○ Prognosis is better for non–cirrhotic portal HTN
- ○ Treatment of variceal hemorrhage is banding
- ○ Safety of octreotide is unknown; avoid vasopressin
- ○ Possible use os non–selective beta blockers (Grade C)
- ○ Minimize second part of labor; avoid excessive fluids

Hepatic Adenomas

- ○ Accelerated growth from high estrogen levels
- ○ Complications
  - – Hemorrhage and intraperitoneal rupture
- ○ Adenomas > 5 cm or symptomatic or intra–lesional bleeding should be considered for surgical resection before contraception

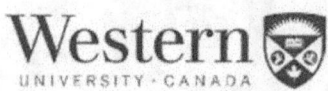

Nutrition Assessment in Liver Cirrhosis

Lynne Sinclair

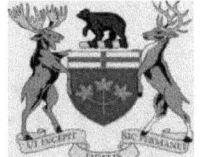

The nutritional management of hepatic encephalopathy in patients with cirrhosis: International Society for Hepatic Encephalopathy and Nitrogen Metabolism Consensus†

Amodio, P., *et al. Hepatology* 2013, 58:325-36.

Detection of Malnutrition in Cirrhosis

o   Hand Grip Strength
  - Correlate with muscle mass, protein visceral status and severity of the disease
  - Standards that identifies malnutrition with good sensitivity
    - HG < 30 kg (men)
    - HG < 14 kg (women)

Protein Energy Malnutrition

o   Independent predictor of morbidity and mortality in patients with cirrhosis

o   Underdiagnosed

o   Potentially reversible

Sarcopenia – An Objective Nutritional Assessment Tool That May Facilitate Prioritization of Liver Transplant Candidates

AASLD LiverLearning®. Tandon, P. Nov 5, 2011;12987.
Topic: Liver Transplant and Surgery

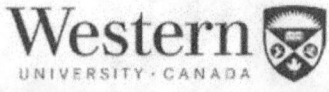

Predictor of Sarcopenia (logistic regression analysis)

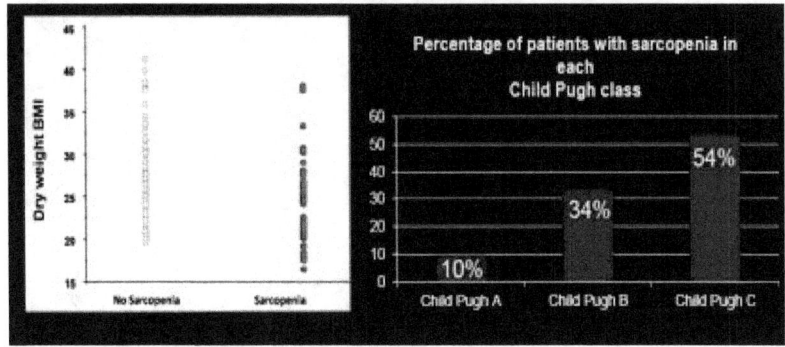

Adapted from: Tandon, P. Liver Transplant and Surgery. AASLD Liver Learning®; Nov 5, 2011:12987.

Characteristics	Odds ratio (95% CI)	P value
o Male gender	7.54 (2.79 – 20.4)	0.001
o Child Pugh C cirrhosis (vs Child Pugh A)	23.2 (1.73 – 311)	0.018
o Dry weight	0.97 (0.95 – 1.00)	0.027

Characteristics	Hazard ratio (95% CI)	P value
o Sarcopenia	2.93 (0.85 – 10.1)	0.09
o Age	1.06 (1.01 – 1.12)	0.02
o MELD score	1.13 (1.08 – 1.19)	0.001
o Sodium (mEq/L)	0.92 (0.84 – 1.00)	0.048

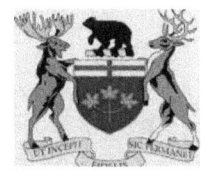

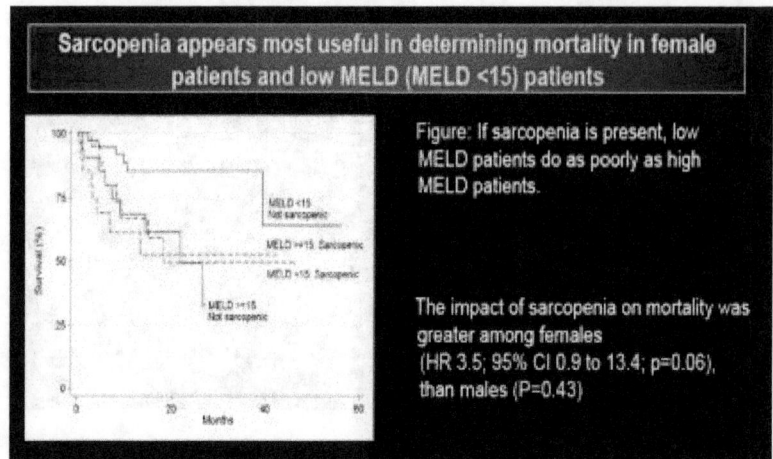

Adapted from: Tandon, P. Liver Transplant and Surgery. AASLD LiverLearning®; Nov 5, 2011:12987.

Detection of Malnutrition in Cirrhosis

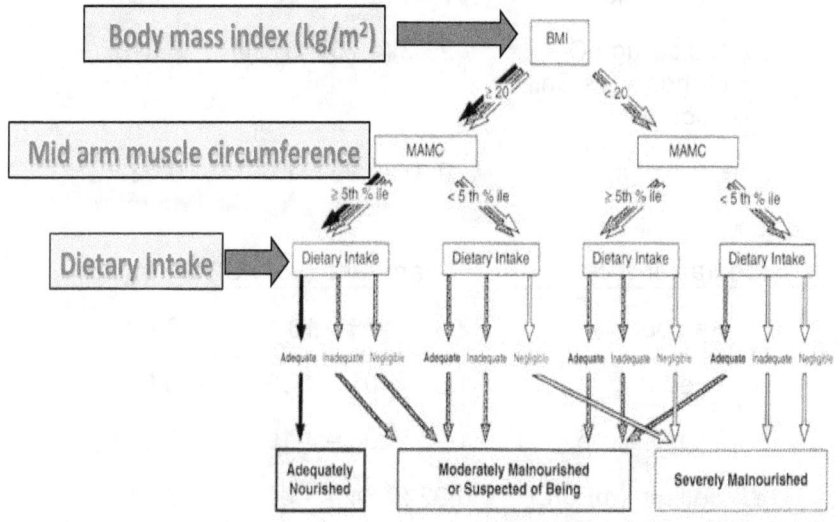

Printed with permission: Morgan, M.Y., et al. *Hepatology* 2006, 44:823-35.

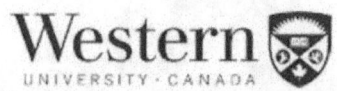

Fuel Use: Respiratory Quotient (RQ)

- Gold standard – indirect calorimetry (IC)

$$RQ = \frac{V_{CO_2}}{V_{O_2}}$$

- Ratio of carbon dioxide produced to oxygen consumption
- Indirect measure of substrate utilization
  - Carbohydrate, fats and protein
- Patients with cirrhosis who fasted for 24 hours had a continued decline in RQ, which did not change in controls

Nakaya, Y., *et al. J Gastronentrol* 2002; 37(7):531-6.

In Liver Transplant Candidates, MELD Score does not Correlate with Nutritional Needs

- Mean mREE was ~ 20% lower in the BMI ≥ 25 group than in BMI < 25 (0.0042)
- Mean pREE was 26% lower than mean mREE in the hypermetabolic (> 120% HBE) group

Protein

- Muscle tissue plays a key role in glutamine synthesis providing an alternate detoxification pathway for the removal of ammonia (NH_3)
- Stable cirrhotic patients can retain nitrogen and form lean body mass if adequately fed and exercised

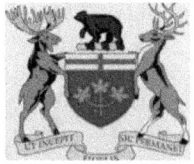

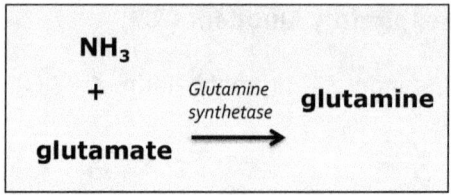

Lean body mass (LBM) **loss associated with bed rest or hospitalization**

Group diet	Loss of lean body leg mass (g)
o Inactivity	
– Healthy young	20
– Healthy elders	110
o Hospitalization	
– Healthy elders	300

Paddon-Jones, D., *et al. Curr Opin Clin Nutr Metab Care.* 2009; 12(1):86–90.

- o Insufficient protein intake is associated with increased mortality in 630 patients with cirrhosis awaiting liver transplantation (Ney, M., *et al. Nutr Clin Pract* 2015 30: 530-6)

- o Amount of protein consumed did not influence the course of hepatic encephalopathy (Cordoba, J., *et al, J Hepatol.* 2004; 41(1):38-43.)

- o Very low protein intake (< 0.8g/kg per day) with
  - – Worse liver disease severity (per Child-Pugh or MELD)
  - – Independent predictor of malnutrition and transplant waiting list mortality

- o Thus, no reason to restrict protein

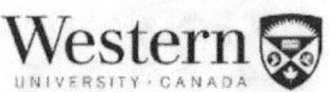

Recommendations regarding energy and protein provision in patients with cirrhosis and HE

- o Optimal daily
  - – Energy 35 – 40 kcal/kg ideal   1A
    body weight
  - – Protein 1.2 – 1.5 g/kg ideal   1A
    body weight

- o Small meals are evenly   1A
  distributed throughout the day
  and a late night snack

- o Encourage ingestion of a diet   2B
  rich in vegetable and dairy
  protein

- o BCAA supplementation might   2B
  allow recommended nitrogen
  intakes to be attained and
  maintained in patients who are
  intolerant of dietary protein

Abbreviation: BCAA, branched chain amino acids

Lipids

- o In cirrhosis, plasma clearance of lipids is not reduced
  - – Avoid fat restriction, if possible

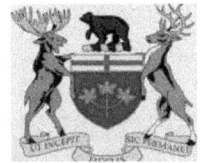

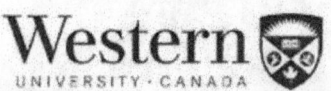

Gallstone Disease

Benson Thomas

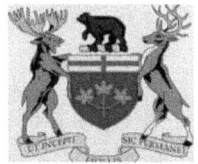

Gallstone Disease

➢ Definition and Types

   ○ Types:
- Cholesterol
  - Mixed (need 50% of cholesterol by weight) or pure
- Pigments
  - Black, brown
- Rare
  - Calcium carbonate, fatty acids, calcium

   ○ Location
- Gallbladder
- Intrahepatic
- Bile duct (hepatic or common bile duct)

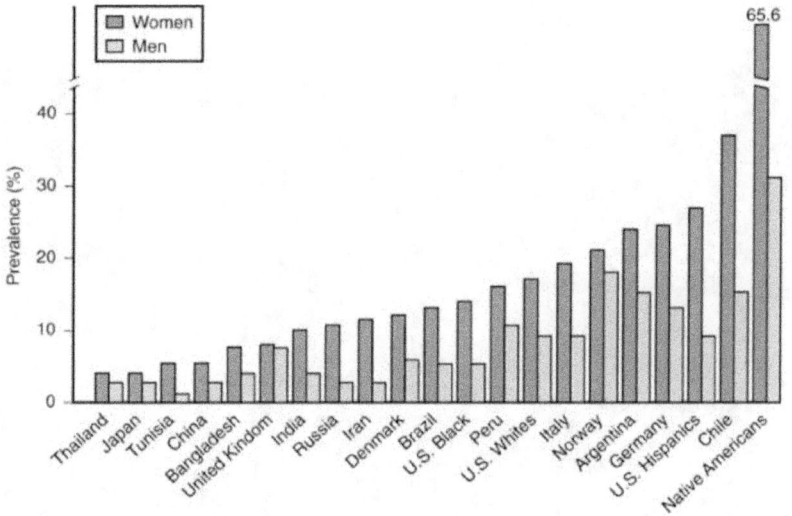

➢ Risk factors

   ○ Age (older), Gender (F > M)

   ○ Total Parenteral Nutrition (as early as 3 weeks)

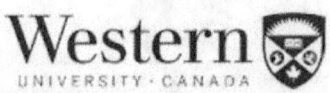

- o Diet

- o Rapid weight loss

- o Pregnancy and parity

- o Drugs (i.e. estrogen, octreotide, ceftriaxone)

- o Systemic disease (i.e. obesity, DM, lipid disorders, ileal disease, spinal cord injuries)

➢ Composition of bile

- o Lipid components
  - – Cholesterol
  - – Phospholipids
  - – Bile salts

- o Protein elements
  - – Albumin
  - – Immunoglobulins
  - – Apolipoproteins

➢ Pathophysiology

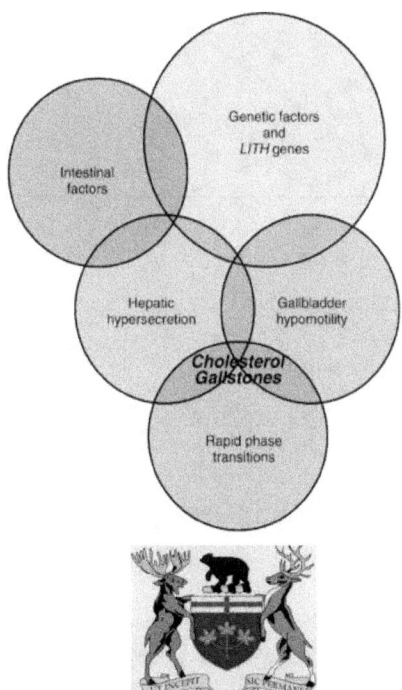

➢ Hepatic Hypersecretion of Biliary Cholesterol

   o Supersaturated bile
     – Contains cholesterol that cannot be solubilized by bile salts and phospholipids at equilibrium

   o Cholesterol Supersaturation
     – ↑ hepatic secretion of biliary cholesterol
     – ↓ bile salt or phospholipids secretion into bile
     – ↑ cholesterol and hyposecretion of solubilizing lipids

   o More likely for cholesterol to form crystals

➢ Rapid Transition

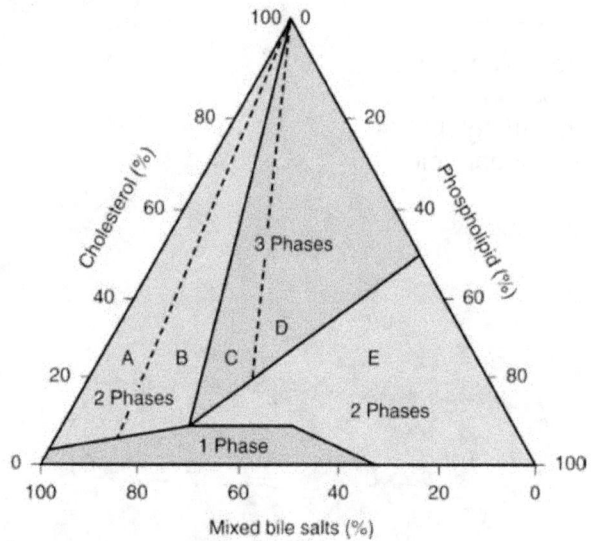

   o Nidation factors in bile

➢ Gallbladder Dysmotility

   o ↑ fasting gallbladder volume

   o ↓ emptying

   o ↑ residual gallbladder volume

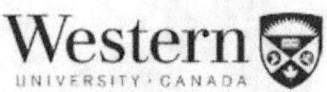

- o Abnormalities: binding of agonists, i.e. CCK, to plasma membrane CCK–1 receptors, during contraction of isolated smooth muscle cells and decreased contractility of isolated smooth muscle strips

➤ Intestinal Factors
- o ↑ cholesterol absorption
  - – ↓ impaired small bowel transit
- o Intestinal resection and TI disease (i.e. Crohn's disease)
  - – ↓ enterohepatic circulation, reduced bile salt secretion
- o Chronic Intestinal Infection – *Helicobacter* species (not *H. pylori* though)

➤ Genetic
- o Gallstones are more frequent by a ratio of 3:1 in siblings and other family members of affected patients than in spouses or unrelated controls

Pigment Stones

- Black Stones
  - o Formed in uninfected gallbladders, typically in patients with the following:
    - – Chronic hemolytic anemia
      - ▪ β–thalassemia
      - ▪ Hereditary spherocytosis
      - ▪ Sickle cell disease
    - – Cirrhosis
  - o Composed of either of the following:
    - – Pure calcium bilirubinate
    - – Polymer–like complexes consisting of unconjugated bilirubin, calcium bilirubinate, calcium and copper

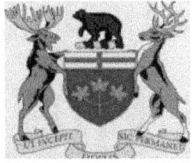

- Brown Stones
  - o Composed mainly of calcium salts of unconjugated bilirubin with varying amounts of cholesterol, fatty acids, pigment fraction and mucin glycoproteins, as well as small amounts of bile salts, phospholipids, and residues
  - o Formed in the gallbladder and biliary tree
  - o Formation requires stasis and infection
    - Clonorchis sinensis
    - E. Coli

Formation of Brown Pigment Stones

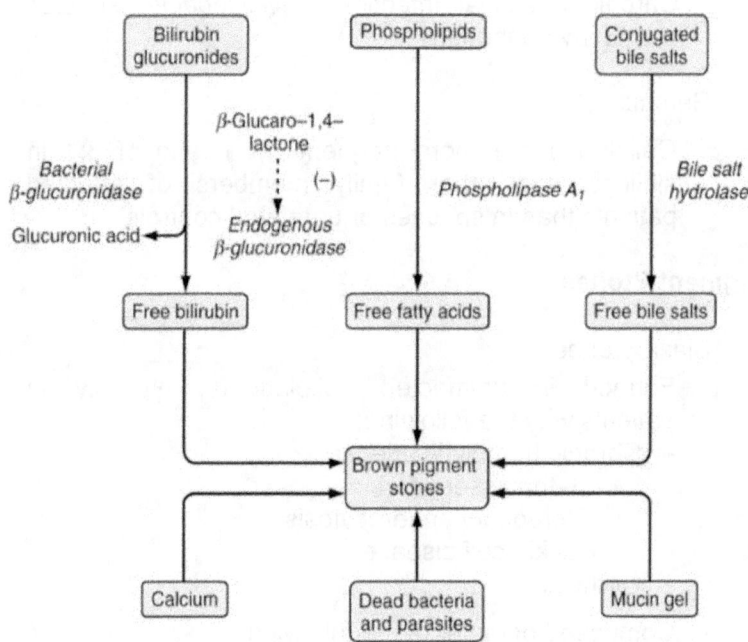

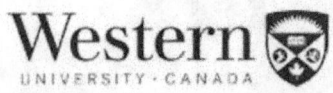

Natural History

- Asymptomatic Stones

2 Studies – that shaped our view

- o Michigan – Gracie and Ransohoff
  - – At 5, 10, and 15 years of follow–up, 10%, 15%, and 18% of patients, respectively, become symptomatic, and none had experienced serious complications (Michigan)
- o The Group for Epidemiology and Prevention of Cholelithiasis (GREPCO) in Rome
  - – Biliary pain was 12% in 2 years, 17% in 4 years, and 26% in 10 years, and the cummulative rate of biliary complication was 3% in 10 years

- Symptomatic Stones
  - o More aggressive course
  - o 30 – 50% of those who have had biliary pain with recurrent episodes
  - o 1 – 2% biliary complication per year, does not increase over time

- ➢ Diagnostic imaging
  - o Abdominal ultrasound (US)
    - – Sensitivity rate is > 95% for stones > 2 mm
    - – Specificity rate is > 95% for stones with acoustic shadows
    - – Best single test for stones in the gallbladder
    - – US Murphy Sign - positive predictive value of > 90% in detecting acute cholecystitis when stones are seen
    - – Can confirm, but not exclude, BD stones

Abbreviation: BD, bile duct

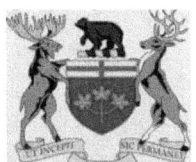

- o EUS
  - Highly accurate in excluding or confirming stones in the BD
  - Specificity rate is ≈ 97%
  - Positive predictive value of ≈ 99%, negative predictive value of ≈ 98%, accuracy rate is ≈ 97%
  - *Considered in patients with a low–to–moderate clinical probability of choledocholithiasis*

- o Cholescintigraphy
  - Assesses patency of the cystic duct
  - Positive result is defined as non–visualization of the gallbladder with preserved hepatic excretion of radionuclide into the BD or small bowel
  - Sensitivity rate is ≈ 95% and specificity rate is ≈ 90%, with false–positive results seen in fasted, critically ill patients (*Normal scan result virtually excludes acute cholecystitis*)
  - With cholecystokinin stimulation, gallbladder "ejection fraction" can be determined and may help evaluate patients with acalculous biliary pain

- o ERCP
  - ERCP is the standard diagnostic test for stones in the BD with sensitivity and specificity rates of ≈ 95%, respectively
  - Recommended for patients with high clinical probability of choledocholithiasis
  - Use of ERCP to extract stones (or at least to drain infected bile) is lifesaving in severe cholangitis and reduces the need for BD exploration at the time of cholecystectomy

- o MRCP
  - Sensitivity rate is ≈ 93% and specificity rate is ≈ 94%, comparable with those for ERCP
  - Evaluate pancreas, liver, etc.
  - *Recommended for patients with a low–to–moderate clinical probability of choledocholithiasis*

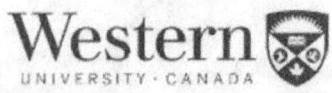

- *A little about CT scan – good to evaluate the complications but other than that is useless*

➢ Clinical Disorders
  o Biliary pain
  o Cholangitis
  o Choledocholithiasis
  o Acute cholecystitis (*pain lasting for > 6 hours)

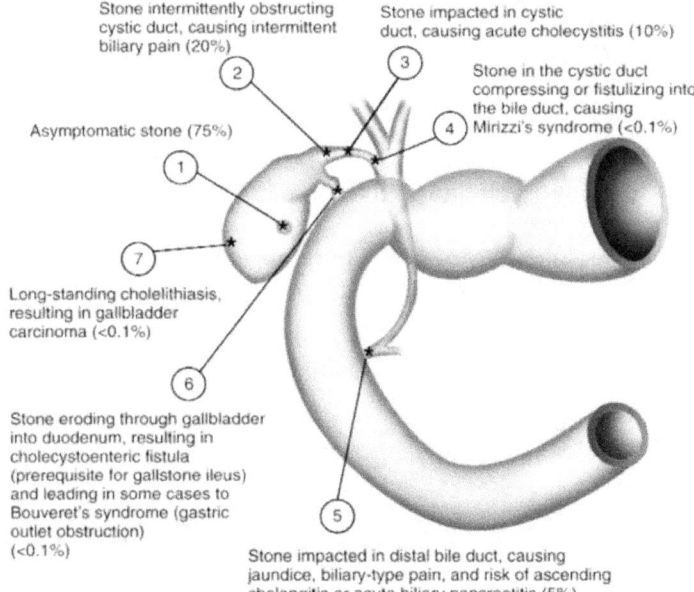

Stone intermittently obstructing cystic duct, causing intermittent biliary pain (20%)

Stone impacted in cystic duct, causing acute cholecystitis (10%)

Stone in the cystic duct compressing or fistulizing into the bile duct, causing Mirizzi's syndrome (<0.1%)

Asymptomatic stone (75%)

Long-standing cholelithiasis, resulting in gallbladder carcinoma (<0.1%)

Stone eroding through gallbladder into duodenum, resulting in cholecystoenteric fistula (prerequisite for gallstone ileus) and leading in some cases to Bouveret's syndrome (gastric outlet obstruction) (<0.1%)

Stone impacted in distal bile duct, causing jaundice, biliary-type pain, and risk of ascending cholangitis or acute biliary pancreatitis (5%)

➢ Uncommon complications

  o Emphysematous cholecystitis
    - Secondary infection of gallbladder wall with gas–forming organisms (*Clostridium welchii*, *E. coli*, anaerobic *Strep.*) – diabetics, elderly, can occur without stones

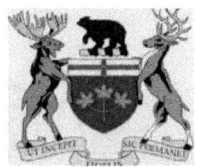

o   Mirizzi syndrome

o   Porcelain gallbladder
    - Intramural calcification of the gallbladder wall
    - ↑ risk of progression to carcinoma

o   Cholecystoenteric fistula

➢   Treatment

o   Stones
    - Small
    - Multiple
    - Radiopaque
    - Functioning gallbladder

o   Medical
    - Ursodeoxycholic acid oral dissolution should be considered for:
      ▪ Patients with uncomplicated gallstone disease, including those with mild, infrequent biliary pain

o   Extracorporeal shockwave lithotripsy

o   Endoscopic ERCP
    - +/- sphincterotomy
    - +/- stone removal

o   Surgical – open or laparoscopic cholecystectomy, ERCP

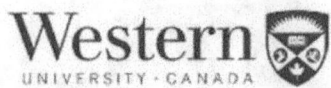

COMPLICATIONS

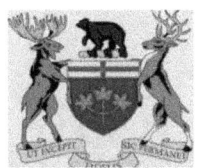

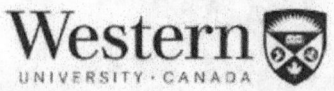

Hepatic Encephalopathy

Ngoc Han Quang Le

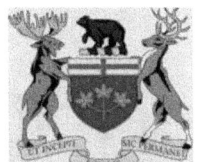

➢ Definition

- o "Hepatic encephalopathy [HE] is a brain dysfunction caused by liver insufficiency and/or portosystemic shunting (PSS); it manifests as a wide spectrum of neurological or psychiatric abnormalities ranging from subclinical alterations to coma."

Vilstrup, H., *et al. Hepatology* 2014; 60(2):715-35.

➢ Demography

- o Prevalence
  - – OHE:
    - ▪ 30 – 40% in all cirrhotics
    - ▪ 10 – 50% post–TIPS (cummulative 1–year incidence)
  - – MHE or CHE:
    - ▪ 20 – 80%
- o Recurrence
  - – Cummulative risk in 1 year is 40%
  - – Another 40% cummulative risk of recurrent OHE in 6 months (with secondary prophylaxis)
- o Survival
  - – At 1 year, 42%
  - – At 3 years, 23%

Abbreviations: CHE, covert hepatic encephalopathy; MHE, minimal hepatic encephalopathy; OHE, overt hepatic encephalopathy

Sharma, *et al. Am J Gastroenterol* 2013; 108:1458-63.

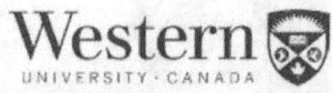

➢ Classification

HE description

Type	Grade		Time course	Spontaneous or precipitated
A	MHE	Covert	Episodic	Spontaneous
	1		Recurrent	
B	2	Overt		Precipitate (specific)
	3		Persistent	
C	4			

Abbreviation: MHE, minimal hepatic encephalopathy

Printed with permission: Vilstrup, H., *et al. Hepatology* 2014; 60(2):715-35.

- o Time course
  - – Episodic HE
  - – Recurrent HE
    - ▪ Bouts of HE that occur within a time interval of 6 months or less
  - – Persistent HE
    - ▪ A pattern of behavioral alterations that are always present and are interspersed with relapses of overt HE
- o Underlying disease
  - – Grade and severity
  - – Time course
  - – Precipitating factors

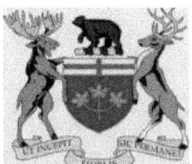

Types	Causes
A	Acute liver failure (ALF)
B	Portosystemic bypass and shunt
C	Cirrhosis

o Clinical severity

WHC and clinical description

WHC including MHE	ISHEN	Description	Suggested Operative Criteria	Comments
o Unimpaired		– No encephalopathy – No history of HE	Tested and proven to be normal	
o Minimal Covert		– Psychometric or neuropsychological alterations of tests exploiting psychomotor speed or executive functions or neurophysiological alterations without clinical evidence of mental changes	▪ Abnormal results of established psychometric or neuro-psychologic tests without clinical manifestations	- No universal criteria for diagnosis - Local standards and expertise required
o Grade I		– Trivial lack of awareness – Euphoria or anxiety – Shortened attention span – Impairment of addition or subtraction – Altered sleep rhythm	▪ Despite oriented in time and space (see below), patient appears to have some cognitive or behavioral delay with respect to his or her standards on clinical examination or to the caregivers	- Clinical findings usually not re-producible

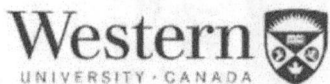

WHC including MHE	ISHEN	Description	Suggested Operative Criteria	Comments
○ Grade II	Overt	– Lethargy or apathy – Disorientation for time – Obvious personality changes – Inappropriate behavior – Dyspraxia – Asterixis	▪ Disoriented for time (at least 3 of the following are wrong: day of the month, day of the week, month, season, or year) ± the other mentioned symptoms	- Clinical findings variable, but re-producible to some extent
○ Grade III		– Somnolence to semistupor – Responsive to stimuli – Confused – Gross disorientation – Bizarre behavior	▪ Disoriented for space (at least 3 of the following wrongly reported: country, state [or region], city, or place) ± the other mentioned symptoms	
○ Grade IV		– Coma	▪ Does not respond even to painful stimuli	- Comatose state usually re-producible

Printed with permission: Vilstrup, H., *et al. Hepatology* 2014; 60(2):715-35.

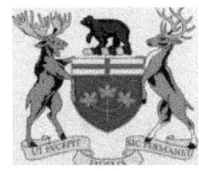

➢ Pathophysiology

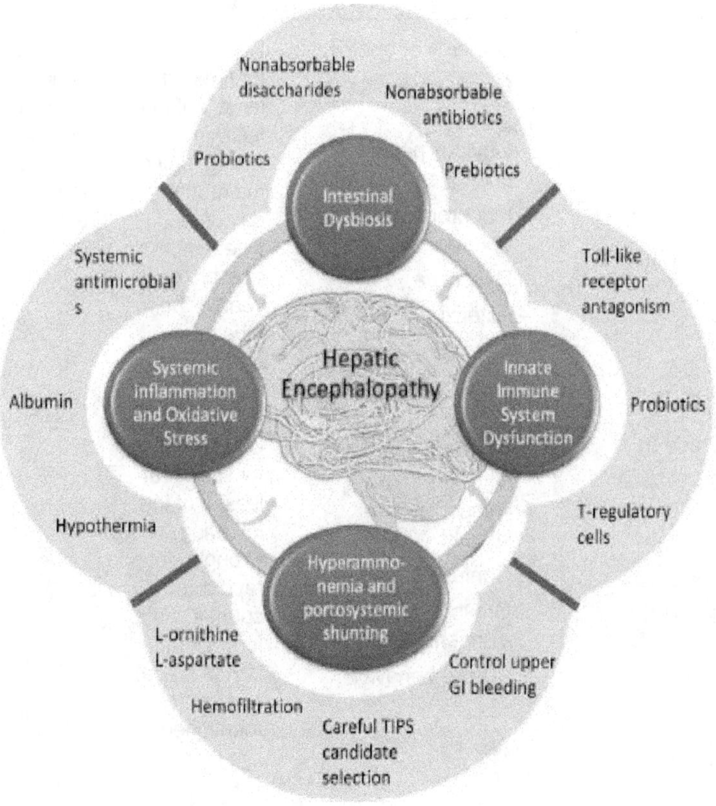

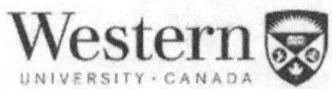

Printed with permission: Tranah, T.H., *et al*. Clinical Liver Disease 2015; 5(3): 59-63.

- Hyperammonia

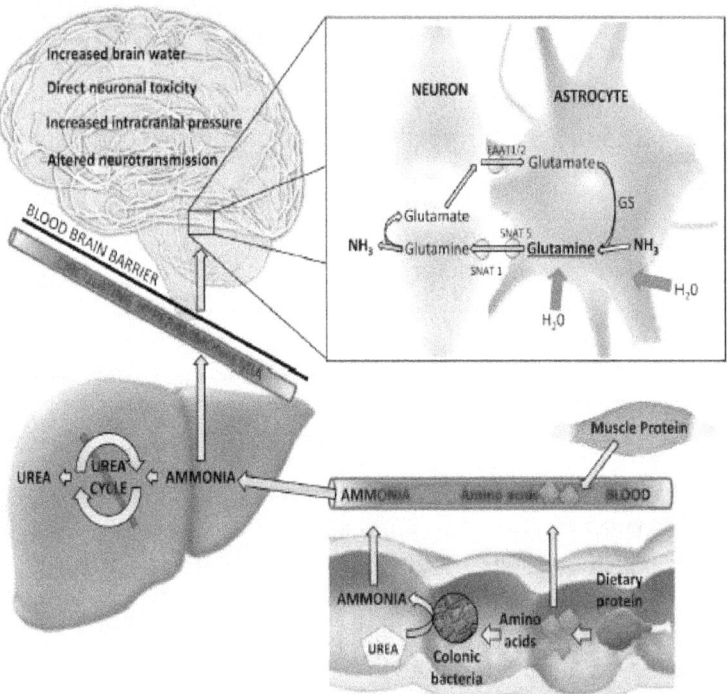

Printed with permission: Tranah, T.H., *et al.* Clinical Liver Disease 2015; 5(3):59-63.

- Other pathways
  - o Inflammatory theory and endotoxemia
    - – Proinflammatory state → cerebral hyperemia with increased ammonia delivery → oxidative stress
  - o Intestinal microbiome
  - o Increased tryptophan (precursor of serotonin)
    - – Sleep–wake cycle
  - o Zinc deficiency (needed in urea cycle)

Tranah, T.H., *et al. Clinical Liver Disease* 2015; 5(3):59-63.

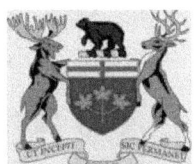

- Outline the functions of the small and large intestines, liver, skeletal muscles, kidneys and brain in patients with liver failure and HE.

  o Small and large intestines
    - Dietary amino acids and urease–positive bacteria → glutamine

---

glutaminase (deamination)

glutamine   →   glutamate + NH_3

← glutamine synthetase (amination)

    - Activity of the gut glutaminase is increased in liver disease
    - Uptake of glutamine

  o Liver
    - Portosystemic shunting, by–passing the portovenous system with less hepatic detoxification of ammonia via the urea cycle
    - NH_3 → urea, periportal hepatocytes → glutamine, perivenous hepatocytes
    - In the presence of hyponatremia, myoinositol falls, with less compensation for ↑ intracellular glutamine

  o Skeletal muscles
    - Normally responsible for the uptake of 50% of NH_3
    - In cirrhosis, atrophy of skeletal muscles → ↓ muscle synthesis of glutamine

  o Kidney
    - ↑ NH_3 production in the presence of hypokalemia

  o Brain
    - NH_3 and glutamate are normally converted and detoxified to glutamine by glutamine synthetase in astrocytes

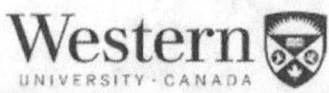

- In cirrhosis, the following are seen:
  - ↑ brain blood flow
  - ↑ blood brain barrier permeability → ↑ brain NH_3 and glutamate → astrocytes swelling
- In the presence of hypokalemia and metabolic alkalosis, NH_4 → NH_3, which crosses the BBB
- Plasma NH_3 > 150 μmol is associated with brain herniation
- Abnormal form and functions of astrocytes, with reduced glutamine synthetase and peripheral type benzodiazepine receptors (PTBR)
  - ↑ mitochondrial permeability → ↑ astrocyte swelling → ↑ brain edema
- ↑ NH_3 activates N–methyl–D–aspartate–nitric oxide–C–guanylate cyclase (NMDA–NO–CGMP) signal transduction pathway → impairment of:
  - Memory
  - Learning
  - Sleep

Neurotransmitter system	Findings in HE
○ ↑ GABA, ↑ serotonin	- ↑ serotonin turnover, synaptic defect
○ ↑ endogenous BZs	- Neuro–inhibition
○ Glutamate (neuro–excitation)	- ↓ receptors → ↓ uptake of glutamate
	- ↓ glutamatergic neurotransmitter function
○ Dopamine and noradrenaline (motor and cognitive)	- ↓ false neurotransmitters

Abbreviations: BZ, benzodiazepine; GABA, γ–aminobutyric acid

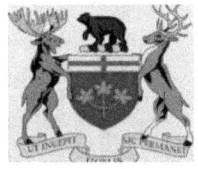

- o Brain
  - – ↑ BB permeability → ↑ NH_3 uptake
  - – ↑ NH_3 taken up into the following:
    - Cerebellum
    - Basal ganglia
    - ↑ brain edema
    - ↑ swelling of astrocytes → ↑ neurosteroids → ↑ activity of GABA–benzodiazepine system
    - ↑ benzodiazepine system
    - ↑ production of glutamine by the astrocytes

- ➢ Clinical
  - o Wide spectrum
  - o MHE or CHE
    - – ↓ attention
    - – ↓ working memory
    - – ↓ psychomotor speed
    - – ↓ visuospatial ability
  - o OHE
    - – AMS
      - Personality changes
      - Sleep–wake cycle
      - Confusional state
      - Stupor
      - Coma
    - – Neurological signs
      - Asterixis
      - Hypertonia
      - Babinski sign
      - Pyramidal and extrapyramidal signs
      - Focal neurological deficits

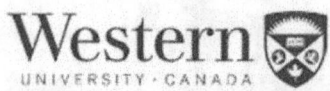

- Give the clinical neurological deficits in MHE.
  - Affect and emotion
  - Behavior
  - Cognition, memory and attention
  - Note: language and verbal skills are relatively spared in HE

- Give the important areas in the assessment of patient with possible MHE.
  - Exclude other causes of metabolic encephalopathy
  - Exclude other possible precipitating factors of HE
  - Neuropsychiatric testing
  - Number connection tests (Trail making)
  - Visuomotor skills
  - Mental tracking and concentration
  - Digit symbol test
  - Block design test
  - Standardized test battery, the psychometric HE score (PHES)
  - Digit span test (Weschler adult intelligence scale – passive auditory, working attention)
  - Critical flicker frequency (correlates with PHES)
  - Quality of life measures: SE – 36, chronic liver disease questionnaire (CLDQ)

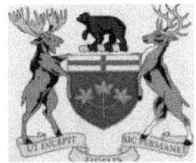

- Give a grading of the mental state of persons with HE.

Stage 0   –   No clinical findings, but abnormal psychometric tests may progress to higher stages of HE

Stage 1   –   Minor changes in the following are seen:
- Affect
- Sleep
- Concentration
    –   Trivial lack of awareness
    –   Euphoria or anxiety
    –   Shortened attention span
    –   Impaired performance of addition; sleep–wake disorder; tremor

Stage 2   –   Drowsiness
    –   Disorientation
    –   Confusion
    –   Lethargy or apathy
    –   Minimal disorientation of time or place
    –   Subtle personality changes
    –   Inappropriate behavior
    –   Impaired performance of subtraction

Stage 3   –   Somnolence
    –   Incoherence
    –   Somnolence to semi–stupor, but responsive to verbal stimuli
    –   Confusion
    –   Gross disorientation

Stage 4   –   Coma (unresponsiveness to verbal or noxious stimuli), with the following:
- Minimal response (4a)
- No response (4b)

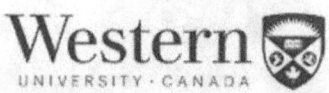

Adapted from: Nevah, M.I. and Fallon, M.B. *Sleisenger & Fordtran's Gastrointestinal and Liver Disease: Pathophysiology / Diagnosis / Management* 10th Ed. 2016, table 94-1, page 1579.

Patients with stage 0 to 2 HE and who can coorperate with the physical examination will present with tremor and asterixis. Patients with stage 3 or 4 may not be able to cooperate for the clinical testing of these signs.

- Give the upper motor neuron (UMN) signs seen in stage 3 or 4 HE demonstrable even without the patient's cooperation.

  o Hyperreflexia

  o Clonus

  o Hyperigidity

  o Positive Babinski sign

Clinical Tips when Assessing Risks of HE

"The absence of papilledema on fundoscopy and other typical features of cerebral edema on computer tomography (CT) of the head do not preclude the presence of cerebal edema complicating and worsening encephalopathy" (Feldman, M., *et al. Sleisenger and Fordtran's Gastrointestinal and Liver Disease.* 9th Edition. Saunders/Elsevier 2010, page 1601).

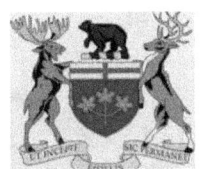

➢ Histopathology

➢ Laboratory
  o Rule out possible precipitants and investigate for the differential diagnosis
  o Ammonia
    – "does not add diagnostic, staging or prognostic values"
  o Possible role as negative predictive marker

The finding of an elevated serum ammonia concentration is not specific for the diagnosis of hepatic encephalopathy.

• Give the causes of hyperammonemia.
  o Liver and GI tract
    – Acute liver failure
    – Cirrhosis
    – Gastrointestinal bleeding
  o Renal
    – Chronic kidney disease
  o Inborn errors of metabolism
    – Proline metabolism disorders

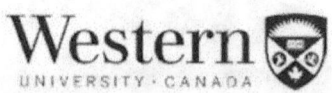

- Urea cycle disorders (i.e. carbamoyl phosphate synthetase I deficiency, ornithine transcarbamylase deficiency, argininosuccinate lyase deficiency, N-acetyl glutamate synthetase deficiency)

o Medications
- Alcohol
- Diuretics (i.e. acetazolamide)
- Narcotics
- Valproic acid

o Muscle exertion and ischemia

o Blood sampling
- Tourniquet use
- High body temperature
- High protein diet

o Diet

o Cigarette smoking

Adapted from: Nevah M.I. and Fallon M.B. *Sleisenger and Fordtran's Gastrointestinal and Liver Disease. Pathophysiology/Diagnosis/ Management.* 10th Ed, 2016, Box 94-1, page 1579.

➢ Diagnostic imaging
o CT of the head to rule out other pathologies

• Special tests
o Portosystemic Encephalopathy Syndrome Test (PSE)
- Paper and pencil test: 5 components (15 minutes)
    ▪ Digit symbol test
    ▪ Number connection tests A and B
    ▪ Serial dotting test
    ▪ Line tracing test
- Results between -18 to 6, if less than -4: abnormal

Lauridsen, M.M., *et al. Clinical Liver Disease* 2015; 5(3):71-4.

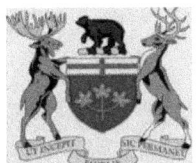

> Diagnosis

- o Exclude other causes of metabolic encephalopathy
- o Exclude possible precipitating factors of HE
- o Clinical examination
- o Altered neuropsychiatric testing
  - – Number connection tests (Trail making)
  - – Visuomotor skills
  - – Mental tracking and concentration
  - – Digit symbol test
  - – Block design test
  - – Standardized test battery, the psychometric HE score (PHES)
  - – Digit span test (Weschler adult intelligence scale – passive auditory, working attention)
  - – Critical flicker frequency (correlates with PHES)
  - – Quality of life measures: SE–36, chronic liver disease questionnaire (CLDQ)
- o Scoring systems
  - – PSET (portosystemic encephalopathy syndrome test)
  - – Psychometric tests
- o Blood concentrations of NH_3
  - – Arterial or venous NH_3 concentrations are neither sensitive nor specific – please see Feldman, M., et al. *Sleisenger and Fordtran's Gastrointestinal and Liver Disease*. 9th Edition. Saunders/Elsevier, Philadelphia, 2010, Table 92.1, for the Differential Diagnosis of Hyperammonemia.
  - – Arterial hyperammonemia in 90% of HE
  - – Arterial NH3 ≥ 200 mg/L predicts brain edema and herniation of the brain stem
  - – MRI–based techniques

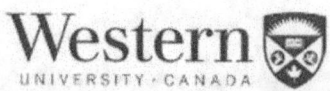

- o EEG abnormalities
    - – Bilateral slow wave activity
    - – Neither sensitive nor specific

Clinical caution:

- o Vitamin E deficiency is common in patients with cirrhosis (cholestasis → ↓ absorption of fat soluble vitamins → vitamin E deficiency)

- o Neurological signs of vitamin E deficiency are similar to HE.

- o Don't confuse the two; when in doubt, give vitamin E (tocopherol 1000 IU/day) to patients with HE.

➤ Testing for MHE and CHE
- o Who to test?
    - – Prognosticate OHE development
    - – Indicate ↓ QOL and ↓ work productivity
- o Risk factors of OHE
    - – Correlation of hepatic encephalopathy with baseline parameter

Parameters	Pearson's coefficient (r)	P values
o MELD score	0.012	0.877
o Child score	- 0.180	0.02
o Ammonia	- 0.252	0.001
o CFF	0.200	0.01
o Two or more abnormal psychometry	0.375	0.001
o Serum sodium	- 0.142	0.07
o Serum creatinine	- 0.053	0.504

Abbreviations: CFF, critical flicker frequency; MELD, model for end–stage liver disease

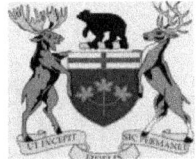

➢ Evaluation of MHE and CHE

- o Continuous reaction time test (CRT)
  - – Measure of motor reaction to sensory stimuli
  - – CRT index: intrapersonal reaction time stability
- o Inhibitory control task test
  - – Tests attention and response inhibition
  - – Visual stimulus
    - ▪ Press only if there is flashing "X" or "Y"
- o Stroop Test (App)
  - – Tests psychomotor speed and cognitive flexibility
  - – Reaction time and cognitive flexibility to the colored field and written names of color
- o Critical Flicker Frequency test (CFF)
  - – When fused lights start to flicker to the observer, he needs to press the handgrip button
  - – Metabolic state of retina which reflects to the functioning astrocytes
- o If tests are normal
  - – Recommend repeating in 6 months

Lauridsen, M.M. and Vilstrup, H. *Clinical Liver Disease.* 2015; 5(3):71-4.

➢ Treatment: AASLD Guidelines

- o Lactulose is the first choice for the treatment of episodic OHE (grade II-1, B, I)

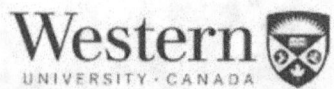

Diagnosis of hepatic encephalopathy

Rule out other causes of encephalopathy

- Drugs
  - Sensitivity to CNS drugs
  - Drug intoxication

- CNS
  - Prior seizure or stroke (postictal confusion)
  - Delirium tremens
  - Wernicke-Korsakoff syndrome
  - Intracerebral hemorrhage
  - CNS sepsis
  - Cerebral edema and/or intracranial hypertension*

- Lung
  - Hypoxia
  - Hypercapnia
  - Acidosis

- Kidney
  - Gross electrolyte changes
  - Uremia

- Endocrine
  - Hypoglycemia*
  - Pancreatic encephalopathy

Identify precipitating causes of hepatic encephalopathy

- Gastrointestinal hemorrhage
- Constipation and dietary protein overload
- Poor compliance with lactulose therapy
- Recent anesthesia
- Bowel obstruction or ileus

- Liver
  - Prior portal decompression procedure (i.e. TIPS)*
  - Superimposed hepatic injury*
  - Development of hepatocellular carcinoma
  - Dehydration
  - Hypokalemia and alkalosis
  - Uremia

- CNS
  - CNS active drugs
  - Sepsis

Initiate empiric treatment for hepatic encephalopathy

- Lactulose, oral dose of 1-30 ml 2x daily
- Rifaximin, oral dose of 550 mg 2x daily
- Neomycin, oral dose of 500 mg 4x daily (use high doses with caution)
- Metronidazole, oral dose of 250 mg four times daily
- Vancomycin, oral dose of 250 mg 4x daily
- Sodium benzoate, oral dose 5 g 2x daily (not approved for use in the USA)
- Flumazenil, intravenous injection of 1-3 mg (potentially effective, but very short duration of action)

Abbreviation: AB, acid base

*Predominantly observed in patients with acute liver failure

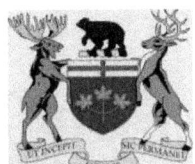

➢ Treat precipitants
- Infections, i.e. SBP, aspiration, RTI
- Increased ammonia production
  - Excessive protein intake
  - Constipation
  - GI bleed, 20%
  - Azotemia, 30%
  - Hypokalemia
- Increased protein catabolism – surgery, diuretics, arterial hypotension and hypovolemia
- Malnutrition
  - Skeletal muscle wasting (less muscle metabolism of NH_3)
  - Treat the zinc deficiency
- Increased diffusion across the BBB (alkalosis)
- Synergistic effects of cytokines – infection (SBP) (10%)
- Altered brain function – sedative drugs, psychotropics, analgesics, benzodiazepines, hyponatremia, astrocyte swelling
- Dehydration – fluid restriction, diuretics, excessive paracentesis, vomiting, diarrhea (mechanism unknown)
- Hypoxia, anemia, fever, sepsis
- Metabolic: $\downarrow$ K^+ in 50%, hyperglycemia, alkalosis, $\downarrow$ hypoxemia, thyroid, dehydration
- Drugs, 30%: benzodiazapines, analgesics, interferon, alcohol, NSAIDs, acetaminophen
- Surgery
  - Shunting, anesthetic, TIPS
- Liver decompensation
  - HCC, PVT

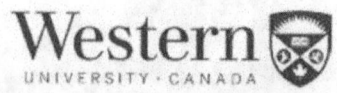

- Lactulose (β–galactosidofructose), lacitol β–galactosidosorbitol (traps NH_3)

  o Enters the colon, broken down by the colonic bacteria to lactic acid and acetic acid, with acidification of stool pH at < 5

  $$\begin{array}{c} pH < 5 \\ NH_3 \quad \rightarrow \quad NH_4^+ \text{ (non–absorbable)} \end{array}$$

  o Lactulose enemas (300 mL in 1L of water) in patients who are unable to take lactulose *po*

  o Lactulose 30 mL *po* every 1 – 2 hours until bowel evacuation, then adjust to a dose that will result in 2 – 3 formed bowel movements per day (usually 15 – 30 mL *po bid*)

  o Lactulose can be discontinued once the precipitating factor has been resolved

- Hyperosmolar purgation (including lactulose)

  o ↑ stool volume

  o ↑ loss of nitrogen compounds

- Acarbose

  o α–glucosidic inhibitor → ↓ glucose absorption → ↑ saccharolytic bacteria and ↓ proteolytic urea producing luminal microbiotica → ↓ NH_3

- Antibiotics (pre–, pro– and synbiotics)

  o ↑ *Lactobacillus spp.*, ↓ urease–containing bacteria → ↓ NH_3 production

  o ↑ bacterial NH_3 utilization

  o ↓ pro–inflammatory response

  o ↓ gut permeability

  o ↓ bacterial translocation

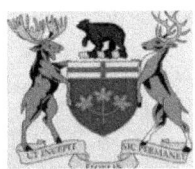

- L–ornithine –L–aspartate (LOLA)
  - Activate the urea cycle $\rightarrow$ $\uparrow$ NH_3 clearance
  - Improves grade 3 or 4 HE in ~ 25% of patients

- Neurotransmitters: flumazenil (a competitive GABA–benzodiazepine receptor antagonist) or bromocriptine

- Nutrition
  - Treat malnutrition, including EN (enteral nutrition), and TPN (total parental nutrition)
  - Treat the associated zinc deficiency
  - Branched chain amino acids
  - Short term (< 72 hours) protein restriction may be considered in severe HE, but is not used for mild to moderate HE
  - No long term protein restriction

- Intracranial pressure (ICP) monitoring
  - Transcranial doppler
  - Jugular venous oximetry
  - 45° elevation of head of the bed
  - Moderate hypothermia to
    - $\downarrow$ ICP and cerebral blood flow (CBF)
    - $\downarrow$ arterial NH_3
    - $\downarrow$ cerebral NH_3 uptake
  - IV mannitol
    - $\downarrow$ ICP
  - Hyperventilation
    - Vasoconstriction $\rightarrow$ $\downarrow$ CBF

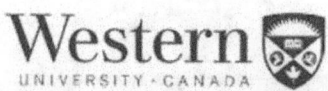

- Manage the circulatory effects
  - Fluid management, consider central venous pressure (CVP) monitoring
  - Manage the lactic acidosis and sepsis
  - Perform short synacthen test, and give GCS if adrenal insufficiency is present
  - Inotropes: terlipressin (a vasopressin analog) or norepinephrine
  - Albumin

- Extracorporeal liver assist devices (ELADs)
  - MARS (molecular adsorbent recirculating system): providing countercurrent hemodialysis against albumin and bicarbonate circuits
  - SPAD (single–pass albumin dialysis): countercurrent albumin dialysis against high blood flow in a fiber hemodin filter, and continuous venovenous hemofiltration
  - Prometheus R system, direct albumin adsorption through a specific polysulfur filter
  - Enteral feeding and TPN

- Orthoptic liver transplantation
  - Removes shunted (non–detoxified blood)
  - ↓ production of potentially toxic SCFA (propionate, butyrate, valerate)

Adapted from: Fitz, G.J. *Sleisenger and Fordtran's Gastrointestinal and Liver Disease: Pathophysiology/ Diagnosis/Management* 2006 pg. 1971-1972.

Note: Osmotic agents (i.e. lactulose) and antibiotics (i.e. metronidazole, neomycin, rifaximin) help relieve symptoms, but do not change the mortality rate

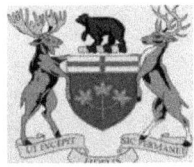

- Sedation (i.e. for EGD and EVL)
  - Propofol is safe in cirrhosis with no Δ cognition
  - Midazolam or fentanyl worsens HE
    - NCT (number connecting time), i.e. ↑ severity of HE score
    - ↑ agitation
  - Titrate sedation to the point where patient's speech is slurred

- Non–absorbable disaccharides for hepatic encephalopathy: systemic review of randomized trials (Als-Nielsen, B., *et al. BMJ.* 2004; 328:1046-50)
  - 22 randomized controlled trials (RCTs)
  - Median duration of treatmetn: 15 days and no follow-up
  - Non–absorbable disaccharides (NAD) *vs* placebo or no intervention
    - High quality studies
      - No significant in the overall effect (P = 0.85)
    - Low quality studies
      - Overall effect of non–absorbable disaccharides (P = 0.003)
    - All studies (P = 0.002)
  - Antibiotics *vs* NAD
    - Aminoglycoside favored *vs* NAD   NO P = 0.16
    - Rifaximin   YES P = 0.04

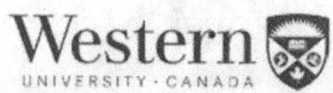

- Lactulose *vs* polyethylene glycol 3350–electrolyte solution for the treatment of vertical hepatic encephalopathy

The HELP randomized clinical trial

- o RCT of 50 patients
  - – 25 in each arm
  - – 4 L PEG lyte in 4 hours *vs* standard of care with lactulose
- o Primary outcome
  - – 1 grade ↓ HE
    - ▪ 91% in PEG (21 of 23 patients) *vs* 52% (13 of 25 patients) in lactulose group
- o Secondary outcome:
  - – Time of resolution: 1 *vs* 2 days, respectively
  - – LOS (P = 0.07)
  - – 6– to 24–hour ammonia concentration difference (P = 0.03)

➢ Summary of Guidelines for the Treatment of Acute OHE

- o Rifaximin is an effective add–on therapy of lactulose for the prevention of OHE recurrence (Grade I, A, 1)
- o Oral BCAAs can be used as an alternative or additional agent to treat patients who are non–responsive to conventional therapy (Grade, B, 2)
- o IV LOLA can be used as an alternative or additional agent to treat patients who are non–responsive to conventional therapy (Grade I, B, 2)
- o Neomycin is an alternative choice for the treatment of OHE (Grade II-1, B, 2)
- o Metronidazole is an alternative choice for the treatment of OHE (Grade II-3, B, 2)

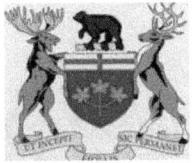

- Rifaximin treatment in hepatic encephalopathy (Bass, N.M., *et al. N Engl J Med* 2010; 362:1071-81)
    - RCT of Rifaximin (140 patients) *vs* placebo (159 patients) for secondary prophylaxis of OHE for 6 months
    - Inclusion criteria:
        - 2 prior episodes of HE within the past 6 months
        - Of note: 90% of patients in each arm were on lactulose maintenance
    - Primary outcome
        - Time to first breakthrough HE episode
            - RIF, 22%
            - PL, 46%

Hazard ratio (NR) with RIF 0.42 (95% CI, 0.28 – 0.64) RRR, 58% NNT, 4

    - Secondary outcome
        - Time of first HE–related hospitalization
            - RIF, 14%
            - PL, 23%

HR with RIF 10.50 (95% CI, 0.29 – 0.87) RRR, 50% NNT, 9

- Rifaximin *vs* non–absorbable disaccharides (NAD) for the management of hepatic encephalopathy: a meta–analysis (Jiang, Q., *et al. Eur J Gastroenterol Hepatol.* 2008; 20(11):1064-70)

    - Comparison with the standard of care for the treatment of acute and chronic hepatic encephalopathy (HE)

    - Only retained studies are looking at clinical efficacy
        - i.e. improvement of HE by passing to a lower stage of HE grading or significant decrease in portosystemic encephalopathy index
        - Left with 5 RCTs (264 patients)

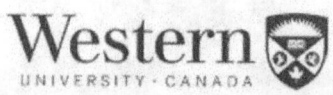

- o Clinical efficacy
  - – RIF *vs* NAD (P = 0.53)
- o Adverse effects
  - – Abdominal pain
    - ▪ RIF *vs* NAD (P = 0.04)
  - – Diarrhea
    - ▪ RIF vs NAD (P = 0.90)
- o Conclusion
  - – "Rifaximin is not superior [to NAD] but with better tolerability [abdominal pain, but no diarrhea]"

- • Secondary prevention
  - o Lactulose is recommended for the prevention of recurrent episodes of HE after the initial episode (Grade II-1, A, 1)

- • Probiotics are as efficacious as lactulose *vs* no therapy for secondary prevention of OHE
  - o Rifaximin as an add–on to lactulose is recommended for the prevention of recurrent episodes of HE after the second episode (Grade I, A, 1)
    - – Breakthrough OHE over 12 months of follow–up
    - – Secondary prophylaxis of HE in cirrhosis: an open–label, randomized controlled trial of lactulose, probiotics and no therapy (Agrawal, A., et al. Am J Gastroentrol. 2012; 107(7):1043-50)

Lactulose + Rifaximin for HE

- • A randomized, double–blind, controlled trial comparing rifaximin plus lactulose with lactulose alone for the treatment of overt hepatic encephalopathy (Sharma, B.C., et al. Am J Gastroenterol. 2013; 108(9):1458-63)

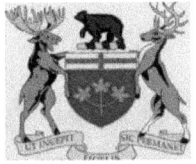

o RCT, N = 120 with overt HE

o Lactulose 30 – 60 mL *tid* (to effect 2 – 3 semisoft BM daily) *vs* lactulose + rifaximin 400 mg *tid*

o Primary endpoint: complete reversal of HE

o Secondary endpoints: mortality, LOS

o 84% of patients: alcohol, HCV, HBV

o Child–Pugh Class: B (31%), Calss C (69%) mean MELD 25

o Encephalopathy grade (West Haven): 2 (18%), 3 (33%), 4 (48%)

Outcomes	Lac + Rif	Lac alone	NNT
– Complete reversal of HE	76%	44%	4
– Mortality	24%	49%	4
– LOS (d)	5.8	8.2	

o Review from Annalytics of Pharmacotherapy (Mohammad, R.A., *et al*, *Ann Pharmacother*. 2012; 46(11):1559-63)

  – 6 studies for combination therapy

  – Aside from RIF and lactulose, no evidence for other combination therapy either for prevention or treatment

• Prevention of post–TIPS HE
o Routine prophylactic therapy (lactulose or rifaximin) is not recommended for the prevention of post–TIPS HE (grade III, B, 1)

Bai, Y., *et al. J Gastroenterol Hepatol.* 2011; 26:678-82.

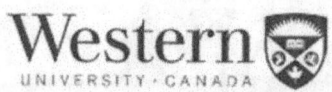

➢   Prognosis

• Give the survival rates and etiological factors for the types of
  hepatic encephalopathy (i.e. acute liver failure, cirrhosis with
  precipitant and chronic HE).

Types of HE	Approximate Survival	Etiological factors
o Acute liver failure	~ 20%	– Viral hepatitis – Alcoholic hepatitis – Drug reactions and overdose

o Cirrhosis with precipitant	~ 80%	– Drugs and toxins
		  ▪ Diuretics
		  ▪ Alcoholic excess
		  ▪ Sedatives
		– Infection
		  ▪ Any type, including SBP
		– Volume loss
		  ▪ Hemorrhage
		  ▪ Paracentesis
		  ▪ Diarrhea and vomiting
		– Surgery
		– Constipation

o Chronic HE	~ 100%	– Portosystemic shunting – ↑ dietary protein intake – Intestinal bacteria

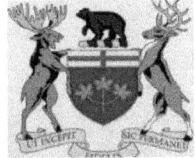

SO YOU WANT TO BE A HEPATOLOGIST!

A patient with cirrhosis develops HE is treated with antibiotics, and their MELD score rises.

- Explain the mechanism of deterioration in HE with antibiotics.
    - Antibiotics for HE reduce the intestinal microbiota
    - The ↓ in microbiotica → ↓ bacterial synthesis of vitamin K
    - ↓ bacterial vitamin K available for absorption and production of coagulation factors (II, VII, IX, X, protein C), the INR rises
    - ↑ INR contributes points to ↑ MELD score

"There are two ways of spreading light:
to be the candle or the mirror that
reflects it".

Edith Wharton

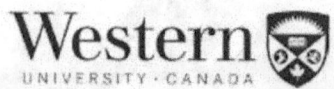

Congenital and Acquired Portosystemic Shunts (PSS)

Yaqoub Alawadh

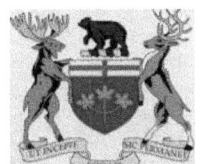

- ➢ Definition
  - ○ A connection between hepatic portal system and the venous part of the systemic circulation
    - – Congenital
    - – Acquired
- ➢ Demography
  - ○ Overall prevalence rate is ~ 1:30,000 births
  - ○ Prevalence of permanent CPSS is ~ 1:50,000

Abbreviation: CPSS, congenital portosystemic shunts

McElhinney, D.B., *et al. Congenit Heart Dis.* 2011; 6(1):28-40.

- ➢ Causes and associations
  - ○ Congenital shunts
    - – Extrahepatic
      - ▪ Type 1 (end–to–end) congenital absence of the portal vein with complete diversion of the portal blood into the systemic veins (the inferior vena cava or renal or iliac veins
      - ▪ Type Ia: separate drainage of the superior mesenteric and splenic veins into the systemic veins
      - ▪ Type Ib: superior mesenteric and splenic veins join to form a short extrahepatic portal vein which drains into a systemic vein
      - ▪ Type 2: (side–to–side), there is a hypoplastic portal vein with portal blood diversion into the vena cava through a side–to–side, extrahepatic communication
    - – Intrahepatic
      - ▪ Are located inside the liver and were classified into four categories.
      - ▪ Intrahepatic shunts located between the portal veins or 1 or several of its branches, and the inferior vena cava or a hepatic vein on the other, including ductus venosus

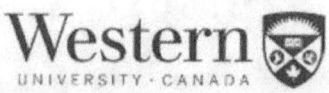

- Hepatic rapidly involuting congenital hemangioma

o Acquired shunts
  - Hepatic hemangioma
  - Hereditary heemorhagic telangiectasia (HHT)
  - Splenic artery steal syndrome (SASS)
  - TIPS
  - Surgical Shunts

Morgan, G. and Superina, R. *J Pediatr Surg.* 1994; 29(9):1239-41.

SO YOU WANT TO BE A HEPATOLOGIST!

- In extrahepatic congenital portosystemic shunt, define extrahepatic "Abernethy malformation".

  o Abernathy malformation is a congenital anomaly of the splanchnic vasculature in which the portal venous blood is diverted into the inferior vena cava.

Collardeau-Frachon, S. and Scoazec, J.Y. *Anat Rec* (Hoboken) 2008; 291(6): 614-27.

---

o Type I
  - single large shunt with a constant diameter connects the right portal vein to the inferior vena cava; the most common site

o Type II
  - localized peripheral shunt with single or multiple communications found between the peripheral branches of the portal and hepatic veins in one hepatic segment

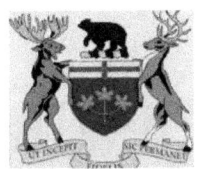

- o Type III
  - – peripheral portal and hepatic veins connected through an aneurysm

- o Type IV
  - – multiple communications between the peripheral portal and hepatic veins seen diffusely in both lobes

Congenital Portosystemic Shunts

- ➤ Clinical presentations
  - o Neonatal
    - – Abnormal galactosemia tests
    - – Congenital heart disease
    - – Neonatal cholestasis

  - o After 1 month of age
    - – Complication of shunt (HE, pulmonary HTN, tumors, HPS)
    - – Abnormal liver tests
      - ▪ Hepatic encephalopathy
      - ▪ Pulmonary hypertension
      - ▪ Hepatopulmonary syndrome

Franchi-Abella, S., *et al. J Pediatr Gastroenterol Nutr.* 2010; 51(3):322-330

- ➤ Laboratory
  - o Serum transaminases and γ–glutamyltransferase activities
  - o Coagulation studies
  - o Pre– and postprandial ammonemia and glycemia
  - o Fasting serum total bile acid concentration
  - o Blood manganese concentration
  - o Serum α–fetoprotein concentration (in case of liver tumor)

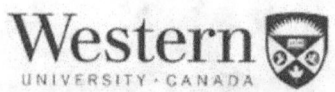

➢ Diagnostic Imaging
  ○ Abdominal color doppler ultrasonography
  ○ Multidetector CT and/or MRI with contrast injection
  ○ Angiography of shunts with or w/o occlusion test
  ○ Echocardiography
  ○ Brain MRI
  ○ Per rectum scintigraphy

➢ Prognosis
  ○ Small intrahepatic PSS
    – Disappear spontaneously by age 1 – 2 years
  ○ Large shunts, as well as the communications involving the extrahepatic portal veins and ductus venosus
    – Persist throughout life and carry risks of complications

Franchi-Abella, S., *et al. J Pediatr Gastroenterol Nutr.* 2010; 51(3):322-330

Hepatic Rapidly Involuting Congenital Hemangioma (RICH)

➢ Definition
  ○ Benign neoplasm occuring in many locations in the body
  ○ Present as an abdominal mass in an otherwise healthy infant

➢ Clinical
  ○ Transient thrombocytopenia and anemia are observed in infants, presumably due to intralesional thrombosis
  ○ Arteriovenous shunting results to heart failure

Andreu-Barasoain, M., *et al. Int J Dermatol.* 2013; 52(8):1025.

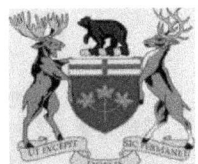

- ➢ Diagnostic imaging
  - o Abdominal ultrasonography
    - – A well–circumscribed vascular mass
    - – Large feeding and draining vessels
    - – Coarse subcapsular calcifications seen after involution

- ➢ Treatment
  - o Infants with heart failure
    - – Treat medically
  - o Perform embolization when medical treatment fails

Rapidly involuting congenital haemangioma of the liver Derek Roebuck, Neil Sebire, Eldon Lehmann, Alex Barnacle March 2012, Volume 42, Issue 3, pages 308-314.

- • Acquired Shunts
  - o Hepatic hemangioma
  - o HHT
  - o SASS
  - o TIPS
  - o Surgical Shunts

Hepatic Hemangioma

- ➢ Demography
  - o Prevalence 0.4 – 20%
  - o 60 – 80% in patients who are between the ages of 30 and 50 years
  - o More frequently in women with a ratio of 3:1

Farges, O., *et al. World J Surg.* 1995; 19(1):19.
Gandolfi, L., *et al. Gut.* 1991; 32(6): 677.

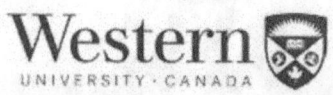

➢ Pathogenesis

o Incompletely understood

o Vascular malformations or hamartomas of congenital origin that enlarge by ectasia rather than by hyperplasia or hypertrophy

o Hormonal influence over tumor growth is suggested by any of the following:
   - Enlargement during pregnancy and estrogen and progesterone therapy
   - Regression after withdrawal of therapy

DuPre, C.T., *et al.* Case report: cavernous hemangioma of the liver. *Am J Med Sci.* 1992;303(4):241.

➢ Pathology

• Gross

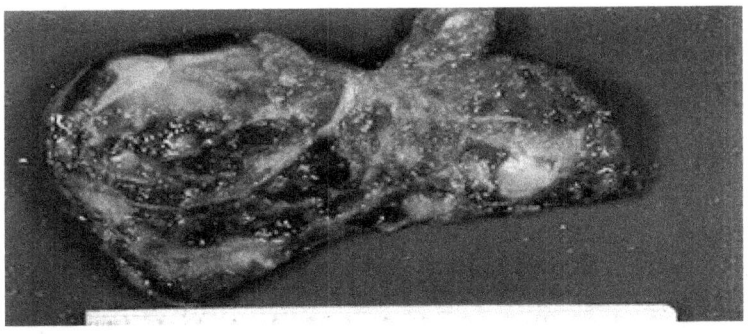

Cut surface demonstrates a brown to red appearance with areas of focal hemorrhages and fibrosis.

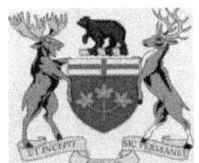

- Histopathology
  - o Multiple vascular channels of various sizes lined by a single layer of flattened endothelium supported by a thin fibrous septae (hematoxylin and eosin).

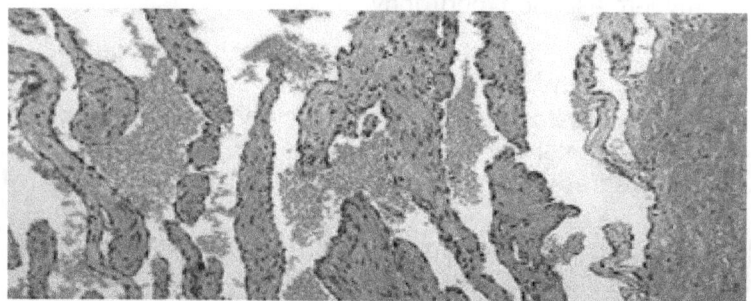

- ➢ Clinical Features
  - o Typically discovered incidentally in a laparotomy, autopsy, or during an imaging test performed for unrelated conditions.
  - o Lesions > 4 cm are more likely to cause symptoms such as:
    - – Abdominal pain
    - – RUQ discomfort or fullness
  - o High output cardiac failure may occur

Kristidis, P., *et al.* Infantile hepatic haemangioma: investigation and treatment. *J Paediatr Child Health.* 1991; 27(1):57.

- ➢ Diagnostic Imaging
  - o Plain radiograph
    - – Shows calcification within the tumor
    - – Calcification is not specific for hemangiomas

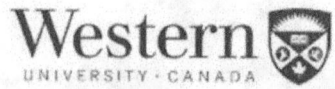

o Ultrasound
  - Typically reveals a well–demarcated homogeneous hyperechoic mass
  - The diagnosis can be strongly suggested by an ultrasound in approximately 80% of patients with lesions measuring < 6 cm
  - Blood flow is demonstrated by a color Doppler in only 10 – 50% of hemangiomas
    ▪ Thus, does not improve the accuracy of ultrasound
  - Some malignant liver lesions have similar acoustic patterns, and therefore, other imaging modalities are usually required for confirmation

Tanaka, S., *et al.* Color Doppler flow imaging of liver tumors. *Am J Roentgenol.* 1990; 154(3):509.

o Computed tomography
  - Non–contrast enhanced
  - A well–demarcated hypodense mass
  - Calcifications are seen in approximately 10% of cases
  - Administration of contrast results in the following:
    ▪ Peripheral nodular enhancement in the early phase
    ▪ Centripetal pattern or "filling in" during the late phase
    ▪ Peripheral nodular or globular enhancement representing venous lakes are seen in up to 94% of hemangiomas measuring > 4 cm in size

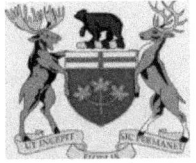

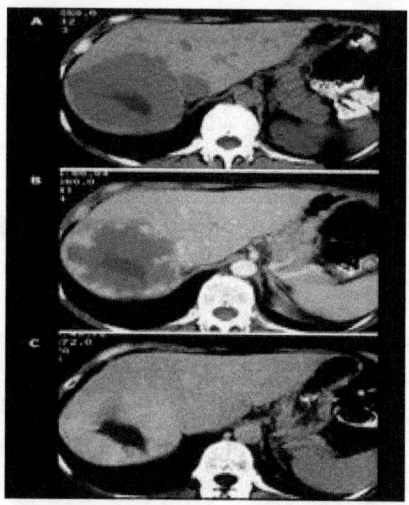

- Panel A: well–demarcated hypodense lesion on non–contrast scan (panel A) in the posterior right lobe of the liver
- Panel B: early phase of contrast enhancement demonstrating peripheral nodular enhancement with gradual "filling in" of the lesion; center of the lesion remains hypodense
- Panel C: the post–contrast delayed image, demonstrating an isodense lesion characteristic of hepatic hemangioma

o Magnetic resonance imaging
  - Sensitivity of approximately 90%
  - Specificity of 91 – 99 %
  - Smooth, well–demarcated homogeneous mass
    ▪ Low signal intensity on T1–weighted images
    ▪ Hyperintense on T2–weighted images

Hepatic hemangiomas and malignant tumors: improved differentiation with heavily T2–weighted conventional spin–echo MR imaging. McFarland, E.G., et al. Radiology. 1994; 193(1):43.

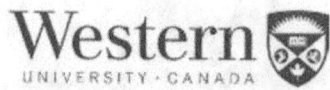

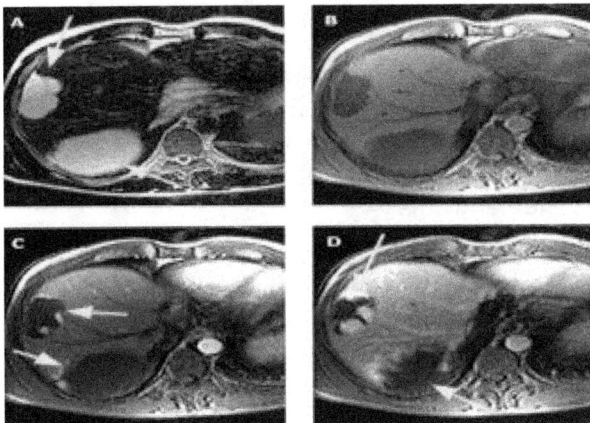

- Panel A: heavily T2–weighted MR image shows the masses (arrows) as very high signal intensity
- Panels B–D: dynamic T1–weighted gradient–echo MR images before (B), during the arterial–phase of gadolinium chelate-enhancement (C), and during the portal phase of enhancement (D) show initial nodular peripheral enhancement (arrowheads) that starts filling the hemangiomas (arrows)

o Technetium–99m pertechnetate–labeled red blood cell pool study:
  - Sensitivity (lesions > 2 cm)
    ▪ 69 – 92%
  - Specificity approximates 100%
  - False negatives
    ▪ Can occur due to the presence of fibrosis or thrombosis

o Angiography
  - Angiography is rarely used for the diagnosis
  - Reserved for atypical tumors that cannot be diagnosed definitively after multiple non–invasive imaging tests

Belli, L., *et al. Surg Gynecol Obstet.* 1992; 174(6):474.

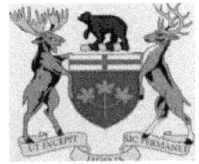

Pathology

- o Percutaneous needle biopsy
  - – Associated with fatal hemorrhage
  - – Needle aspiration or biopsy
  - – Not recommend for the evaluation of possible hemangioma

Terriff, B.A., *et al. Am J Roentgenol.* 1990; 154(1):203.

- ➤ Management
  - o Asymptomatic, particularly lesions < 1.5 cm
    - – Observe
    - – Hemangiomas ≤ 5 cm in size
      - ▪ No follow–up imaging
    - – Lesions > 5 cm
      - ▪ Repeat imaging in 6 to 12 months for such lesions using the modality that best showed the hemangioma previously (CT or MRI)
      - ▪ If there is no changes in the size of the lesion, then no additional imaging is needed
  - o Patients who have pain or symptoms suggestive of extrinsic compression of adjacent structures
    - – Considered for surgical resection
    - – Has similar results for liver resection *vs* enucleation
    - – Risk of bleeding is related more to the large size hemangioma than to the type of surgery (resection or enucleation)
      - ▪ Enucleation
      - ▪ Liver transplantation
  - o Mortality from resection is negligible in specialized hepatobiliary centers
  - o OLTx has also been used successfully to treat symptomatic patients with unresectable giant hemangiomas and hemangiomas associated with Kasabach–Merritt syndrome

Longeville, J.H., *et al. HPB Surg.* 1997; 10(3):159-62.

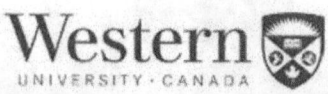

o   Non–surgical treatments
  - Arterial embolization used to control acute bleeding, to manage symptoms, and to shrink hemangiomas prior to surgical resection
  - Radiotherapy
    ▪ Reserved for the treatment of childhood hemangiomas associated with Kasabach–Merritt syndrome
    ▪ It is rarely considered a first line therapy because of its known effects on the growth and the risk of secondary malignancy
  - Interferon α–2a has been used in infants with life–threatening hemangiomas in extrahepatic sites, although success are not uniform

Hereditary hemorrhagic telangiectasia (HHT, Osler–Weber–Rendu syndrome)

➢ Definition

  o   An autosomal dominant vascular disorder

➢ Demography

  o   ~ 1:5000 to 1:8000

➢ Causes

  o   Among the most common are epistaxis, GIB and iron deficiency anemia, along with a characteristic mucocutaneous telangiectasia

➢ Pathology

  o   (AVMs) commonly occur in the pulmonary, hepatic, and cerebral circulations

  o   Liver biopsy is **not** recommended
    - Not useful in the diagnosis of HHT
    - May be complicated by bleeding

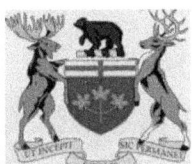

- ➢ Clinical features
  - ○ Asymptomatic in ~ 75%
  - ○ Large AVMs between the hepatic artery and vein can cause a significant left–to–right (L → R) shunt with ↑ cardiac output → high–output heart failure
  - ○ Include portal hypertension and biliary disease, reflecting different patterns of vascular involvement
  - ○ Hepatomegaly, a liver bruit or abnormal liver enzymes
- ➢ Diagnostic imaging
  - ○ Computed tomography
  - ○ MRI
  - ○ Doppler ultrasonography
  - ○ Angiography
- ➢ Treatment
  - ○ Treatment–associated complications
    - – Heart failure
    - – Complications of portal hypertension
    - – Biliary disease
  - ○ Liver transplantation
    - – Medical management fails in acute hepatic failure and acute biliary necrosis syndrome
  - ○ Under study
    - – Bevacizumab (angiogenesis inhibitor)
    - – Not yet replaced liver transplantation due to the very short follow–up available for bevacizumab–treated patients

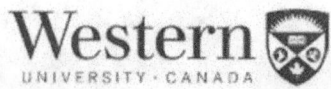

> Treatment Alert
> - o Embolization is no longer recommended because of higher morbidity and mortality compared with transplantation.

Splenic Artery Steel Syndrome (SASS)

➢ Definition
- o Arterial hypoperfusion of the graft caused by a shift of the blood flow into the splenic or gastroduodenal arteries

➢ Demography
- o Up to 6% of liver transplant recipients develop SASS

➢ Clinical features
- o Occurs within days or weeks after transplantation
- o ↑ liver function enzymes
- o Allograft dysfunction
- o Cholestasis
- o Graft loss

Sevmis, S., *et al. Transplant Proc.* 2006; 38:3651.

➢ Diagnostic Imaging
- o Doppler US
- o Angiography

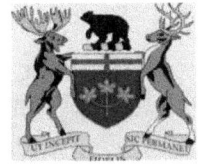

➤ Treatment
   ○ ↓ SA flow by:
      - Partial splenic embolization (PSE)
         ▪ Metal coils via the Seldinger technique
      - Stenosis of the SA
         ▪ Endoluminal stent or suture (banding)
      - Splenectomy

Quintini. C., *et al. Liver Transpl.* 2008;14:374-9.; Nüssler, N.C., *et al. Liver Transpl.* 2003; 9:596-602.

Hepatic Artery Aneurysm (HAA)

➤ Pathophysiology
• Give why "Ischemic" or "Hypoxic" hepatitis may not be a satisfactory term.
   ○ Reduced hepatic blood flow from any cause, such as congestive heart failure, respiratory failure, systemic hypotension, cause the following pathological changes:
      - Very little inflammatory infiltrates (i.e. no "hepatitis")
      - Centrilobular necrosis
      - Loss of hepatocytes
      - RBC in the sinusoids
      - May progress to centrilobular fibrosis

➤ Laboratory
• Give laboratory measures that suggest ischemic hepatitis.
   ○ ↑ AST
   ○ ↑↑ LDH
   ○ ALT-to-LDH ratio of < 1.5
   ○ Rapid fall of LDH and AST, usually within 4 days
   ○ In congestive hepatopathy
      - ↑ SAAG
      - ↑ protein in ascites

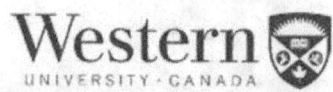

➤ Pathology

- In chronic centrilobular vascular congestion, define "reverse lobulation".

    o Reverse lobulation is the formation of bridging necrosis between central veins, (the reverse of bridging necrosis between portal tracts), a characteristic of cardiac cirrhosis.

Note: Same answer for different question: Give the pathological feature distinguishing portal cirrhosis from cardiac cirrhosis.

➤ Causes
    o Atherosclerosis (may cause hepatic infarction)
    o Mycotic infection
    o Vasculitis
    o Pseudoaneurysms
        - Liver biopsy
        - Percutaneous transhepatic cholangiogram
        - Liver transplantation

SO YOU WANT TO BE A HEPATOLOGIST!

Atherosclerosis may involve the hepatic artery causing hepatic artery aneurysm (HAA), which may rupture, and is associated with a 30% mortality rate.

- Give other chronic hepatobiliary complication of artherosclerosis of the hepatic artery.
    o Slow obstruction of the hepatic artery reduces the blood supply to the bile duct (common bile duct), leading to:
        - Ischemic cholangiopathy of:
            ▪ CBD strictures
            ▪ Obstruction

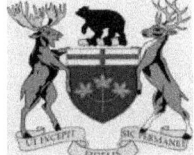

➢ Clinical

- Give physical findings on the abdominal wall of patients with cirrhosis suggest hepatic bruit coming from the recanalization of the umbilical vein.

  ○ The presence of caput medusa suggests ↑ blood flow in the abdominal wall veins, arising from the recanalization of the umbilical vein, producing the C–B (Cruveilhier–Baumgarten) murmur.

Other patients with ascites, despite salt restriction and compliant in taking the appropriate diuretics, loses ascites when hepatic bruit develops.

- Name the bruit and explain the mechanism of the spontaneous clearance of ascites.

  ○ C–B (Cruveilhier–Baumgarten) murmur

  ○ Development of spontaneous portosystemic shunt, as a result of portal hypertension, helps to partially bypass the liver blood flow blocked by the cirrhotic nodules resulting to ↓ PHT and ↓ ascites

➢ Treatment

Abdominal ultrasound demonstrates cystic mass and CT confirms an HAA (hepatic artery aneurysm).

- Give the surgical management for HAA.

  ○ Extrahepatic
    - Proximal to gastroduodenal artery
      ▪ Proximal and distal ligation of HA (collateral blood supply still occurs in the gastroduodenal artery)
    - Distal to gastroduodenal resection artery
  ○ Intrahepatic
    - Partial hepatic resection

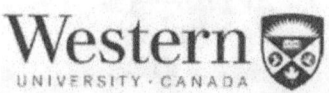

Primary Resection and Salvage Transplantation For HCC

Ibrahim Al Hasan

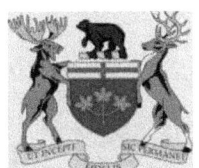

- ➢ Risk Factors
    - ○ Hepatitis B
    - ○ Hepatitis C
    - ○ Aflatoxins
    - ○ Hemochromatosis
    - ○ Cirrhosis (any etiology)
    - ○ Alcohol
    - ○ Anabolic steroids

- ➢ Treatment Options
    - ○ Transplantation
    - ○ Resection
    - ○ Radiofrequency ablation, Microwave and Knano Knife
    - ○ Percutaneous ethanol ablation
    - ○ Cryoablation
    - ○ TACE
    - ○ Radioembolization
    - ○ Systemic chemotherapy and molecularly targeted therapies

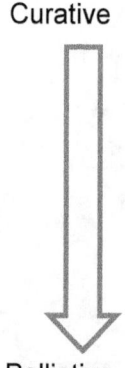

Curative

Palliative

- ➢ Staging
    - ○ Liver Disease
        - – Child–Pugh
        - – MELD

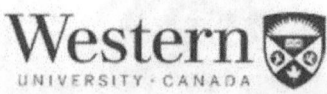

o Hepatocellular carcinoma
   - TNM
   - Okuda
   - Cancer Liver Italian Program (CLIP)
   - Barcelona Clinic Liver Cancer (BCLC) System

The BCLC Staging System and Treatment Algorithm

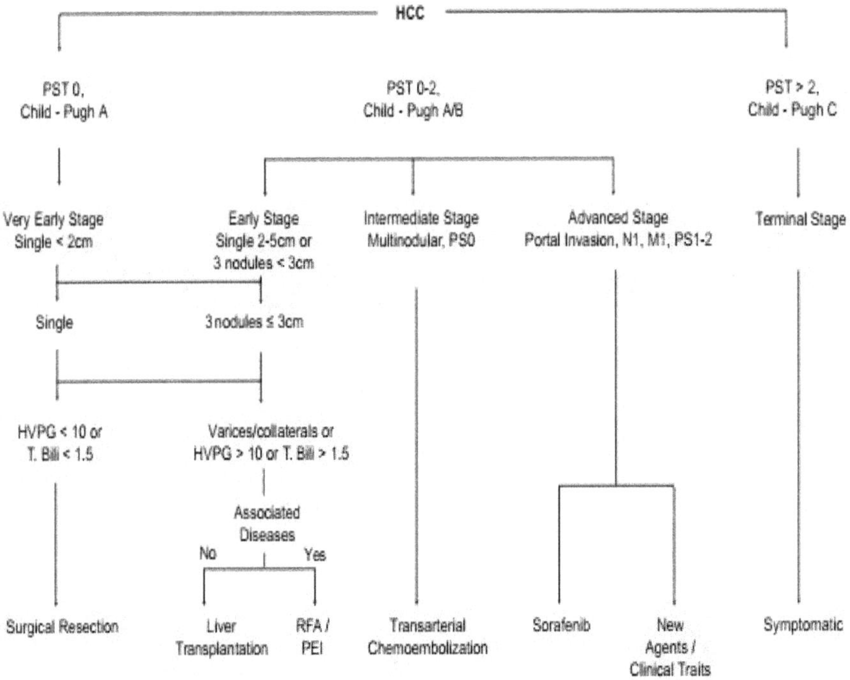

```
                                      HCC
  ┌────────────────────────────────────┴──────────────────────────────────┐
  │                                                                         │

PST 0,                         PST 0-2,                              PST > 2,
Child - Pugh A                 Child - Pugh A/B                      Child - Pugh C

  │                    ┌──────────────┴──────────────┐                      │

Very Early Stage      Early Stage         Intermediate Stage    Advanced Stage        Terminal Stage
Single < 2cm          Single 2-5cm or     Multinodular, PS0     Portal Invasion,      
                      3 nodules < 3cm                           N1, M1, PS1-2

  ┌──────────────────────┴──────────┐
Single              3 nodules ≤ 3cm

  ┌──────────────────────────────────┐
HVPG < 10 or          Varices/collaterals or
T. Bili < 1.5         HVPG > 10 or T. Bili > 1.5

                           Associated
                           Diseases
                      No    │    Yes

Surgical Resection    Liver       RFA /    Transarterial      Sorafenib    New          Symptomatic
                      Transplantation PEI  Chemoembolization                Agents /
                                                                            Clinical Traits
```

Printed with permission: Llovet, J.M., *et al. Semin Liver Dis.*
1999; 19:329-38.

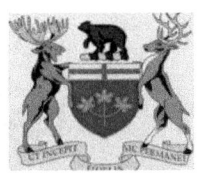

Multidisciplinary Canadian consensus recommendations for the management and treatment of hepatocellular carcinoma.

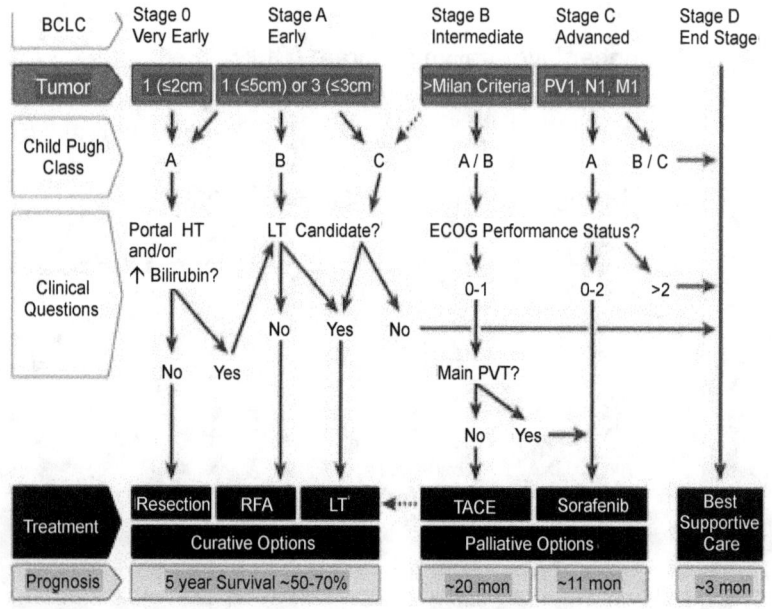

Printed with permission: Sherman, M., *et al. Curr Oncol.* 2011; 18(5):228-40.

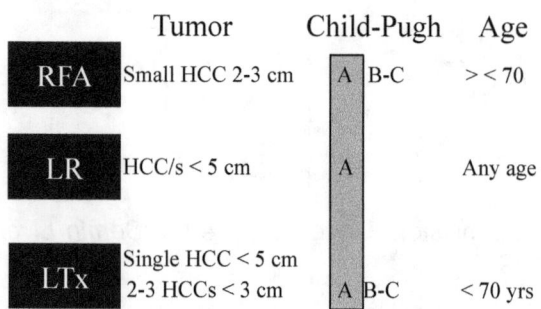

Abbreviations: LR, liver resection; LTx, liver transplantation; RFA, radiofrequency ablation

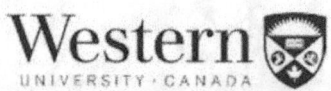

Liver Resection For HCC

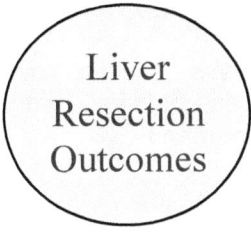

Mortality and Morbidity 1-12%	Survival and Tumour Recurrence	Pros & Cons

- o Factors ↓ survival
  - – PHT
    - ▪ platelets < 150,000
    - ▪ bilirubin > 1.1 mg/dL

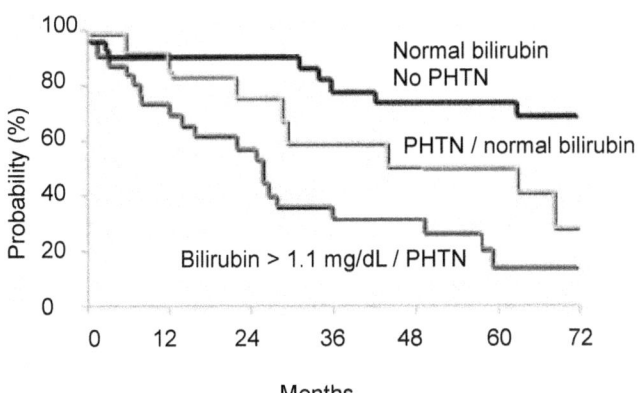

Months

Abbreviation: PHT, portal hypertension

Printed with permission: Llovet, J.M., *et al. Hepatology.*
1999; 30:1434-40.

- o Unisegmentectomy in a small shrunken cirrhotic liver
  - – Major procedure

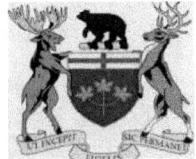

➤ Variable response
- Give the minor liver resection for one patient that can be a major resection to another.
  o Inability to accurately predict the functional liver reserve → imbalance between remnant liver function and ↑ metabolic demand

➤ Laparoscopic Liver Resection
  o Peripheral hepatocellular carcinoma in patients with chronic liver disease
    - 3 –year survival
      ▪ Overall, 93%
      ▪ Disease–free, 64%

Cherqui, D., *et al. Annals Surg.* 2006; 243:499–506.

Liver resection for early hepatocellular carcinoma within the Milan criteria

  o Of 152 studies reviewed, 2 randomized clinical trials and 27 retrospective case series were eligible for inclusion
  o The 5–year overall survival rate after resection of HCC ranged from 27 – 81% (median 67%)
  o Median disease–free survival rate from 21 – 57% (median 37%)
  o There was a trend towards improved overall survival in recent years; operative mortality rate ranged from 0 – 5% (median 0.7%)

Lim, K.C., *et al. British J Surg.* 2012; 99:1622-9..

In CTP class A patients with HCC ≤ 5 cm, the cummulative mortality rates in 5 years are disappointing
    - Overall, 30%
    - Disease–free, 60%

Poon, R.T.P., *et al. Annals Surg.* 2002; 235:373-82.

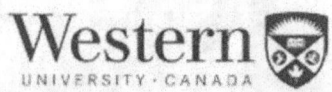

o Overall, the cummulative intrahepatic recurrence rate of 5–year after resection of hepatocellular carcinoma in cirrhotic patients is ~ 95%

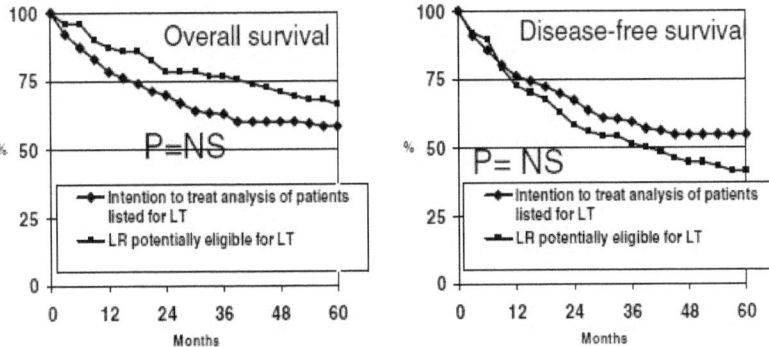

Abbreviations: LR, liver resection; LT, liver transplantation

Printed with permission: Del Gaudio, M., *et al. Am J Transpl.* 2008; 8(6):1177-85.

o Resection is more easily performed and more available to all acceptable–risk patients than transplantation.

o Assumed that the lesions are identified, preoperatively represent the entire extent of tumor (may be often incorrect).

o Livers of patients thought to harbor single HCC < 5 cm found that in 39%, there were other unrecognized foci of the disease.

o < 1/3 of lesions smaller than 1 cm are identified preoperatively, even with the best imaging modalities.

o Some post–resection recurrence is in fact progression of established HCCs that were present at the time of resection, but were undetected on preoperative imaging.

Burrel, M., *et al. Hepatology.* 2003; 38:1034-42.; Krinsky, G.A., *et al. Liver Transpl.* 2002; 8:1156-64.

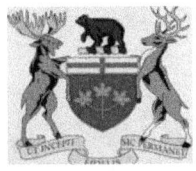

Liver Transplantation for HCC

- o Indication and diagnosis of LT influence survival
- o The United Network for organ Sharing liver allocation policy has given extra priority to patients with hepatocellular carcinoma (HCC) who meet the specific medical criteria
- o Under the current allocation system, transplantation for HCC results in excellent recurrence–free survival (RFS)

Post–LT	RFS	PS
1	96	86%
3	89	72%
5	84	62%

- o Patient survival (PS) is also very good and depends on factors other than the HCC
- o AFP level is associated with an increased risk of HCC recurrence after transplantation
- o Liver transplantation (LT) is superior to liver resection (LR) for HCC
- o 1, 3, and 5–year overall survival (OS) after LR was 89%, 75% and 56%, respectively, compared with 90%, 70% and 64% for OLT (P = 0.84)
- o Only patients who waited < 4 months for OLT had better survival than those who underwent LR (P = 0.05)
- o Patients who waited longer than 4 months for OLT had a 2.5x higher risk of death (Cox multivariate model [odd ratio (OR) 2.5; 95% confidence interval (CI): 1.3-5; P = 0.07)
- o On multivariant analysis, the relative risk (RR) was 9.2, if there was macrovascular invasion
- o For small HCC, LT was superior to LR in terms of 5–year (appoximal values) overall survival (OS) and recurrence–free survival (RFS)

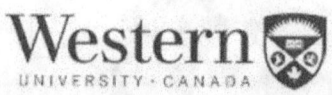

Overall survival and recurrence–free survival time of patients with hepatocellular carcinoma within Milan criteria A: Overall survival curve; B: Recurrence–free survival curve. Overall survival and recurrence–free survival time of patients with hepatocellular carcinoma beyond Milan criteria; C: Overall survival curve; D: Recurrence–free survival curve

Overall survival recurrence–free survival

OS	LT = LR
RFS	LT > LR
REC	LR > LT (52% *vs* 30%)
Post REC	LT = LR

- LT should be considered as the primary treatment in patients with HCC within Milan criteria
- LR is recommended for patients with HCC beyond the Milan criteria; LT group showed a significant lower recurrence rate than the LR group

Printed with permission: Lee, K.K., *et al. J Surg Oncol.* 2010; 101:47-53.

- The number of patients on the waiting list for liver transplantation has risen in a linear manner from 20,000 in 1982 to over 100,000 in 2009
- Results of LT are far better at 5 years for overall survival (OS) and for a disease–free (HCC recurrence free) survival
- The issue remains the very long waiting list, with ~ ½ listed patients dying before LT
- Possibly, some hyperselected patients could benefit from resection of the following:
  - Small HCC
  - HCC recurring after LT
  - "bridge" to LT
  - Untransplantable patients are ideal candidates

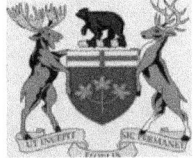

- o Resection for single, small (≤ 5 cm) HCC in patients with preserved liver function
- o Outcomes
  - – Resection become a strategy for salvage transplantation

Cumulative survival rates after resection for HCC ≤ 5 cm

Year	OS	DFS
1	90%	74%
3	76%	50%
5	70%	36%
10	35%	22%

Abbreviations: OS, overall survival; DFS, disease–free survival

Poon, P.T.P., *et al. Ann Surg.* 2002; 235(3):373-82.

- o While there is usually a high recurrence rate of HCC after liver resection, recurrence–free survival for > 10 years, is associated with the following:
  - – Single HCC
  - – Small ≤ 5 cm
  - – Simple nodular
  - – No vascular invasion
  - – No intrahepatic metastases
  - – Low levels of tumor markers

Eguchi, S., *et al. Br J Surg.* 2011; 98:552-7.

- o Better outcomes with primary transplantation (PLT) than with secondary liver transplantation (SLT), i.e. LT after initial resection

Adam, R., *et al. Ann Surg.* 2003; 238(4):508-18.

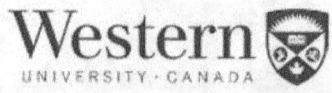

Comparison of Outcome of Primary and Secondary Transplantation for HCC

	Secondary LT	Primary LT	P
o Tumor recurrence	54%	18%	0.001
o Extrahepatic resection	23%	0%	< 0.0001
− OS			
1−year	71%	80%	
3−year	53%	68%	0.03
5−year	41%	61%	
− DFS			
1−year	47%	76%	
3−year	29%	64%	0.003
5−year	29%	58%	

Adam, R., *et al. Ann Surg.* 2003; 238(4):508-18.

- o Survival of cirrhotic patients with HCC. Primary LT should therefore remain the ideal choice of treatment for cirrhotic patients with HCC, even when the tumor is resectable.
- o There is a high risk of failure of salvage transplantation after initial LR for HCC

Fuks, D., *et al. Hepatology.* 2012; 55:132-40.

- o Some authors report meta−analysis of 14 studies that there was no difference in 5−year overall survival between SLT and PLT 2.

Belghiti, J., *et al. Ann Surg.* 2003; 238(6):885-93.

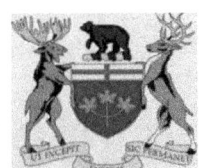

> Liver Transplantation (LT) after Liver Resection (LR)
>   o A best (80%) and a worst scenario (40%) (Majno, *et al. Hepatology*. 2000; 31:899-906.)
>   o A 79% transplantability rate from analysis of the mode of recurrence of HCC (Poon, R.T., *et al. Ann Surg*. 2002; 236(5):602-11.)

> Resection for HCC Possible Role
>   o Primary
>   - Liver transplantation as "**salvage**" for recurrence and liver failure

> Conclusion
>   o Resection and LT represent the components of a combined strategy for the management of HCC in cirrhosis.
>
>   o The choice of a particular treatment option should depend upon the individual risk factors and the availability of a donor organ.
>
>   o LT is overall the best option at long term and on a disease–free basis.
>   - Resection provides similar survival only for single HCC < 3 cm.
>
>   o Liver resection may provide good survival benefit to hyperselected patients.
>
>   o Salvage transplantation could be a solution after recurrence.
>
>   o Resection, as a selection tool, needs to be validated.

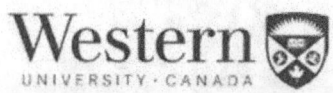

Pre – Op Assessment For Cirrhosis: Can We Predict Morbidity And Mortality?

Mark A. Levstik And Puneeta Tandon

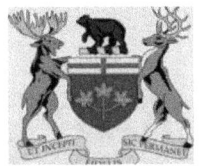

- Give the management considerations in the pre– and post–operative care for patients with advanced liver disease.

➢ Risk stratification

➢ Prevention of HE
- o Hepatic encephalopathy
- o Correction of reversible metabolic factors (i.e. hyponatremia, hypocalcemia)
- o Oral lactulose administration, titrated to ~ 3 – 4 bowel movements per day
- o Administration of non–absorbable antibiotics
- o Avoidance of nephrotoxic insults (i.e. NSAIDs, narcotics, benzodiazepines)
- o Supportive care
- o Correction of reversible metabolic factors

➢ Treat the complications of portal hypertension (PHT)
- o Ascites, peripheral edema
- o Oral diuretic therapy with spironolactone and/or furesomide
- o Fluid restriction (if sodium concentration is < 120 mmol/L)
- o Avoidance of excessive saline administration
- o Albumin infusion (with paracentesis volumes > 5 l)
  - Antibiotics for spontaneous bacterial peritonitis
  - Steroids, as indicated

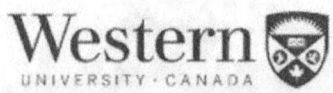

- o Coagulopathy
    - – Vitamin K supplementation (oral or parenteral)
    - – Fresh, frozen plasma transfusions
    - – Intravenous administration of cryoprecipitate
    - – Intravenous administration of recombinant factor VIIa
    - – Platelet transfusions
- o Paracentesis with analysis of ascitic fluid as evidence of infection

➢ Diet

- o Maintenance of an adequate protein intake (1 – 1.5 g/kg per day)
- o Promotion of a balanced diet
- o Dietary sodium restriction (< 2 g daily)

➢ Pain control

- o Dilaudid
- o Avoid benzodiazepines, NSAIDs and narcotics

➢ Assess pulmonary function

- o Supplemental oxygen

Adapted from: Hanje, A.J., and Pate, T. *Nature Clinical Practice Gastroenterology & Hepatology* 2007; 4: page 272.

Post–operative Hepatic Dysfunction is Common, please see: Shah, V.H. and Kamath P.S. *Sleisenger and Fordtran's Gastrointestinal and Liver Disease.* 10th Ed. Saunders/Elsevier, Philadelphia, 2016, page 1536-1543.

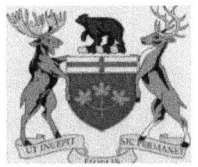

> Summary approach in predicting post–operative mortality
  o Child–Pugh classification
  o MELD (model for end–stage liver disease) score
  o Presence of PHT (portal hypertension)
  o Comorbidities
  o For high risk surgery, consider performing the surgery at a center with hepatobiliary experience, including liver transplantation (L–Tx)
  o Consider pre–operative assessment for L–Tx (liver transplantation), in case the patient does not do well post–operatively

- Give the **Child–Pugh classification** of liver disease.

Parameters	1	2	3
– Ascites	None	Slight	Mod/severe
– Encephalopathy	None	Slight/mod (1-2)	Mod/severe (3-4)
– Bilirubin (mg/dl)	< 2 (< 34)	2-3 (34-50)	> 3 (> 50)
– Albumin (mg/dl)	> 3.5 (> 35)	2.8-3.5 (28-35)	< 2.8 (< 28) > 6 (> 2.2)
– PT (INR)	1-3 (< 1.7)	4-6 (1.7-2.2)	

Total scores	Child–Pugh classification
5-6	A
7-9	B
10-15	C

Adapted from: Kim, W.R., *et al. Hepatology* 1999; 29(6):1643-8.; Durand, F. and Valla, D. *J Hepatol.* 2005; 42.

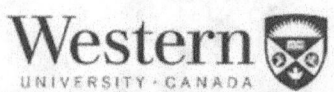

- Give the peri–operative mortality rates (MR) of patients with cirrhosis.

Child's	Surgical MR (%)
A	5-10
B	30
C	70-80

  o 30–day peri–operative mortality, 30% (total):
    - Worsening Ascites, 7%
    - Pneumonia, 8%
    - Infection, 8%
    - Bleeding, 10%

Source: Sterling, R.K. *ACG Annual Scientific Meeting Symposia Sessions.* 2009; 71-77.

- Give the uses of **MELD score** in predicting peri–operative complications.

  ➤ MELD score   5-20   1% increase in mortality with each 1 point increase

           > 20   2% increase in MR for each MELD point increase

  o If MELD < 11 (especially < 8), acceptable risks

  o If MELD > 20, elective surgery should be postponed

  o If MELD 12 – 20, complete L–TX evaluation in case of deterioration

  o Derived from creatinine, bilirubin, INR

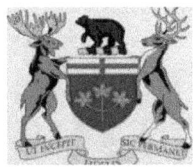

- o Correlates with mortality rate for the following:
  - – Liver transplantation
  - – Liver resection
  - – Other abdominal operations
  - – Cardiac surgery

➢ Summary of findings: "MELD Plus"

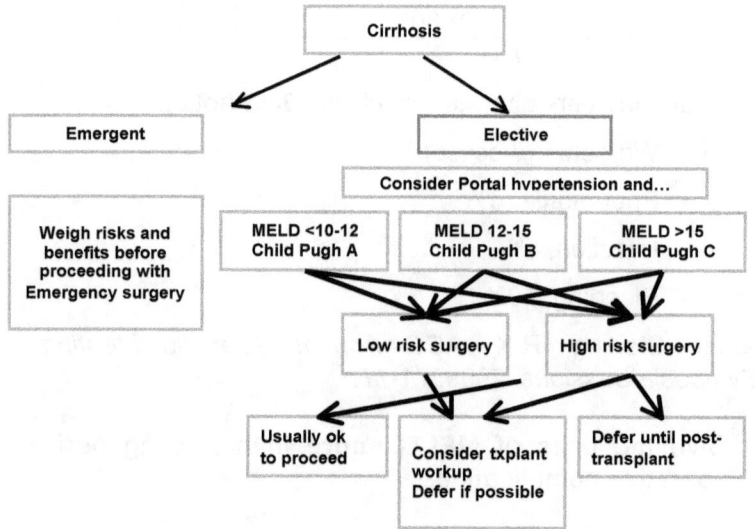

Adapted from SM Malik, Mclin Nam 2009

- o MELD, ASA class, and age are most important
  - – www.mayoclinic.org/meld/mayomodel9.html
  - – C–statistic is 0.80 (30–day) and 0.84 (90–day)

- o Emergency surgery predicted duration of hospitalization (p < 0.001) but not mortality

- o ASA class V best to predict 7–day mortality

- o MELD is best beyond 7 days

Adapted from: Teh, S.H., *et al.* Risk factors for mortality after surgery in patients with Cirrhosis. *Gastroenterology* 2007; 132:1261-9.

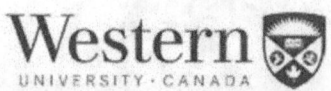

Assessment of Liver Function

➢ Child–Pugh score
  o Subjective, non–shunt intra–abdominal surgery

	Child–Pugh A	Child–Pugh B	Child–Pugh C
Garrison RN N = 100 Abdominal	10%	31%	76%
Mansour A N = 92 Abdominal	10%	30%	82%

➢ MELD score
  o Retrospective study of 772 cirrhotic patients
    – Major digestive, orthopedic, cardiovascular surgery
    – Independent predictors of 30– and 90–day mortality
      ▪ MELD score
      ▪ American Association of Anesthesiologists class (ASA)
        – III – severe systemic disease
        – IV – severe systemic disease, constant threat to life
        – V – moribund, not expected to survive within 24 hours
      ▪ Age
        – Only extremes of age influence mortality
  o MELD score

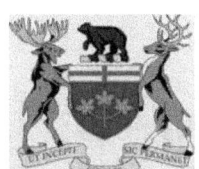

Relationship between MELD score and post–operative mortality

MELD score	Mortality, % (No. of patients at risk)			
	7 days	30 days	90 days	1 year
0-7 (n=351)	1.9 (314)	5.7 (301)	9.7 (287)	19.2 (252)
8-11 (n=257)	3.3 (236)	10.3 (219)	17.7 (200)	28.9 (170)
12-15 (n=106)	7.7 (94)	25.4 (78)	32.3 (69)	45.0 (56)
16-20 (n=35)	14.6 (29)	44.0 (19)	55.8 (15)	70.5 (10)
21-25 (n=13)	23.0 (7)	53.8 (4)	66.7 (3)	84.6 (2)
≥ 26 (n=10)	30.0 (6)	90.0 (1)	90.0 (1)	100 (0)

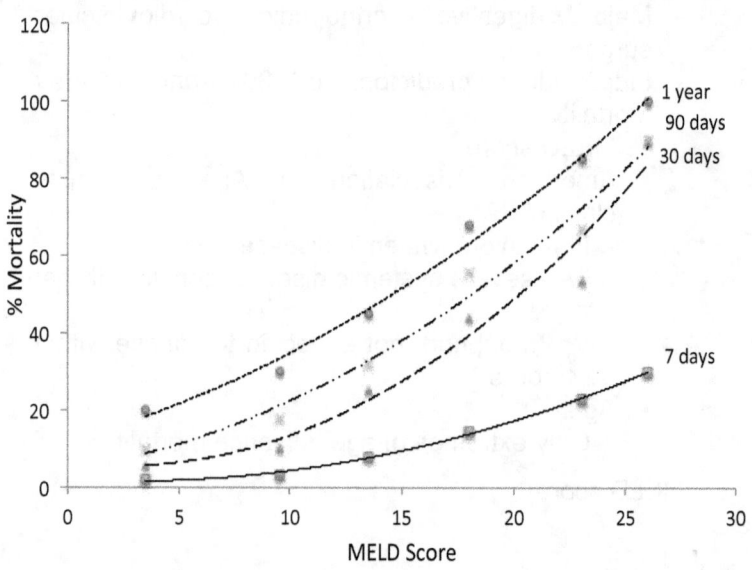

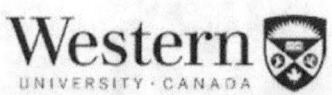

Post-operative Mortality Risk in Patients with Cirrhosis

To determine the risk of post-operative mortality for all types of major surgery, especially gastro-intestinal, orthopedic and cardiac surgery (includes open-heart procedures), please enter the following variables:

ASA score

III – severe systemic dz

IV – severe systemic dz, constant threat to life

V – moribund, not expected to survive 24 hours

What is the age?	60	
What is the ASA score?	4	(use 1-5)
What is the bilirubin?	4.1	(mg/dl)
What is the creatinine?	1.7	(mg/dl)
What is the INR?	2.0	
What is the etiology of cirrhosis?	○ Alcoholic or Cholestatic	
	◉ Viral/Other	

[Compute]   [Reset form]

Probability of Mortality

7 days	30 days	90 days	1 year	5 years
25.699 %	70.442 %	86.034 %	82.363 %	99.181 %

http://www.mayoclinic.org/meld/mayomodel9.html

Outcomes with Hernia Repair

- o Hernia surgery included in the "minor surgery control group" of the Teh, *et al.* study
- o Limited data were available
  - – 21 patients (6 CPB, 13 CPC)
  - – 71% for incarcerated hernias

  - – Peri–operative morbidity, 71%, mortality, 5%
  - – Majority of ruptured hernia patients had peri–operative TIPS procedure

- o **Case 2**
- o Would the predicted mortality with surgery have been the same if this was cardiac surgery? A hip pinning for a fracture?

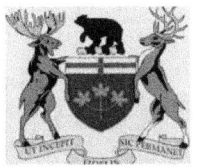

Post-operative Mortality Risk in Patients with Cirrhosis

To determine the risk of post-operative mortality for all types of major surgery, especially gastro-intestinal, orthopedic and cardiac surgery (includes open-heart procedures), please enter the following variables:

Mortality Risk Models

The MELD Model
The MELD-Na Model
The MELD Model, UNOS modification
MELD score and 90-day mortality rate for alcoholic hepatitis
Post-operative Mortality Risk in Patients with Cirrhosis
Other mathematical models for liver disease patients

What is the age? `45`

What is the ASA score? `4` (use 1-5)

What is the bilirubin? `2.3` (mg/dl)

What is the creatinine? `1` (mg/dl)

What is the INR? `1.6`

What is the etiology of cirrhosis? ⊙ Alcoholic or Cholestatic
                                     ○ Viral/Other

[Compute] [Reset form]

Probability of Mortality

7 days	30 days	90 days	1 year	5 years
2.758 %	10.84 %	16.916 %	28.052 %	59.814 %

Portal Hypertension

- Limited data – 29 patients with Child–Pugh A cirrhosis and HCC undergoing hepatic resection
    - Pre-operative hepatic venous pressure gradient
    - HVPG < 10 mm Hg → no decompensation
    - HVPG ≥ 10 mm Hg → 73% decompensation 3 months after surgery

What problems do cirrhotic patients run into post–operatively?

- Hepatic dysfunction (ascites, HE, shock liver)
- Renal failure
- Coagulopathy
- Wound complications (infection, dehiscence)

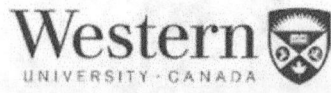

Why do these problems occur?
- o Susceptibility to hypoxemia
  - Impaired baseline hepatic perfusion
  - Co–existing vasoactive drugs, hemorrhage, liver–lung syndromes (PPH, HPS)
  - Anesthesia reduces hepatic blood flow by 30%
  - Positive pressure ventilation, pneumoperitoneum with laparoscopic surgery → decrease hepatic blood flow
  - Traction on the abdominal viscera → dilatation of the splanchnic capacitance vessels
- o Impaired clearance of medications
  - Anesthetic agents
  - Benzodiazepines
  - Narcotics

Source: O'Leary, J.G. *Clin Liver Dis.* 2009; 13(2):211-31.

Perioperative Care
- o Coagulopathy
  - Vitamin K for 10 mg/day x 1 – 3 days +/- FFP +/- cryoprecipitate
  - Platelet transfusion, if platelets < 50,000/mm^3
- o Ascites and hydrothorax
  - Peri–operative control without impacting renal function
- o Renal function
  - Avoid nephrotoxic agents
  - Close monitoring of volume status and urine output
  - HRS is a terminal diagnosis without transplant
- o Hepatic encephalopathy
  - Avoid surgery until this is controlled as there are many precipitants in the peri–operative period
  - Lactulose, rifaximin
- o Gastroesophageal varices
  - Peri–operative β–blockade, ligation
  - +/- TIPS

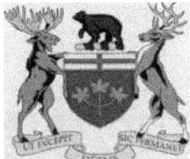

- o Nutritional deficiency
  - − Poor nutritional status adversely impacts prognosis
  - − Oral or enteral nutritional supplementation

Elective Surgery for

- o Alcoholic hepatitis
- o Mortality rate, 58%, if open liver biopsy is done *vs* 10% if percutaneous liver biopsy is done
  - − Can get significant improvements in liver function in a short period of time; if possible, delay the interventions for at least 12 weeks
- o Acute hepatitis
- o Acute liver failure

Type of Surgery

- o Emergency surgery *vs* elective surgery
  - − Emergency surgery − higher mortality rate
  - − Mansour, 1997
    - ▪ Child−Pugh A − 22% *vs* 10% mortality
    - ▪ Child−Pugh B − 38% *vs* 30% mortality
    - ▪ Child−Pugh C − 100% *vs* 82% mortality
  - − Teh, 2007
    - ▪ Emergency surgery not an independent predictor of mortality as patients had a higher MELD score
    - ▪ Was an independent predictor of a longer duration of hospitalization post operatively

Source: Mansour, A., *et al. Surgery.* 1997; 122(4):730-5.; Teh, S.H., *et al. Gastroenterology.* 2007; 132(4):1261-9.

Umbilical Hernia Repair

- o Umbilical hernias occur in up to 20% of patients with end−stage liver disease
- o Ascites control is paramount

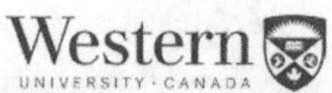

Suggested Reading

Arvaniti, V., *et al*. Infections in patients with cirrhosis increase mortality four fold and should be used in determining prognosis. *Gastroenterology.* 2010; 139:1246-56.

Berzigott, A., *et al*. Obesity is an independent risk factor for clinical decompensation in patients with cirrhosis. *Hepatology.* 2011; 54:555-61.

Kanwal, F., *et al*. An explicit quality indicator set for measurement of quality of care in patients with cirrhosis. *Clinical Gastroenterology and Hepatology.* 2010; 8:709.

Macaron, C., *et al*. Safety of cardiac surgery for patients with cirrhosis and Child-Pugh scores less than 8. *Clin Gastroenterol Hepatol.* 2012; 10(5):535-539.

Violi, F., *et al*. Patients with liver cirrhosis suffer from primary haemostatic defects? Fact or fiction? *J Hepatol.* 2011; 55(6):1415-27.

Volk, M.L., *et al*. Hospital readmissions among patients with decompensated cirrhosis. *Am J Gastroenterol.* 2012; 107(2):247-52.

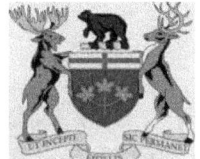

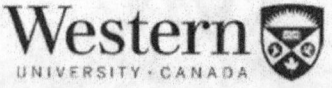

Approach to Patients With Hepatic Mass

Anouar Teriaky

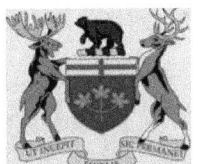

HEPATIC TUMORS

Benign Lesions

- Give the causes of hepatic mass seen on abdominal ultrasound.
    - Tumors
        - Primary and secondary metastases
    - Benign lesions (usually require no further treatment)
        - Cavernous hemangioma
        - Focal fatty liver areas
        - Focal nodular hyperplasia (reaction to an arterial malformation; the telangiectatic subtype of FNH is associated with estrogen use; 10% multiple, 20% associated with cavernous hemangioma)
        - Simple liver cysts
        - Hepatic adenoma (associated with the use of OCA; require further follow–up)
    - Malignant lesions
        - Cholangiocarcinoma (CA 19–9)
        - Cystadenocarcinoma
        - Epithelioid angiomyolipoma
        - Hemangioendotheliomatosis
        - Liver metastases
        - Lymphomas
        - Mixed epithelial and stromal tumors
        - Mixed hepatocellular–cholangiocarcinoma
        - Primary hepatocellular carcinoma
        - Sarcomas
    - Abscesses
        - Amebic liver abscess
        - Biliary cystadenoma
        - Echinococcal cysts
        - Granulomatous abscesses
        - Inflammatory pseudotumor
        - Nodular regenerative hyperplasia
        - Pyogenic liver abscess

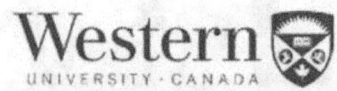

Abbreviation: OCA, oral contraceptive agents

Adapted from: Roberts, L.R. *2008. AGA Annual Postgraduate Course Syllabus*: page 245.

- o When a mass is identified in the liver of patient with or without chronic liver disease, a triple phase CT or MRI with gadolinium is performed

- o Nuclear scintigraphy with sulphur colloid is taken up by the Kupffer cells; uptake is increased with metastatic lesions (thyroid, breast, lung, pancreas, colon), hemangioma or cysts, and is reduced in hepatic adenomas and HCC

- o Radionucleotide scanning with RBC identifies hepatic mass as a hemangioma

- Give an algorithm for the evaluation of hepatic mass in patient with and without chronic liver disease.

   o   Without Cirrhosis

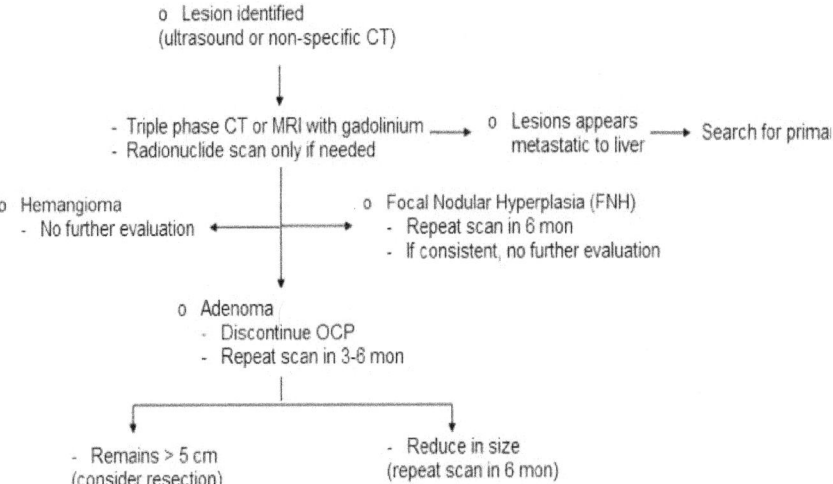

Abbreviation: OCP, oral contraceptive pill

o   With Cirrhosis

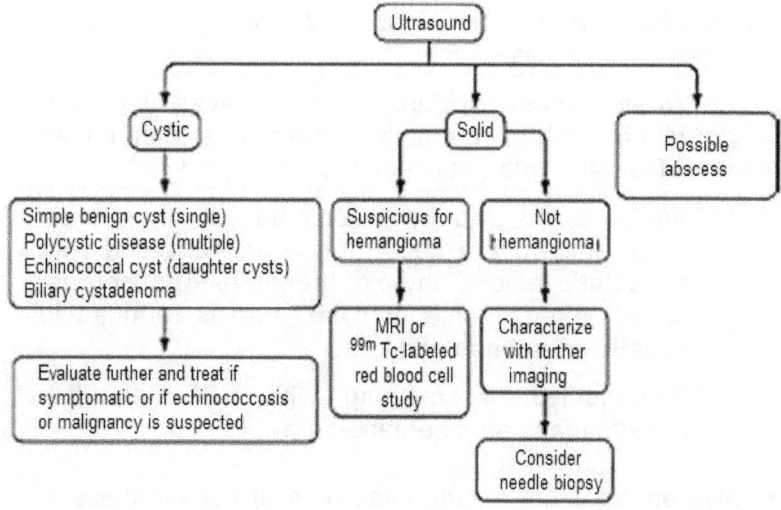

Hepatic Cysts

- Classification hepatic cysts.
    - o Simple hepatic cysts
    - o < 5 cm, and up to 3 cysts before PCLD (polycystic liver disease) needs to be considered
    - o Polycystic liver disease
    - o ADPKD (autosomal dominant polycystic kidney disease)
    - o Biliary microhamartomas
    - o Caroli disease (type V choledochal cyst)
    - o Congenital hepatic fibrosis
    - o Type IV choledochal cysts

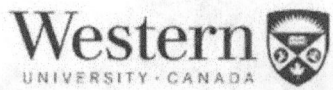

- Give features seen on diagnostic imaging which differentiate the nature of the hepatic tumor and cyst.
  - Cysts containing daughter cysts (hydatid)
  - Partly cystic and partly solid
    - Biliary
      - Cystadenoma
      - Cystadenocarcinoma
  - Hyperechoic lesion with interspersed hypoechoic areas
    - Areas of:
      - Necrosis
      - Hemorrhage
      - Fat
  - Vascular
    - Hemangiomas
    - Metastasis from NET (neuroendocrine tumor)

- ➤ Simple Hepatic Cysts
  - Present in > 2% of the population and felt to be congenital in origin
  - Generally < 5 cm and ≤ 3 cysts
  - Usually asymptomatic, and an incidental finding
  - Complications when symptomatic, include:
    - Bleeding
    - Infection
    - Rupture
    - Compression
  - US, CT, or MRI provides the diagnosis
  - Should be left alone, if asymptomatic
  - Treatment includes:
    - Percutaneous drainage
    - Surgery

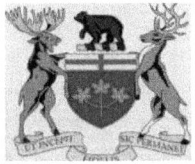

Liver Abscesses

- Pyogenic liver abscess
- Amebic liver abscess

Hepatic Mass: an Approach

- Was the lesion detected incidentally or was the individual symptomatic?
- What are the characteristics (age, gender, HPx, FHx, meds) of the patient?
- Is there a history of risk factors for chronic liver disease or cirrhosis?
- Is there a travel history or features suggesting amebic or pyogenic abscess?

Abbreviations: FHx, family history; HPx, history and physical examination

Malignant Hepatic Neoplasms

- Primary
  - Hepatocellular carcinoma (HCC)
  - Intrahepatic cholangiocarcinoma
  - Hepatoblastoma
  - Hemangiosarcoma
  - Epithelioid hemangioendothelioma
  - Cystadenocarcinoma
- Secondary
  - Metastasis

Benign

- Hepatocellular adenoma
- Cavernous hemangioma
- Infantile hemangioendothelioma

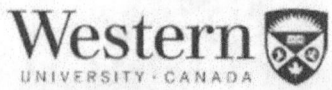

Hepatocellular Carcinoma (HCC)

➢ Demography
  o Most common primary malignant liver tumor
  o 5th most common cancer in men and 8th in women
  o Ranks fourth in the annual cancer mortality rates
  o Men are generally more susceptible than women
  o Hepatocellular carcinoma (HCC) is one of the most common malignant tumors worldwide and incidence is increased in industrialized countries
  o M:F 2:1 – 4:1; increased BMI, androgenic hormones
  o 70 – 90% of HCC occur against the background of hepatic fibrosis grades 3 to 4, or cirrhosis, 1 – 4% per year (El-Serag, H.B., Rudolph, K.L. *Gastroenterology* 2007:2557-2576); the remainder is associated with HBV and hemochromatosis (HCV in Japan)

➢ Causes and risk factors
  o 70 – 90% of HCC occur against the background of hepatic fibrosis grades 3 to 4, or cirrhosis, 1 – 4% per year (El-Serag, H.B., Rudolph, K.L. *Gastroenterology* 2007:2557-2576); the remainder is associated with HBV and hemochromatosis (HCV in Japan)

• Give risk factors for the development of HCC.
  o Patient
    – M:F 2:1 – 4.1
    – Africans > 20 years (HBV⁺)
    – Asian males > 40 years / females > 50 years (HBV⁺)
    – Family history of HCC
    – Dietary aflatoxin exposure
    – Obesity
    – Tobacco, marijuana smoking
    – Oral contraceptive pill
    – Androgenic hormones

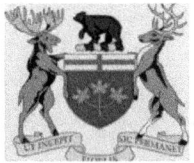

- o Without cirrhosis
    - Chronic HBV infection (even without cirrhosis)
    - Chronic HCV infection (Japan; all others, HCV cirrhosis)
    - Hepatic adenoma
    - Hemochromatosis
    - Aflatoxin B1
    - Congenital and familial
    - Previously resected HCC
- o With cirrhosis
    - HCV
    - HCV + ALD + obesity (accelerated)
    - EtOH
    - Hemochromatosis: dietary Fe overload in patients of African ancestry; HH
    - PBC
    - Alpha–1–antitrypsin deficiency
    - NASH
    - Autoimmune hepatitis
    - Wilson's disease
    - Type 1 hereditary tyrosinemia
    - Type 1 and type 2 glycogen storage disease
    - Hypercitrulinemia
    - Ataxia–telangiectasia

- o Medications
    - Exposure to OCAs (oral contraceptives)

Abbreviations: ALD, alcoholic liver disease; FH, family history; NASH, non–alcoholic steatohepatitis; PBC, primary biliary cirrhosis

Adapted from: Di Bisceglie A.M. and Befeler A.S. *Sleisenger & Fordtran's Gastrointestinal and Liver Disease: Pathophysiology/Diagnosis/Management.* 10th Ed. 2016, Box 96-1, page 1604.

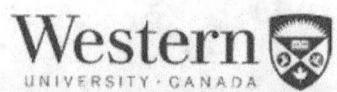

Major Etiologies

- o Chronic hepatitis B, C or D

- o Toxins (i.e. alcohol, tobacco, aflatoxins)

- o Hereditary metabolic liver diseases (i.e. hemochromatosis, α–1–antitrypsin deficiency)

- o Autoimmune hepatitis

- o Obesity (males)

- o Diabetes mellitus

- o Non–alcoholic steatohepatitis (NASH)

- o Non–alcoholic fatty liver disease (NAFLD)

Printed with permission: Macmillan Publishers Ltd: Spangenberg, *et al*, Nat.Rev. *Gastroenterol Hepatol* 2009; 6:423-432.

- Explain the **mechanism** for the ↑ risk of HCC in HBV, even without the presence of cirrhosis.
  - o There is ↑ risk of HCC with HBV infection. The mechanisms include:
    - HBV is incorporated into cellular DNA (in 90% of HCC patients)
    - Chromosomal insertion is random
    - HBV is indirectly and directly carcinogenic
    - Cis–activation of cellular genes
    - Transcriptional activation of HBV x protein
    - Viral mutations
    - Activation of the following:
      - MAP (mitogen–activated protein kinase)
      - JAK/STAT pathways (Janus kinase–signal transducer and activator of transcription)
  - o Risk of developing HCC
    - HBV: ~ 4/100 patient–years

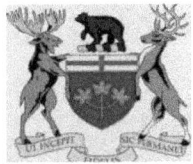

- Give the risk factors of **HCC in HBV**.
  - o Patient
    - Presence of cirrhosis
    - Young age of acquisition
    - Asian or African race
    - Male gender
    - Older age
    - Family history of HCC
    - Exposure to aflatoxin, alcohol and tobacco
    - Long duration of HCV
    - Hepatitis B co–infection with HBV, HIV
    - Heavy alcohol intake
    - Obesity +/- NASH
  - o Infection
    - Co–infection with HCV, HDV, and possibly, HIV
    - Active replication of HBV
    - Genotype C

Adapted from: Gores, G.J. *AGA Institute Post Graduate course book* 2006: page 251-2.

- Give the risk factors of **HCC in HCV**.
  - o Patient
    - Alcohol drinking (heavy > 50 gm/d)
    - Male gender
    - Increased BMI
  - o Liver
    - Degree of hepatic fibrosis
    - Associated iron overload (hereditary hemochromatosis)
  - o Infection
    - HCV infection for > 25 years
    - Failure of HCV to respond to IFN (interferon)
    - Older age of HCV onset and diagnosis
    - Absence of previous HCV treatment
    - HBV co–infection
    - HIV co–infection
    - Long duration of active disease

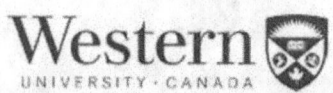

➢ Clinical

    o Usually seen in patients with cirrhosis but also with non–cirrhosis, if HBV, HCV in Japan, hereditary hemochromatosis, α1–AT deficiency, and NAFLD and NASH.

Symptoms	Frequency (%)
– Abdominal pain	59-95
– Weight loss	34-71
– Weakness	22-53
– Abdominal swelling	28-43
– Non–specific GI symptoms	25-28
– Hepatomegaly	54-98
– Ascites	35-61
– Fever	11-54
– Splenomegaly	27-42
– Wasting	25-42
– Jaundice	4-35
– Hepatic bruit	6-25

➢ Paraneoplastic Syndromes Associated with HCC

o Carcinoid syndrome	o Polymyositis
o Hypercalcemia	o Porphyria
o Hypertrophic osteoarthropathy	o Sexual changes (gynecomastia)
o Hypoglycemia	o Systemic arterial hypertension
o Neuropathy	o Thyrotoxicosis
o Osteoporosis	o Thrombophlebitis migrans
o Polycythemia	o Watery diarrhea syndrome

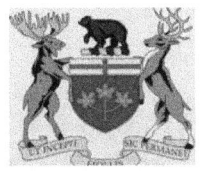

> Screening

- Screening recommendations for HCC patients
  - Hepatitis B carriers
    - African > 20 years
    - Asian males > 40
    - Asian females > 50
    - Family history of HCC
    - All patients with cirrhosis
  - Non HBV non–cirrhosis
    - Hepatitis C (in Japan)
    - Hereditary hemochromatosis
    - Alpha–1 antitrypsin deficiency
    - NASH
    - Autoimmune hepatitis

Adapted from: El-serag, H.B. *2009 ACG Annual Postgraduate Course*: pages 39-43.

SO YOU WANT TO BE A HEPATOLOGIST!

Approximately, what proportion of patients with HCC or pancreatic cancer suggests the primary lesion is resectable will the tumor turn out to be non–resectable as defined by diagnostic laparoscopy and laparoscopic ultrasound?

- About one third of patients with HCC, or pancreatic cancer, will have their resectability status downgraded to a non–resectable by diagnostic laparoscopy and laparoscopic ultrasonography.

> Pathology
  - Risk of seeding from tumor biopsy is ~ 3%
  - Not necessary to biopsy the liver to diagnose HCC

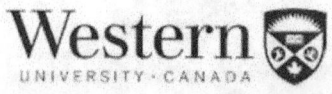

- Give the pathological findings of hepatocellular (HCC).

  - Gross
    - Nodules
    - Large circumscribed mass
    - Diffuse infiltration
  - Microscopic
    - Well–differentiated
      - Trabecular form (thick trabeculae)
        - Hepatocytes – polygonal
        - Cytoplasm – ↓ eosinophils
        - Nuclei
          - Large
          - Hyperdramatic
        - Nucleoli are prominent
        - Bile production
      - Acinar (pseudoglandular) form
        - Glandular structures around the bile canaliculus containing bile
    - Moderately differentiated
      - Pleomorphic, multinucleated giant cells
      - Cell nests
      - Central ischemic necrosis
      - Little bile in the connective tissue
    - Differentiated
      - Pleomorphic cells and nuclei
      - Bizzare giant cells
      - Globular hyaline
      - Mallory hyaline

- ➢ Prognosis and risk stratification or staging

- Give the prognostic factors in HCC.

  - Patient
    - ECOG classification
    - Presence of symptoms

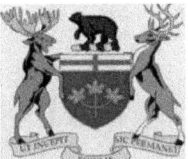

- o Liver function
  - – Child–Pugh class
  - – Serum bilirubin
  - – Albumin levels
  - – Presence or absence of portal hypertension
- o Tumour status
  - – Number and size of nodules
  - – Presence or absence of macrovascular invasion
  - – Presence or absence of extrahepatic spread

Abbreviation: ECOG, Eastern Cooperative Oncology Group

Useful background: The Okuda Staging System of HCC

Criterion	Cut–off
o Tumor size	> 50% (largest cross–sectional area of tumor to largest cross–sectional area of liver) = positive < 50% = negative
o Ascites	Clinically detectable = positive Undetectable = negative
o Serum albumin	< 3 g/dL = positive > 3 g/dL = negative
o Serum bilirubin	< 3 g/dL = positive > 3 g/dL = negative
o Stage	
I	No positive criterion
II	Positive criteria
III	Three positive criteria

Printed with permission: Nguyen, M.H. and Keeffe, E.B. *Best Practice & Research Clinical Gastroenterology*. 2005; 19(1):164.

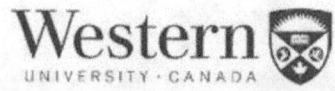

Accurate staging at the time of diagnosis, based on the Barcelona Clinic Liver Cancer classification (BCLC), is central to the choice of the appropriate therapeutic strategy.

- Give the components of **BCLC** staging classification for HCC.
  - o Tumor size and spread
  - o Patient performance status
  - o Child–Pugh class

Please see: Feldman, M., et al. Sleisenger and Fordtran's Gastrointestinal and Liver Disease. 9th Edition. Saunders/Elsevier. 2010; Figure 94.4, page 1576.

➤ Risk Factors for HCC

Major Risk Factors
  - o Liver
    - Chronic Hepatitis B
    - Chronic Hepatitis C
    - Cirrhosis
  - o Diet
    - Dietary exposure to alfatoxin B1

Other Liver Conditions
  - o Alpha–1 antitrypsin deficiency (A$_1$ATD)
  - o Hemochromatosis (HH)
  - o Membranous obstruction of the IVC
  - o Glycogen storage disease (type 1/2)
  - o Type 1 hereditary tyrosinemia
  - o Wilson's disease (WD)

Other Factors
  - o Cigarette smoking
  - o Diabetes mellitus
  - o Oral contraceptive steroids

Inherited conditions (non-liver)
  - o Ataxia–telangiectasia
  - o Hypercitrullinemia

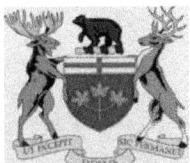

➢ Diagnosis

o Gold standard for the diagnosis of HCC is pathology

o Serum tumor markers may be helpful in conjunction with imaging, but not alone

o Tumor markers include the following:
- AFP
- Fucosylated AFP
- Des–gamma–carboxy prothrombin

➢ Imaging

o Ultrasound
- Detects most of HCC, but may not distinguish from other solid lesions; Sn, 48% and Sp, 97%
- Contrast–enhanced Doppler US aids the diagnosis

o CT
- Dynamic (multiphase) CT is the imaging of choice
- Sn 67.5 and Sp 92.5
- Nodules > 2 cm with classic CT features Sp 100%
- Nodules 1 – 2 cm require a second dynamic imaging study to confirm the diagnosis

o MRI
- Dynamic MRI provides findings on multiphase contrast enhancement similar to those by CT
- Sn, 80.6% and Sp, 84.8%

o Hepatic Angiography
- Diagnostic role has decreased with CT and MRI
- Angiography is essential in delineating the hepatic arterial anatomy prior to embolization

Abbreviations: Sn, sensitivity; Sp, specificity

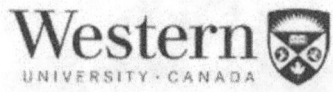

➢ Pathology
  o Gross Appearance
    - Nodular: most commonly co–exists with cirrhosis
    - Massive: large circumscribed mass
    - Diffusely infiltrating: large part of liver is involved

  o Microscopic Apppearance
    - Well–differentiated
    - Most common
    - Organized
    - Moderately–differentiated
      ▪ Solid
      ▪ Scirrhous
      ▪ Clear
    - Undifferentiated: great variety in size and shape

Hepatocellular Cancer (HCC)

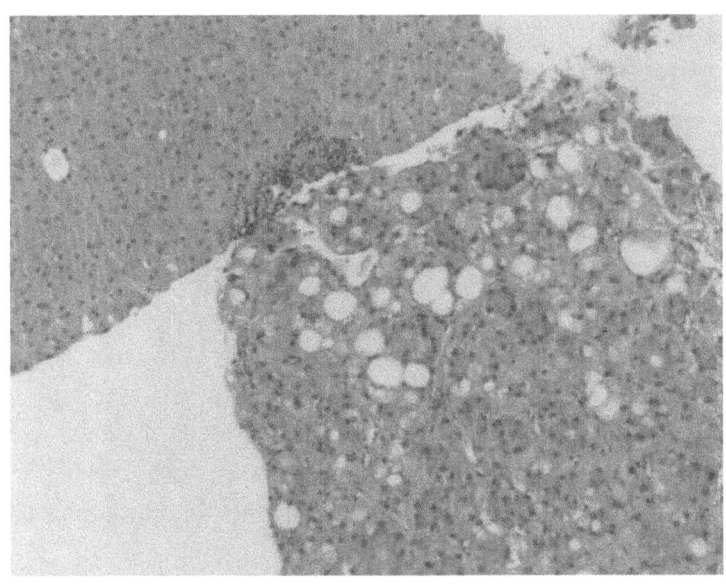

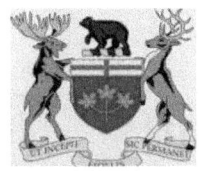

Hepatocellular Cancer (HCC)

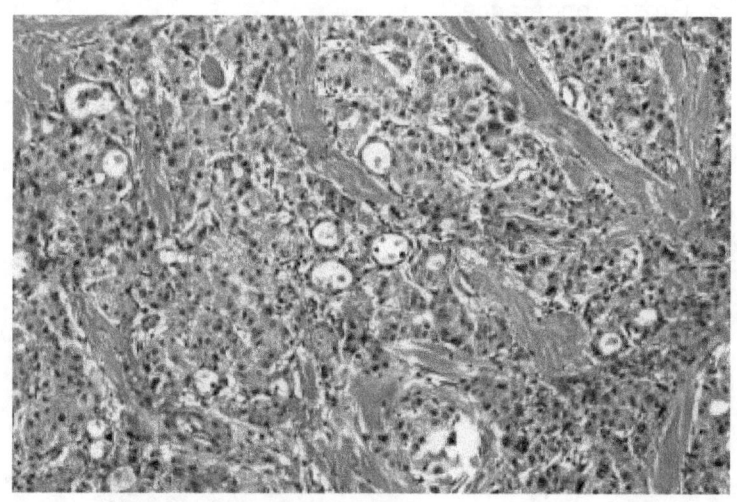

- Give the non–histological diagnostic criteria for hepatocellular cancer (HCC).

    o   Hepatic mass on ultrasound in cirrhotic

    o   Focal lesion > 2 cm with evidence of cirrhosis (if < 2 cm, on 2 imaging modalities – CT angiogram arterial hypervascularization and venous washout MRI (contrast–enhanced ultrasound; MRI – triphasic (hyper–T_2, 150–T_1)

    o   AFP > 200 ng/ml (normal AFP does not rule out HCC)

    o   Sulphur colloid scan – cold (Kupffer cells positive in FNH)

    o   Non–cirrhotic HBV, HCV (Japan), hemochromatosis, α1–AT deficiency

Adapted from: Talwalkar, J.A. and Gores, G.J. *Gastroenterology.* 2004; 127(5 Suppl 1):S126-32.

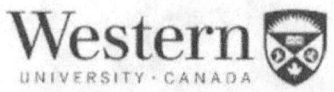

➢ Diagnostic imaging

- Give the diagnostic imaging characteristics on CT, MRI, PET scan and nuclear medicine of hemangioma, focal nodular hyperplasia (FNH), adenoma, HCC and metastases.

  o Hemangioma: nodular, no wash–out at periphery, RBC scan, triphasic CT scan (arterial phase)

  o Focular nodular hyperplasia Central vessel
    - Stellate central scar
    - Homogenous

  o Adenoma
    - Heterogeneous
    - Hemorrhage
    - Fat
    - Necrosis
    - Impaired arteriole (no bile duct) "feeding" lesion

  o HCC
    - Tumor thrombus in the vessels
    - Fat
    - Cirrhosis
    - Capsule heterogeneous
    - Bile production
    - Extrahepatic involvement

  o Metastases
    - Wash–out at periphery
    - Ring enhancement
    - Fat
    - Blood
    - Calcification
    - New or increasing size – may be hyper– or hypovascular

Adapted from: Hussain, S.M. and Semelka, R.C. *Magn Reson Imaging Clin N Am.* 2005; 13(2): 255-75.

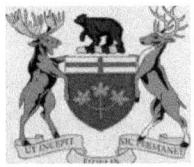

- Non–invasive criteria have been established by the American and European groups (AASLD and EASL) provide a similar sensitivity of about 80% in making the diagnosis of what turns out to be HCC.

  o CT
    - ↓ HA, PV supply
    - Arterial neovascularization
    - Venous wash–out

  o Hypervascularization in the arterial phase followed by wash–out in the venous phase is suggestive of malignancy

  o Dynamic MRI
    - Dynamic MRI, using gadolinium–contrast agents, may be used in association with dynamic CT if the hepatic mass is 1 – 2 cm in size. The findings on the arterial phase of high signal intensity on T2–weighted images, on venous and delayed phases finding central wash–out if with contrast– and capsular enhancement, have a sensitivity and specificity for HCC of 81% and 85%, respectively

  o MRI super–paramagnetic MRI
    - Iron oxide taken up by Kupffer cells are missing in HCC
    - Slows up dark HCC on this test
    - Art phase gives sensitivity
    - Venous phase gives specificity

- Give the imaging criteria applied in confirming HCC to patients with cirrhosis and a nodule detected by ultrasound.

➢ Ultrasound
  o Lesion has nodular configuration
  o Lesion is at least 1 cm in its longest diameter*

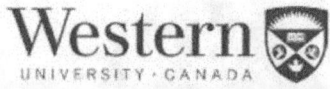

- o Lesion shows arterial hypervascularization:
  - Hyper–enhanced nodule in the arterial phase by two imaging techniques**
  - Hyper–enhanced nodule in the arterial phase and as hypo–enhanced nodule in the portal venous or delayed phase by one imaging technique**
- o In general terms, abdominal ultrasound has a sensitivity of 48% and a specificity of 97% for the detection of HCC.

Algorithm for mass or nodule in cirrhotic liver is seen on abdominal ultrasound (US) in patients at risk for HCC

Diameter	Follow–up
< 1 cm	US every 4 months for 1 year, then every 6 months long term
> 1 cm	4–phase CT and dynamic contrast–enhanced MRI

- Give the differentials of the causes of **hypervascularity** on ultrasound, in addition to HCC.
- o Arterial portal shunts
- o Atypical hemangiomas
- o Aberrant venous drainage
- o Dysplastic nodules
- o Confluent fibrosis
- o Notes:
  - Most sensitive and specific imaging technique for the diagnosis of HCC is Gad-MR (gadolinium magnetic resonance)
  - Other methods include contrast–enhanced ultrasonography, helical–computed tomography, and superparamagnetic iron oxide magnetic resonance
  - Hepatic nodules smaller than 2 cm in diameter may still contain a focus of HCC

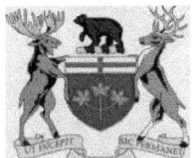

Abbreviation: LT, liver transplantation; RFA, radiofrequency ablation; TACE, transarterial chemoembolization; TACI, transarterial chemotherapy infusion

- Give the performance characteristics of CT and MRI for HCC.

➤ CT

  o Arterial enhancement (hypervascular, supplied by hepatic artery) and wash–out for HCC, sensitivity is 90% and specificityis 95%

➤ MRI

  o Similar performance characteristics as CT, but size of HCC is a factor, with accuracy of > 90% for > 20 mm lesions seen on MRI, but 30% for lesion < 20 mm

  o Biopsy under radiological guidance

Tests	Sensitivity	Specificity
– US	90%	91%
– CT	92%	98%

  o For hyper–enhanced nodule > 1 cm, suspect HCC

*apply to lesions emerged during US surveillance; for lesions detected during the first imaging examination, lesion diameter should be at least 2 cm to allow non–invasive diagnosis of HCC

**imaging techniques include, contrast–enhanced US, contrast–enhanced spiral CT and gadolinium–enhanced MRI

Source: El-Serag, H.B. 2009. *ACG Annual Postgraduate Course*: 39-43.

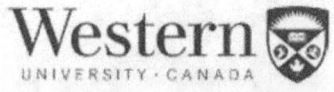

➤ Screening and surveillance

- Categorize patients with chronic liver disease recommended for surveillance for HCC.

  o Non–cirrhotic
    - HBV carriers with
      ▪ Active hepatitis
      ▪ Family history of HCC
    - HCV chronic hepatitis plus fibrosis

  o Cirrhotic
    - C–P A and B
    - C–P C awaiting liver transplantation

Abbreviation: C–P, Child–Pugh

- Give the risk of cirrhosis, hepatocellular carcinoma (HCC) and mortality in hepatitis B and C viruses (HBV/HCV) mono–infected and co–infected patients.

	Cirrhosis[1]	HCC (OR)[2]	Mortality (SMR)[3]
o HBV monoinfection	~ 22%	16-23	1.4-5.3
o HCV monoinfection	~ 30%	8-17	2.4-3.1
o HBV/HCV coinfection	~ 50%	36-165	5.6-49

Abbreviations: HBV, hepatitis B; HCC, hepatocellular carcinoma; HCV, hepatitis C; OR, odds ratio; SMR, standard mortality ratio

[1]Zarski, et al. 1998
[2]Shi, et al. 2005; Donato, et al. 1998
[3]Amin, et al. 2006; Di Marco, et al. 1999

Printed with permission: Wursthorn, et al. Best Practice Res Clin Gastroenterol. 2008; 22:1063-79.

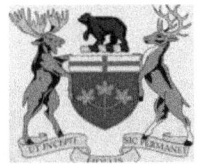

SO YOU WANT TO BE A HEPATOLOGIST!

Multiphasic, dynamic, helical CT is the imaging technique of choice for the diagnosis of HCC. The most helpful features are enhanced arterial phase in the involved area, wash–out (loss of central nodule enhancement composed of uninvolved liver), and enhancement of the capsule in the porto–venous and delayed phases. When the lesion is > 2 cm, diagnostic imaging changes.

- Explain why classical CT changes of HCC disappears as the HCC enlarges.

    o   Arterial enhancement (neoangiogenesis causing hypervascularity)

    o   Shift of blood from primary portal artery

- Give the features of hereditary hemochromatosis patients with ↑ risk of HCC.

    o   Males with iron overload and advanced fibrosis

    o   Dysplastic lesions

    o   Proliferative lesions

    o   Increased number of iron–free foci (IFF, > 50% at risk to develop HCC)

Adapted from: Hytiroglou, P., *et al. Gastroenterol Clin North Am.* 2007; 36(4):867-87.

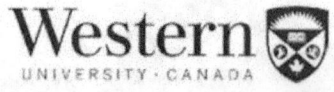

> Staging

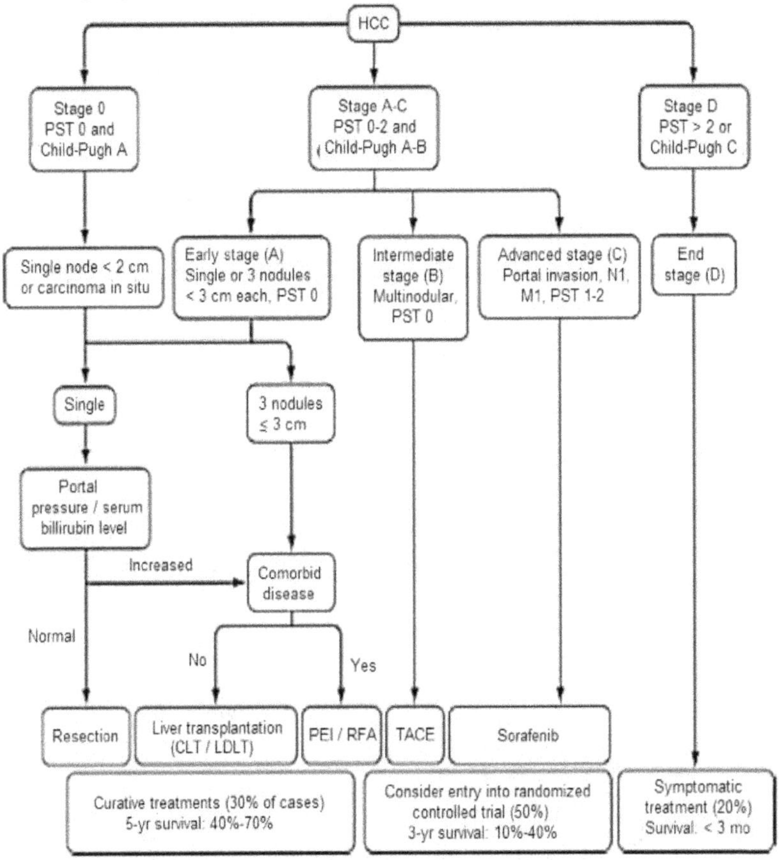

```
                              ┌───────┐
                              │  HCC  │
                              └───┬───┘
        ┌─────────────────────────┼─────────────────────────┐
┌───────────────┐         ┌───────────────┐         ┌───────────────┐
│   Stage 0     │         │  Stage A-C    │         │   Stage D     │
│  PST 0 and    │         │  PST 0-2 and  │         │  PST > 2 or   │
│ Child-Pugh A  │         │ Child-Pugh A-B│         │ Child-Pugh C  │
└───────┬───────┘         └───────┬───────┘         └───────┬───────┘
```

| Single node < 2 cm or carcinoma in situ | Early stage (A) Single or 3 nodules < 3 cm each, PST 0 | Intermediate stage (B) Multinodular, PST 0 | Advanced stage (C) Portal invasion, N1, M1, PST 1-2 | End stage (D) |

```
   ┌─────────┐        ┌──────────┐
   │ Single  │        │ 3 nodules│
   └────┬────┘        │  ≤ 3 cm  │
        │             └────┬─────┘
 ┌──────────────┐          │
 │   Portal     │          │
 │pressure/serum│          │
 │billirubin lvl│     ┌──────────┐
 └──────┬───────┘     │ Comorbid │
        │  Increased  │ disease  │
   Normal│            └──────────┘
         │          No        Yes
```

| Resection | Liver transplantation (CLT / LDLT) | PEI / RFA | TACE | Sorafenib | | Symptomatic treatment (20%) Survival. < 3 mo |

| Curative treatments (30% of cases) 5-yr survival: 40%-70% | Consider entry into randomized controlled trial (50%) 3-yr survival: 10%-40% |

Abbreviations: CLT, cadaveric liver transplantation; LDLT, live donor liver transplantation; PEI, percutaneous ethanol injection; PST, performance status test; RFA, radiofrequency ablation; TACE; transarterial chemoembolization; TAE, transarterial embolization

Printed by permission: Cabibbo, *et al. Nature Clinical Practice Gastroenterology and Hepatology.* 2009; 6(3):159-169, Figure 1, page 160.; and Bruix, J. and Sherman, M. Management of hepatocellular carcinoma: An update. *Hepatology.* 2011; 53(3). Figure 2, 1020–1022.

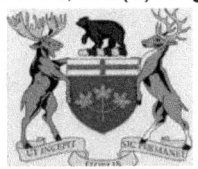

➤ Treatment

- o Accurate staging at the time of diagnosis, based on the Barcelona Clinic Liver Cancer classification, is central to the choice of the appropriate therapeutic strategy

- o Surgical resection
  - Curative, but limited to non–cirrhotic and cirrhotic patients without portal hypertension
  - 5– and 10–year survival rates are 40 and 26%, respectively

- o Liver transplantation
  - Cirrhotics with portal hypertension
  - Successful in selected patients (Milan criteria: 1 lesion ≤ 5 cm or 2 – 3 lesions ≤ 3 cm with no LVI or metastasis)

- o Alcohol injection and radiofrequency ablation (RFA)
  - Potentially curative for small tumors, including multiple tumors
  - High recurrence rate

- o Chemoembolization
  - Palliative treatment for patients with intact hepatic function and tumors that are not amenable for other treatments

- o Chemotherapy
  - Used alone or in combination
  - Sorafenib, an inhibitor of Raf and tyrosine kinase, improves survival

- o Alternative techniques
  - New local ablative techniques (cryoablation, laser)
  - Stereotactic radiotherapy
  - Radiotherapy with Y microspheres

Abbreviation: LVI, liver vascular involvement

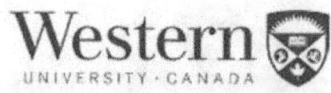

➢ Screening

- o Patients at high risk of HCC should be entered into a surveillance program

- o When to start surveillance is dependent on patient demographics and the cause of CLD

- o Surveillance should be performed using US at 6 – 12 months and AFP should not be used alone unless US is not available

NON–HCC MALIGNANT HEPATIC TUMORS

Fibrolamellar HCC

- o Typically occurs in young adults with equal gender distribution

- o Does not secrete AFP

- o Is not associated with Hepatitis B, C or cirrhosis

- o More often amenable for surgery

- o Doesn't respond well to chemotherapy

Cholangiocarcinoma

➢ Demography

- o Prevalence in North America, $1/10^5$

- o Cholangiocarcinoma is the second most common hepatic malignant tumor

➢ Causes and associations

- Give the factors and associations that increase the risk of cholangiocarcinoma.

  - o Infection   – HCV–associated cirrhosis
                          – *O. viverrini* and *C. sinensis*

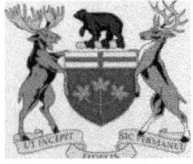

- o Developmental – Caroli disease
  - Choledochal cyst

- o Cholelithiasis, – PSC (primary sclrosing cholangitis)
  intrahepatic – Caroli disease
  - Choledochal cyst
  - Thorotrast contrast dye

➤ Laboratory

- Give the tests used to diagnose cholangiocarcinoma.

  - o Diagnosis – Serology CA 19–9, CEA, CA 19–9
    + CEA, CA–125

  - o Tumor marker CA 19–9

    - – False • Cancer – Stomach
      positives – Pancreas
      - Colon
      - Gynecologic
      - • Acute bacterial cholangitis

    - – False • Lewis blood group–negative
      negatives – With PSC – CA 19 – 9 > 129
      U/mL; sensitivity, 79%;
      specificity, 98%
      – Without PSC > 100 U/mL;
      sensitivity, 53%; specificity, 89%

  - – Performance characteristics

	Sensitivity	NPV	Specificity
CA 19 – 9, biliary obstruction			
• Without PSC	53%	72 – 92%	
• With PSC	38 – 89%		50 – 98%

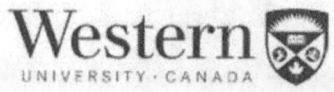

➢ Histopathology
- o Few cells (paucicellular)
- o Brush cytology
- o FNA (fine–needle aspiration)
- o Desmoplastic reaction
- o FISH (fluorescence hybridization)
- o Cytology
  - Acinar or tubular structures
  - Absent bile secretion
  - Desmoplastic reaction
  - Prominent colonization of stroma
  - May be difficult to distinguish from metastatic adenocarcinoma
- o Subtypes
  - Intrahepatic
  - Extrahepatic
  - Hilar (Klatskin tumor)
  - Distal bile duct
  - Four types, by bismuth - Corlette Calssification (Feldman, M., et al. *Sleisenger and Fordtran's Gastrointestinal and Liver Disease*, 9th Edition. Sauders/Elsevier, Philadelphia. 2010. Table 69.3, page 1173., for details of the Diagnostic Criteria for Cholangiocarcinoma)
- o Perihilar cholangiocarcinoma is extrahepatic in location, but the ICD classification considers that this is an intrahepatic tumor

➢ Diagnostic Imaging
- o Locations
  - Hepatic bifurcation (Klatskin tumor)
  - Distal CBD
  - Intrahepatic (5 – 15%)

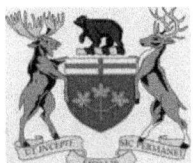

o MRI
- MRI "......is currently the imaging technique for cholangiocarcinoma" (Feldman, M., *et al. Sleisenger and Fordtran's Gastrointestinal and Liver Disease.* 9th Edition. Saunders/Elsevier, Philadelphia. 2010. page 1174).
- IDUS (high frequency intraductal ultrasound)
- CT or PET; sensitivity and specificity; intrahepatic, 93% and 80%, but extrahepatic, 53% and 33%, respectively
- MRCP –
  - T1–weighted, hypodense lesion
  - T2–weighted, intense lesion
- Variable fibrosis and necrosis
- Atrophy
- Capsular retraction
- Biliary duct dilation
- Hypovascular (progressive, delayed hyper–enhancement)

o Endoscopy
- ERCP + cytology
- Choledochoenteroscopy
- ERCP + choledoscopy (for dominant stricture; sensitivity is 92%)

Note: See Feldman, M., *et al. Sleisenger and Fordtran's Gastrointestinal and Liver Disease.* 9th Edition. Saunders/Elsevier, Philadelphia, 2010, Table 69.3, page 1173 for the details of the Diagnostic Criteria for Cholangiocarcinoma.

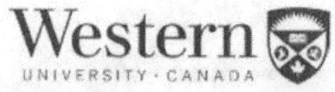

o Cytology

	Sensitivity
– Cytology	30%
– Cytology, brushings and biopsies	40 – 70%

o Symptoms, usually don't occur until the tumor is advanced, i.e.:
   – Malaise
   – Weight loss
   – Abdominal pain
   – Jaundice

o Diagnosis involves the following:
   – LEs abnormal, LFTs
   – CA 19–9
   – AFP
   – Imaging (US/CT/MRI/MRCP/ERCP)

o Treatment, includes:
   – Surgery, if discovered early (rare)
   – Endoscopic or percutaneous drainage
   – Chemotherapy
   – Radiation

Cholangiocarcinoma

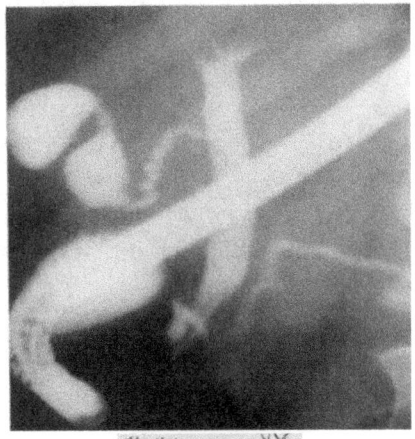

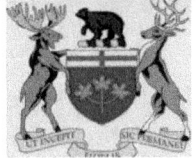

➤ Treatment

- Give the criteria for surgical resection of cholangiocarcinoma.
  - o No extrahepatic metastases
  - o No encasement or invasion
  - o No involvement of both segmental bile ducts
  - o No contralateral lobular atrophy

➤ Prognosis
  - o When not a surgical candidate, survival rates:
    - – 1 year: 28%
    - – 5 year: 5%
  - o Liver transplantation combined with radiation, brachytherapy and chemosensitization
    - – 5–year: 82% survival rate

Hepatoblastoma
  - o Most common hepatic tumor in children
  - o Malignant derivatives of incompletely differentiated hepatocyte precursors
  - o Clinical features, include the following:
    - – Abdominal swelling
    - – FTT
    - – Weight loss
    - – Abdominal pain
    - – Poor appetite
    - – Nausea
    - – Diarrhea
  - o Diagnosis is confirmed with blood work and imaging (US/CT/MRI)
  - o Occurs sporadically or in association with hereditary syndromes
  - o Rapidly progressive tumor

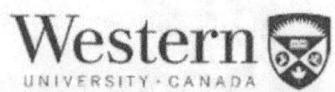

- o Treatment involves the following:
    - – Neoadjuvant chemotherapy, if necessary, followed by surgery
    - – Liver transplantation

Hemangiosarcoma

- o A rare mesenchymal liver tumor
- o More prevalent in the $6^{th}/7^{th}$ decade and in men
- o Risk factors, include:
    - – Thorium dioxide
    - – Arsenic
    - – Vinyl chloride monomer
- o Symptoms include the following:
    - – Upper abdominal pain
    - – Abdominal swelling
    - – Malaise
    - – Weight loss
    - – Poor appetite
    - – Nausea
    - – Jaundice
    - – Ascites
- o Diagnosis is made
    - – When progressive hepatic dysfunction occurs
    - – Mass lesions seen on imaging (US/CT/MRI)
- o Due to rapid growth, prognosis is poor
- o Results of treatment with radiation or chemotherapy are poor and even when surgery is possible, survival is limited

Epithelioid Hemangioendothelioma

- o Rare tumor
- o More common in females
- o Non–specific symptoms

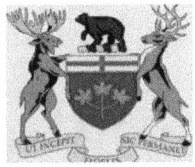

- o Tumor consists of dendritic and epithelioid cells that contain vacuoles
- o Imaging shows a highly vascular mass
- o Low–grade malignant potential
- o Surgical resection or transplantation are effective treatments

Cystadenocarcinoma

- o Found in the elderly
- o Probably arise from malignant transformation of a cystadenoma
- o Multilocular (resemble cystadenomas)
- o A thick wall showing large tissue masses protruding from the internal cyst lining
- o If suspected, treatment should consist of a formal liver resection

Hepatic Metastases

- o Most common malignant tumor of the liver
- o Symptoms:
  - Usually absent
  - Can include abdominal pain, malaise, weight loss, and jaundice
- o Dynamic CT is the most useful imaging technique
- o US and MRI also have a role
- o Treatment depends on the primary malignancy, including the following:
  - Surgery
  - Chemotherapy
  - Radiofrequency
  - Ethanol ablation

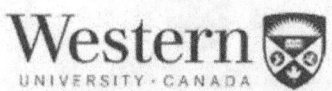

BENIGN HEPATIC NEOPLASMS

Hepatic Cysts

➤ Classification

- Classify hepatic cysts.
  - o Simple hepatic cysts
  - o < 5 cm, and up to 3 cysts before PCLD (polycystic liver disease) need to be considered
  - o Polycystic liver disease
  - o ADPKD (autosomal dominant polycystic kidney disease)
  - o Biliary microhamartomas
  - o Caroli disease (type V choledochal cyst)
  - o Congenital hepatic fibrosis
  - o Type IV choledochal cysts

➤ Diagnostic imaging

- Give the features seen on diagnostic imaging help to differentiate hepatic tumor from cyst.
  - o Cysts contain daughter cysts (hydatid)
  - o Partly cystic and partly solid
    - – Biliary
      - ▪ Cystadenoma
      - ▪ Cystadenocarcinoma
  - o Hyperechoic lesion with interspersed hypoechoic areas
    - – Areas of:
      - ▪ Necrosis
      - ▪ Hemorrhage
      - ▪ Fat

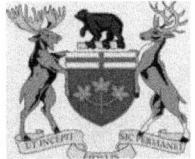

- o Vascular
  - – Hemangiomas
  - – Metastasis from NET (neuroendocrine tumor)

Peliosis Hepatis

- ➤ Definition
  - o Multiple blood–filled cavities distributed randomly throughout the parenchyma of the liver

- ➤ Types
  - o Parenchymal
    - – Cavities lined by hepatocytes
  - o Phlebectatica
    - – Cavities lined by hepatocytes
  - o May progress to any of the following:
    - – Fibrosis
    - – Regenerative nodules
    - – Cirrhosis
    - – Tumors

- ➤ Clinical
  - o Anabolic steroids
  - o *Bartonella* infection in HIV–immunosuppressed patients
  - o Azathioprine
  - o OCA (oral contraceptive agent)
  - o Vitamin A
  - o Hydroxyurea
  - o About 1/3 of patients with severe disease will have a symptomatic, harmless ↑ ALT

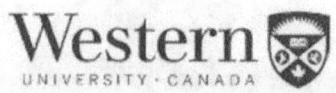

Hepatocellular Adenoma (HA)

➤ Demography
  o Usually seen in $1/10^6$ of women in their childbearing years, and especially if they are on OCA (3x increased risk)
  o Premalignant, with risk of malignancy is increasing with size of adenoma

➤ Causes and associations
  o Estrogen and/or progesterone oral contraceptive agents (OCAs)
  o Anabolic steroids
  o Type I glucagon storage disease

➤ Pathophysiology
  o HNF 1α inactivation, through biallelic mutations of the TCF1 gene
  o β–catenin activation
  o Acute inflammation

➤ Clinical
  o May enlarge
  o When ≥ 5 cm, may undergo with the following:
    – Bleed
    – Malignant degeneration
  o Associated with the use of OCA (oral contraceptive agent)
    – Large, subcapsular lesions may rupture and bleed
    – Resect, if > 5 cm
    – No malignant potential

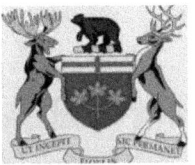

- ➤ Histopathology
  - o 90% single, 10% multiple
  - o Circumscribed, but not encapsulated
  - o Vascular channels of various sizes
  - o Thrombi in vascular channels
  - o Mast cells within hemangiomas
  - o Sclerosis
  - o Sheets of normal, or near–normal looking, hepatocytes
  - o No triads, central vein or bile ducts
  - o Adenomatosis may occur
  - o May undergo malignant transformation
  - o Associated with the use of the following:
    - – OCP
    - – Anabolic steroids
    - – Obesity
    - – Alcohol
    - – Genetic alterations
  - o Clinical features
    - – May be absent
    - – Can include abdominal pain or hemoperitoneum from rupture

- ➤ Laboratory
  - o AFP is usually normal

- ➤ Diagnostic imaging
  - o Multiphase, helical CT or MRI
    - – Definite margin (pseudocapsule)
    - – Vessels enter adenoma at the periphery and pass in a spoke–wheel manner to the center
    - – Focal avascular areas

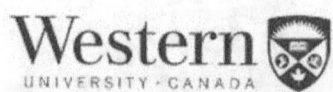

- o Technetium sulfur colloid scan
  - – Features on triphasic CT or gadolinium–enhanced MRI may be difficult to distinguish from HCC
  - – A technetium sulfur colloid scan is needed to show the typical cold lesions (no sulfur colloid uptake)
  - – Serum AFP becomes positive when hepatic adenomas turns malignant
- o US is used for initial imaging, but dynamic CT or MRI may also be used
- o Diameter from 8 – 15 cm
- o Surgical treatment is recommended because of danger of rupture
- o Arterial embolization has been successful in controlling hemorrhage from a ruptured HA
- o HA can rarely undergo malignant transformation into HCC
- o Most common benign liver tumor, and more commonly, found in females
- o Great majority is asymptomatic discovered incidentally
- o US appearance is variable and non–specific
- o SPECT or MRI show tumors to be highly vascular
- o Percutaneous needle biopsy should not be performed due to risk of severe bleeding
- o Multiple tumors occur in 10%
- o Microscopically composed of multiple vascular channels of varying sizes

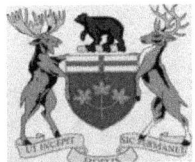

➤ Treatment
- o Great majority can be left untreated
- o If causing severe symptoms, then remove surgically
- o Other treatments include:
  - Irradiation
  - Arterial ligation
  - Arteriographic embolization
  - Systemic glucocorticoids

Cavernous Hemangioma

➤ Causes and associations
- o Caused by the following:
  - Congenital malformation
  - Hamartomatous change
  - Enlarges under influence of estrogens and pregnancy
- o The increased vascularity is of capillary origin

➤ Histopathology
- o Common congenital malformation of the liver vasculature
- o Ectactic blood vessels with no malignant potential and not affected by oral contraceptive hormones
- o Because of tortuous vessels and stasis, thrombosis and pain may occur

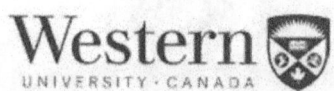

Cavernous Hemangioma

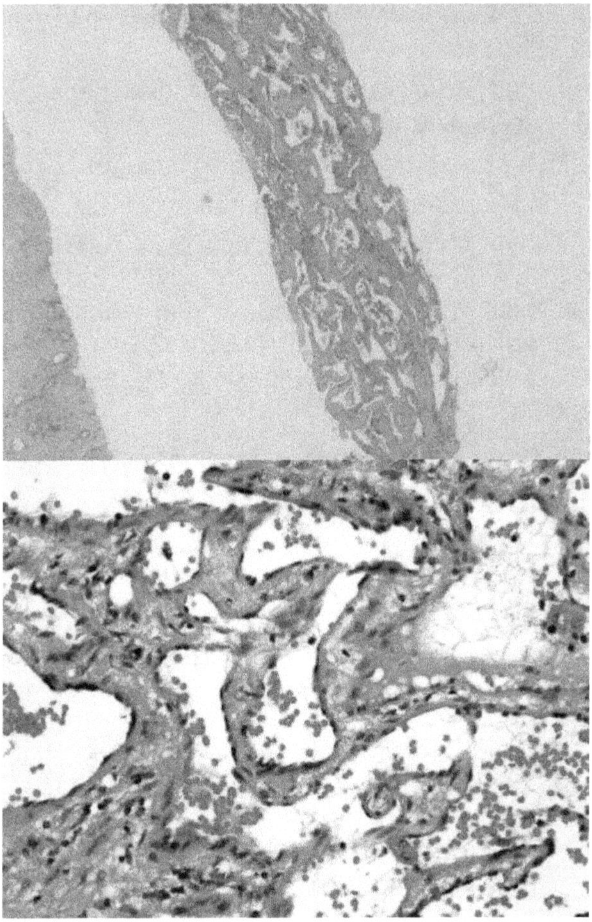

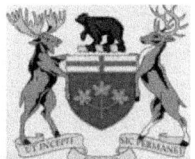

- ➤ Diagnostic imaging
  - o Abdominal ultrasound is echogenic
  - o Bolus–enhanced CT with sequential scans
    - – These show   ▪ Periphery – enhanced
      - ▪ Margin – corrugated
      - ▪ Centre – hypodense

- SPECT (single photon emission computed tomography) with colloid ^{99M}Tc–labelled red blood cells

Note: Enhanced slowly with dynamic studies because the increased vascularity is from capillaries

- MRI may show pathognomonic changes
- Ring– or C–shaped configuration
- Center: fibrous, with no uptake (avascular)

You are sensible and don't want to perform a percutaneous biopsy in patient with large hypoechoic liver lesion on abdominal ultrasound is suggestive of a cavernous hemangioma.

- Give the findings in diagnostic imaging tests suggesting hepatic mass is a cavernous hemangioma.

o CT or MRI contrast–enhanced	– Centipedal filling of contrast (from the periphery to the center)
	– Well circumscribed
o RBC nuclear scan with technetium	– ↑ uptake of labelled RBC on the venous phage
	– ↑ retention on delayed films

SO ho-ho-ho, YOU WANT TO BE A HEPATOLOGIST!

In a large hemangioma, define **Kasabach-Merritt** syndrome.

- Kasabach–Merritt syndrome is a large hemangioma, DIC (disseminated intravascular coagulopathy) and thrombocytopenia resulting from platelets being sequestered and destroyed in the hemangioma.

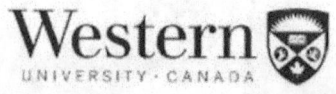

Infantile Hemangioendothelioma

- o Most common liver tumor in infants
- o Manifests in the first 6 months
- o More common in girls
- o Diagnostic triad of the following:
  - – Enlarged liver
  - – CHF
  - – Multiple cutaneous hemangiomas
- o Ultrasound shows one or more echogenic masses
- o Hepatic angiography is helpful
- o Treatment involves treating CHF
- o If these measures fail, use the following:
  - – Embolization
  - – Ligation of the hepatic artery
  - – Surgery
  - – Liver transplantation

Focal Nodular Hyperplasia (FNH)

➤ Definition

- o "Focal nodular hyperplasia is a circumscribed, usually solitary lesion [of the liver] composed of nodules of benign hyperplastic hepatocytes surrounding a central stellate scar" (Di Bisceglie A.M. and Befeler A.S. *Sleisenger and Fordtran's Gastrointestinal and Liver Disease*. 10th Edition. *Saunders/Elsevier* 2016, page 1622).

➤ Demography

- o 2nd only to hemangiomas as a cause of a benign tumor of the liver
- o More common in females
- o Occurs at all ages

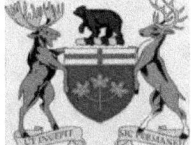

- ➢ Pathophysiology
  - ○ Reaction to arterial malformation

- ➢ Pathology
  - ○ Common congenital malformation of the liver vasculature, with hyperplasia of hepatocytes around the vascular abnormality, leading to a central scar
  - ○ Hyperplastic regenerative nodules separated by fibrosis septae
  - ○ Circumscribed
  - ○ Usually solitary lesion of nodules
  - ○ Benign hyperplastic hepatocytes
  - ○ Microscopically, FNH resembles a focal form of inactive cirrhosis
  - ○ Hepatocytes are indistinguishable from normal liver, but lacks the normal organization

Focal Nodular Hyperplasia (FNH)

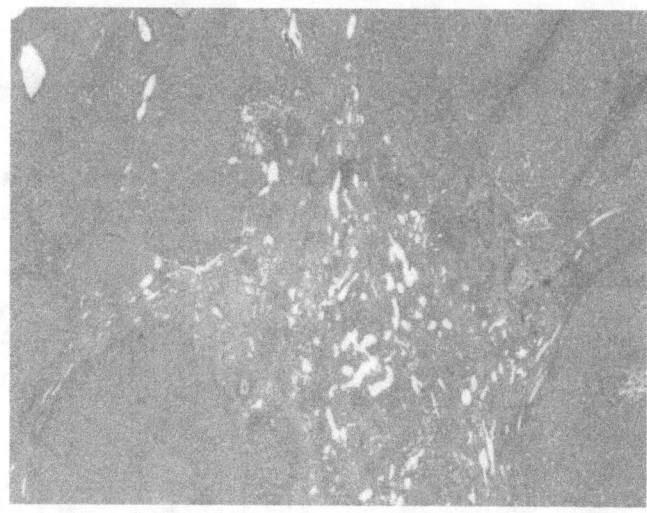

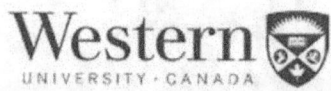

- ➢ Causes and associations
  - o Adenomas
  - o Cavernous hemangiomas (20%)
  - o HHT (hereditary hemorrhagic telangiectasia)
  - o Epithelial hemangioendothelioma
  - o Not caused by OCA (oral contraceptive agents), but may enlarge under the influence of OCA
  - o Vascular malformations may play a role in pathogenesis
  - o Associated with hepatic hemangiomas in 20%

- ➢ Clinical
  - o Patients are usually asymptomatic, but pain may result from bleeding or necrosis
  - o Symptomatic or complicated lesions should be resected or enucleated, but can also be treated with radiofrequency ablation

- ➢ Laboratory
  - o AFP is usually normal

- ➢ Diagnostic Imaging
  - o MRI may be useful for diagnosis as CT and US are not specific
  - o Contract–enhanced CT (triphasic)
    - – Hypodense
    - – Arterial phase
      - ▪ Enhanced
    - – Single lesion
    - – Subcapsular
    - – Enhancement of mass during arterial phase
    - – Fibrous septa
    - – Center
      - ▪ No enhancement
      - ▪ Central stellate scar
      - ▪ Hemorrhage and necrosis

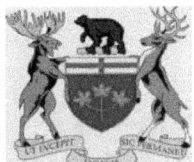

➢ Differential

- **Distinguish focal nodular hyperplasia** (FNH) from **hepatic adenoma** (HA).

Characteristics	FNH	Adenoma
Gender	Female	Female
Hormone therapy	-*	+++
Symptoms	Rare	Occasional
Multiple	About 30%	12 – 30%
Pathological associations	Hemangiomas	Glycogenoses androgens, peliosis
Central arterial scar	Yes Static	No; If stimulated (estrogens, OCA)
Treatment	Conservative	Resection if symptomatic
Malignant potential	-	+

*telangiectatic subtype of FNA is associated with estrogen use

- Give the diagnostic features and imaging modalities that will help distinguish hepatic hemangioma, focal nodular hyperplasia and adenoma.

	Hemangioma	Focal nodular hyperplasia	Adenoma
➢ Ultrasound	o Hyperechoic o Well-defined borders	– Variable appearance well defined borders	– Non diagnostic

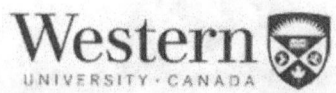

	Hemangioma	Focal nodular hyperplasia	Adenoma
➢ Triple phase CT	o Pre–contrast: hypodense o Centripital globular enhancement o Retained contrast in delayed images	– Pre–contrast: Hypo– or isodense – Homogenous arterial enhancement – Hypodense central scar – Isodense in delayed imaging	▪ Pre–contrast: Hypo– or isodense ▪ Irregular enhancement ▪ Delayed peripheral arterial enhancement during venous phase
➢ MRI	o T1: well circumscribed low signal o T2: Hyperintense signal	– T1: low signal – T2: Hyperintense signal with central scar	▪ T1: Low signal intensity with well defined capsule ▪ T2: Heterogenous enhancement
➢ Gadolinium– enhanced MRI	o Progressive enhancement o Delayed wash–out on venous phase	– Homogenous arterial enhancement – Hypodense central scar – Contrast accumulates in scar on delayed T1	▪ Irregular enhancement with delayed wash–out
➢ Radionuclide scan (tagged RBC)	o ↑ uptake during venous phase o Delayed emptying	– Equal or ↑ uptake compared to surrounding liver	▪ ↓ uptake compared to surrounding liver

Source: Shiffman, M.L. *2009. ACG Annual Postgraduate Course*: 167-71.

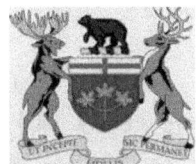

- **Differentiate** the clinical, laboratory and diagnostic imaging features of **FNH** and **FLHCC** (fibrolamellar hepatocellular cancer).

Features	FLHCC	FNH
o Associated with cirrhosis	-	-
o Normal hepatic synthetic function	+	-
o Treated by surgical resection	+	Depends
o Diagnostic imaging		
– Central scan	+	+
– Calcification	+	-
– ↓ intensity (dark, hypointense) on T2–images of MRI	+	-
– Progressive enlargement	+	-
o Histology		
– Large, granular cells	+	-
– Pale bodies	+	-
– Bands of fibrosis	+	-
– Bile duct proliferation	-	+
– Malformed blood vessels in central scan	-	+

➢ Treatment

- o No malignant potential for FNH
  - – No treatment needed

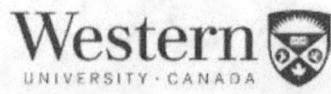

Focal Fatty Liver

➢ Diagnostic imaging

  o Abdominal ultrasound
    – Hyperechoic lesion
      ▪ CT
    – Hypodense lesion
      ▪ MRI
    – T1–weighted positive images
    – No distortion of surrounding architecture

Nodular Regenerative Hyperplasia (NRH)

➢ Definition

  o Regenerative nodules without fibrosis

➢ Pathology

  o Injury to the hepatic vasculature from the following:
    – Autoimmune disorders
    – Myeloproliferative syndromes
    – Antineoplastic medications → remodeling of the surrounding liver tissue into a nodule around portal triads containing liver tissues and no fibrosis

  o Nodular regenerative hyperplasia (NRH)
    – Characterized by nodularity without fibrosis
    – Associated with RA and Felty syndrome

  o Macronodular nodules may occur
    – In advanced cirrhosis
    – After massive hepatic necrosis

  o Inflammatory pseudotumor
    – Rare entity
    – Results from focal infection
    – Can be mistaken for hepatic tumor

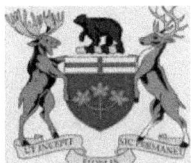

Nodular Regenerative Hyperplasia (NRH)

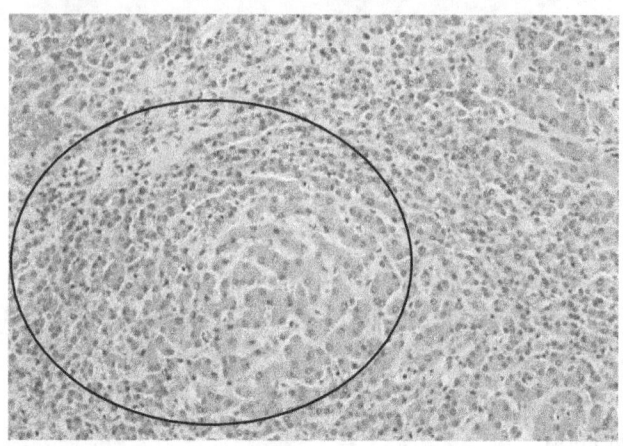

- ➢ Clinical
  - o Nodules of regenerative liver tissue
    - – Compress adjacent hepatic vasculature leading to non–cirrhotic portal hypertension
    - – Compress bile ducts leading to jaundice
  - o Associated conditions
    - – Hematological
      - ▪ Hypercoagulable states
      - ▪ Myelopreliferative disorders
      - ▪ Lymphoproliferative disorders
    - – Drugs
      - ▪ Azathioprine
      - ▪ Chemotherapeutic agents

- ➢ Diagnosis
  - o MRI is the best diagnostic imaging test to distinguish HCC from large cirrhotic nodule

Abbreviation: NRH, nodular regenerative hyperplasia

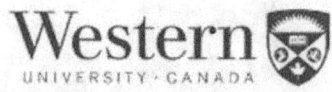

- ➤ Treatment
  - o Stop the offending drug
  - o Treat associated hematological disorders

Polycystic Liver Disease (PCLD)

- ➤ Definition
  - o PCLD alone, or PCLD plus ADPKD (autosomal dominant polycystic kidney disease), or PCLD plus cysts in the pancreas or spleen, arises from ductal plate malformation

- ➤ Demography
  - o Rare condition
  - o Usually presents in association with ADPKD
  - o Women tend to have larger and more numerous cysts

- ➤ Causes and associations
  - o May coexist with the following diseases:
    - – Other fibrocystic liver diseases
    - – Berry aneurysms
    - – MVP
    - – Diverticular disease
    - – Inguinal hernias

- ➤ Pathology
  - o Multiple liver cysts
  - o May transform to squamous cell carcinoma

- ➤ Clinical associations
  - o Cysts rarely cause morbidity

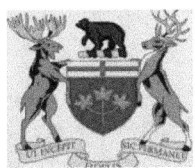

- o Symptomatic presentations
  - – Abdominal discomfort
  - – Distention
  - – Swelling
  - – Dyspnea
  - – Jaundice
- o Complications include the following:
  - – Bleeding
  - – Infection
  - – Rupture
  - – Torsion of cyst
- o CNS
  - – Berry aneurysms
- o CVS
  - – Mitral valve prolapse
- o Biliary tree
  - – Biliary microhamartomas
- o Liver
  - – Congenital hepatic fibrosis
- o Colon
  - – Colonic diverticulosis
- o Inguinal hernias

➤ Laboratory
- o Liver enzymes
  - – Usually normal
  - – ALP and GGT may be elevated

➤ Diagnostic imaging used
- o US, CT, and MRI can confirm diagnosis

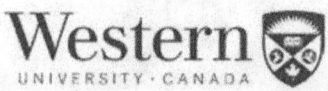

- o MRI
  - – T2–weighted image: bright fluid–filled cysts
- o Multiple complexes of cystically dilated intra– and interlobular bile ducts embedded in fibrous stroma
- o Occurence
  - – Almost all patients with congenital hepatic fibrosis
  - – Ccoexist with Caroli disease or ADPKD
- o Arise as a result of malformation of the ductal plate
- o May be complicated by the development of cholangiocarcinoma

➤ Treatment

- o If required, treatment includes:
  - – Fenestration
  - – Percutaneous injection of sclerosant

Biliary Microhamartomas (von Meyenburg Complexes)

➤ Definition

- o Malformation of ductal plate leading to "cystically dilated intra– and interlobular bile ducts embedded in a fibrous stroma" in or near the portal tracts

Source: Feldman, M., *et al. Sleisenger and Fordtran's Gastrointestinal and Liver Disease.* 9th Edition. *Saunders/Elsevier.* 2010, page 1590.

➤ Clinical

- o Associations
  - – Congenital hepatic fibrosis
  - – Caroli disease
  - – Autosomal dominant polycystic kidney disease (ADPKD) or PCLD, polycystic liver disease
- o May undergo malignant degeneration to cholangiocarcinoma

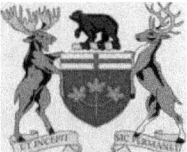

Caroli Disease

➢ Definition

- o Intrauterine malformation of the ductal plate

➢ Demography

- o Rare disorder
- o Characterized by congenital non–obstructive gross dilatation of the segmental intrahepatic bile ducts

➢ Pathogenesis

- o Affects men and women, equally
- o Intra–uterine malformation of the ductal plate
    - – Dilated ducts associated with the following:
        - ▪ Congenital hepatic fibrosis
        - ▪ Medullary sponge kidney
        - ▪ Choledochal cysts, type V
    - – Stones form in the dilated ducts
        - ▪ Cholangitis (~ 33%)
        - ▪ Cholangiocarcinoma (10%)

➢ Clinical

- o Associated with the following:
    - – Medullary sponge kidney
    - – Hepatic fibrosis
- o Patients may develop:
    - – Recurrent cholangitis
    - – Cholangiocarcinoma occurs in 10%

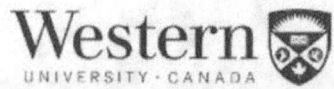

➢ Pathology
  o Dilated ducts associated with:
      – Congenital hepatic fibrosis
      – Medullary sponge kidney
      – Choledochal cysts, type V
  o Stones form in the dilated ducts
      – Cholangitis (~ 33%)
      – Cholangiocarcinoma (10%)

Please see: Di Bisceglie A.M. and Befeler A.S. *Sleisenger and Fordtran's Gastrointestinal and Liver Disease.* 9th Edition. *Saunders/Elsevier.* 10th Ed. 2016. Figure 96-10, page 1626 for Algorithms to use to Approach the Patient with Hepatic Mass Lesion without or with associated cirrhosis.

➢ Treatment
  o ERCP is used to remove stones
  o Liver transplantation may be required in diffused disease

Cystadenoma
  o Rare cystic tumor within the liver parenchyma is more common in females
  o Symptoms include:
      – Abdominal pain
      – Abdominal mass
      – Anorexia
  o US or CT will show complex cysts with loculation and septation
  o Histology is required to confirm the diagnosis

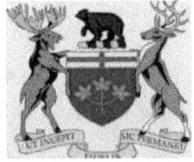

- o Treatment is resection of the cyst due to the risk of malignant transformation

Echinococcal Cyst

- o Caused by the larval form of *Echinococcus granulosus*
- o Fluid–filled structures limited by a parasite–derived membrane
- o Often asymptomatic
- o Treat the active hydatid liver disease with albendazole plus surgical resection

Liver Abscesses

- o Pyogenic
- o Amebic

➤ Pyogenic Liver Abscess
- o Clinical manifestations, include the following:
  - Fever
  - Abdominal pain
  - Nausea
  - Vomiting
  - Weight loss
  - Malaise
  - Anorexia
- o Diagnosis, confirmed by:
  - US or CT
  - Aspiration and culture of the abscess material
- o Pyogenic liver abscesses are polymicrobial

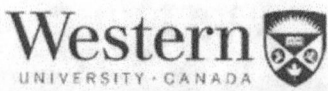

- o Treatment
    - – Antibiotic therapy
    - – Percutaneous or surgical drainage

➤ Amebic Liver Abscess

- o Results from ingestion of cysts of *Entamoeba histolytica*

- o Patients present with a 1 – 2 week history of:
    - – Fever
    - – RUQ pain
    - – Diarrhea

- o Diagnosis confirmation
    - – Imaging
    - – Serological
    - – Antigenic testing
    - – Stool testing

- o Needle aspiration is not usually required

- o Treatment

- o A tissue agent (flagyl)

- o A luminal agent (paromomycin)

"It's not your perfection that makes you an angel; it's your intention."

Alberto Agraso and Mony Dojeiji

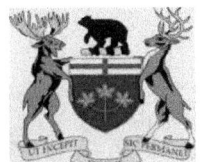

References and Suggested Reading

Abdalla, E.K. Overview of treatment approaches for hepatocellular carcinoma. *UpToDate.* www.uptodate.com 2014.

Cabrera, R., *et al.* The anti-viral effects of sorafenib in hepatitis C-related hepatocellular carcinoma. *Aliment Pharmacol Ther.* 2013; 37(1):91-97.

Curry, M.P. Hepatic adenoma. *UptoDate.* www.uptodate.com 2014.

Schwartz, J.M. Approach to the patient with a focal liver lesion. *UpToDate Online Journal.* www.uptodate.com 2014.

Schwartz, J.M. Clinical features, diagnosis, and screening for primary hepatocellular carcinoma. *UpToDate.* www.uptodate.com 2014.

Schwartz, J.M. Epidemiology and etiologic associations of hepatocellular carcinoma. *UpToDate.* www.uptodate.com 2014.

White, D.L., *et al.* Association between nonalcoholic fatty liver disease and risk for hepatocellular cancer, based on systematic review. *Clin Gastroenterol Hepatol.* 2012; 10(12):1342-1359.

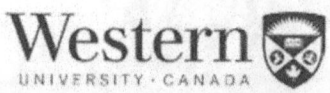

More on Liver Tumors

Yaqoub Alawadh

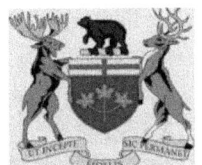

Focal Nodular Hyperplasia (FNH)

➢ Demography

  ○ Most common non–malignant hepatic tumor that is not to have a vascular origin

  ○ Found predominantly in women (in a ratio of 9:1) between the ages of 20 and 50 years

  ○ Most often solitary (80 – 95%)

  ○ Usually less than 5 cm in diameter

➢ Clinical

  ○ Symptoms or signs directly attributable to FNH are infrequent
    - Abdominal discomfort
    - Palpable liver mass

➢ Laboratory

  ○ Normal or minor elevations in aspartate and alanine aminotransferase, alkaline phosphatase and gamma glutamyl transpeptidase

➢ Diagnostic imaging

  ○ Ultrasound
    - Central scar (in 20%) of cases
    - Characterstics of the mass
      ▪ Difficult to distinguish from an adenoma or malignant lesions

  ○ CT with contrast
    - Hyperdense
      ▪ Hepatic arterial phase due to arterial origin of blood supply
    - Isodense
      ▪ Portal venous phase
      ▪ Central scar become hyperdense as the contrast diffuses into the scar

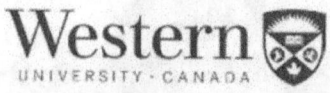

Focal Nodular Hyperplasia (FNH)

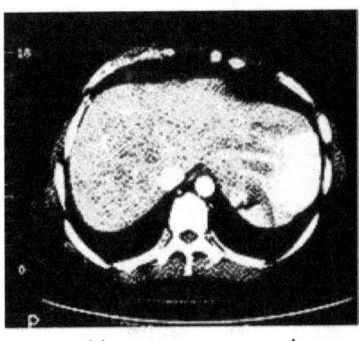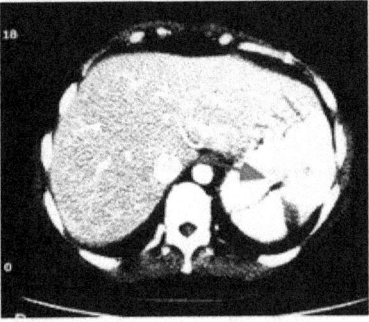

- o Homogenous enhancement seen early in the arterial phase
- o The central scar is seen will not enhance
- o Technetium sulfur colloid scanning —
  - – FNH usually contains Kupffer cells
  - – 80% of lesions show ↑ uptake of technetium sulfur colloid on nuclear medicine scanning
  - – Hepatic adenomas and hepatocellular carcinomas generally show no uptake due to the lack of Kupffer cells

Technetium Sulfur Colloid Scanning

- o Uniform uptake
  - – Indicates focal nodular hyperplasia of the mass that has Kupffer cells

Focal Nodular Hyperplasia (FNH)

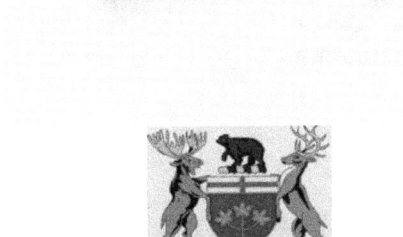

➤ Treatment

   o If FNH is stable and with no complications
- Manage conservatively
- No need for follow–up

Primary Hepatic Lymphoma (PHL)

➤ Definition

   o Primary hepatic lymphoma (PHL) is a lymphoma confined to the liver with no evidence of lymphomatous involvement of the spleen, lymph nodes, bone marrow or other lymphoid structures

➤ Demography

   o Very rare malignancy
- Constitutes about:
  - 0.016% of all cases of non–Hodgkin's lymphoma
  - 0.4% of cases of extranodal NHL

   o Commonly presents at 55 years of age

   o Male to female ratio is 2.3:1

➤ Pathology

   o Majority of cases are diffuse large B–cell lymphoma

   o Other histologies include:
- Diffuse mixed small and large B–cells
- Lymphoblastic
- Diffuse immunoblastic
- Diffuse histiocytic
- Mantle cell
- Small non–cleaved
- Burkitts lymphoma

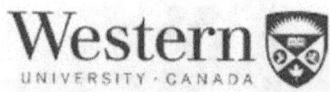

- o Very rare
  - Mucosa–associated lymphoid tissue (MALT) and unclassified small B–cell lymphomas
- o PHL is a pathologic diagnosis
- o Liver biopsy is the most valuable tool for the diagnosis of PHL

➢ Clinical associations

- o ↑ HCV and possibly, HBV
- o In immunocompromised patients
  - EBV
    - Regulatory T–cell function is deficient leading to unchecked B–cell proliferation and possibly, lymphoma
    - Loss of T–cell surveillance and uninhibited B–cell proliferation

➢ Presentation

- o Abdominal pain (70%)
- o "B" symptoms (37%)
- o Anorexia, malaise, nausea, and vomiting (16%)
- o Fatigue
- o Jaundice
- o Heptomegaly
- o Small patients are asymptomatic and are diagnosed incidentally

➢ Laboratory

- o ↑ AP / ↑ ALT (~ 80%)
- o ↑ β2–macroglobulin (~ 90%)
- o Normal α–FP, CEA

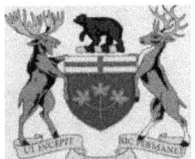

➢ Diagnostic imaging
  ○ Ultrasound
    – Solitary or multiple masses (~ 60%)
      ▪ Especially when α–FP and CEA are normal
  ○ Diffuse hepatic infiltration is uncommon
    – Suggests a worse prognosis
  ○ Lesion is hypoechoic to the surrounding normal liver parenchyma
  ○ CT with contrast
    – Hypo–attenuating lesion(s)
  ○ 50% of PHL lesions do not enhance
  ○ 33% show patchy enhancement
  ○ 16% show a ring of enhancement

Primary Hepatic Lymphoma

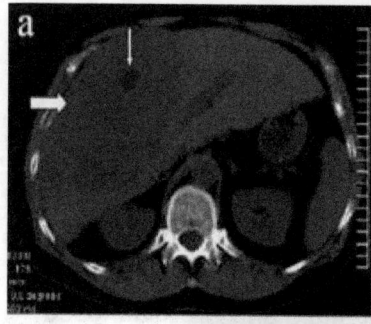
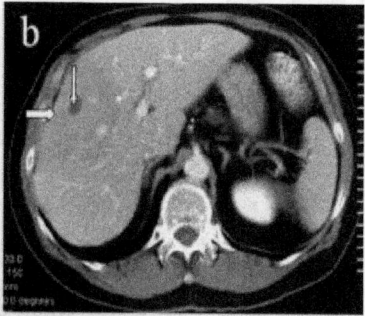
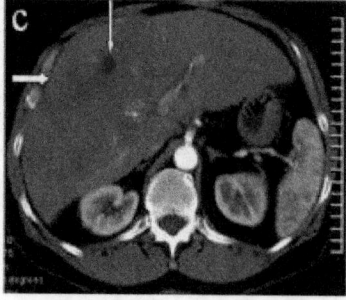

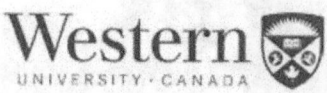

(a) Non–contrast–enhanced CT of the abdomen shows a large geographic hypodense mass in the right lobe of the liver extending to the medial aspect of the left lobe (broad white arrow) with a small central area of lower attenuation (narrow white arrow)

(b) Contrast–enhanced CT scan of the abdomen (early arterial phase) demonstrates hypovascular mass

(c) Contrast–enhanced CT scan of the abdomen in the portal–venous phase shows minimal enhancement of the mass without distortion of the liver anatomy and without portal vein thrombosis

➢ Liver biopsy

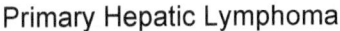
Primary Hepatic Lymphoma

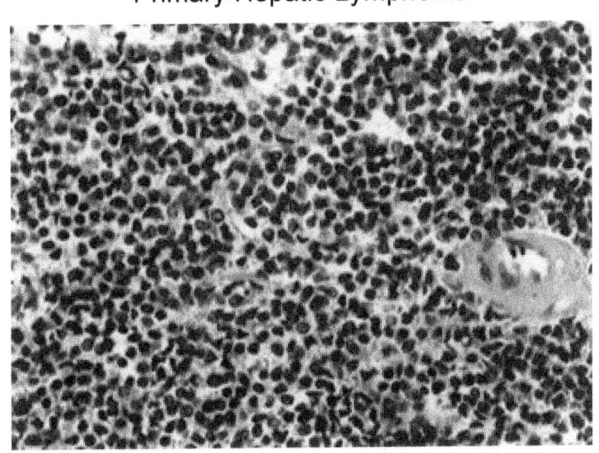

o Monotonous sheets of small lymphocytes replacing normal hepatic parenchyma

o The lymphocytes have the following:
  – Scanty cytoplasm
    ▪ Clumped chromatin pattern
    ▪ Round nuclei

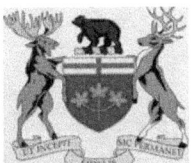

➢ Treatment
- o Options:
  - – Surgery
  - – Chemotherapy
  - – Radiation
- o Chemotherapy
  - – In localized disease
    - ▪ Surgery followed by adjuvant chemotherapy (to prevent disease recurrence)
  - – Unresectable disease
    - ▪ Anthracycline–based combination chemotherapy and surgical resection after completion of chemotherapy

MALT Lymphoma

➢ Definition

- o MALT lymphomas are low grade B–cell lymphoma with indolent behavior

- o Related to chronic immune reactions driven by bacterial, viral or autoimmune stimuli (i.e. *H. pylori* and MALT lymphoma in stomach)

- o Primary hepatic MALT lymphoma cases have significantly better prognosis than primary hepatic DLBCL cases ($p < 0.05$)

- o Has been described in patients with PBC

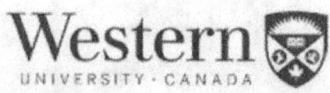

Approach to Liver Lesions

Mansour Alghanem

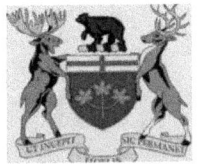

Introduction

- ○ The increased use of diagnostic imaging has led to enhance the discovery of incidental liver masses
- ○ The differential diagnosis for hepatic lesions is extremely wide
- ○ An approach incorporating the clinical picture, laboratory testing and imaging characteristics lead to correct diagnosis in most cases and avoidance of invasive procedures

Cystic Lesions

- • Simple Cysts:
- ➢ Demography
    - ○ Prevalence of 2 – 7%
    - ○ F:M is up to 6:1

- ➢ Pathology
    - ○ Serous contents
    - ○ Lined by cuboidal, biliary–type epithelium
    - ○ No communication with the bile ducts

- ➢ Clinical
    - ○ < 5 cm
        - – Usually asymptomatic
    - ○ ≥ 5 cm
        - – Mass–effect symptoms

- ➢ Diagnostic imaging
    - ○ Ultrasonography
        - – Anechoic mass
        - – With well–defined thin walls
        - – Strong posterior wall echoes

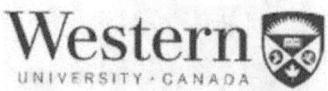

- o CT of the abdomen is non–enhancing well–demarcated lesions isodense to water
- o MRI of the abdomen
  - – Hypointense T1
  - – Hyperintense T2

> Treatment
  - o Usually no need for further intervention or follow–up, unless have the following characteristics:
    - – 4 cm
    - – Follow–up U/S every 6 – 12 months for 3 years
    - – Symptomatic
      - ▪ FNA + sclerosing
      - ▪ Surgical De–roofing

Cystadenoma and Cystadenocarcinoma

> Demography
  - o Rare
  - o Usually elderly
  - o W > M

> Pathology
  - o Size of cystadenomas range from 2 – 28 cm
  - o 75% in the hepatic parenchyma of the right lobe
  - o Multilocular lesions comprising 3 layers of tissue:
    - – Inner epithelium lining containing mucous–secreting cuboidal cells
    - – Middle mesenchymal cells
    - – Outer cells are composed of collagen
  - o Features of malignant transformation
    - – Thick wall showing large tissue masses protruding from the internal cyst lining

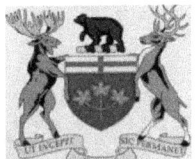

> Clinical

  o Usually asymptomatic

  o Present with abdominal pain and anorexia

> Diagnostic imaging

  o Ultrasonography
    - Anechoic masses
    - Internal septations and irregular walls
    - Hemorrhagic areas within the lesions present as hyperechoic regions

  o CT abdomen
    - Septated cysts
    - Areas of enhancement +/- calcifications

> Treatment

  o Complete surgical resection is recommended for **both** cystadenomas and cystadenocarcinoma

Pyogenic Hepatic abcess:

> Clinical

  o Presentation depends on mode of transmission:
    - Hematogenous spread
    - Biliary obstruction or instrumentation
    - Intra–abdominal sepsis, i.e. diverticulitis
    - Cryptogenic

> Diagnostic imaging

  o U/S of the abdomen
    - Hyperechoic lesion
    - Distinct margins

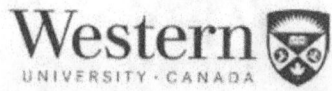

- o CT of the abdomen with contrast
  - – Peripheral enhancement of the abscess wall is virtually diagnostic
  - – Likely cause of abscess in 70%
  - – Cryptogenic abcess
  - – Usually single
  - – Right lobe seen in 70%
  - – Seeding abcess usually measures (microabcess) < 2cm
    - 2 distinct pictures
    - Diffuse miliary (*S. aureus*)
    - Cluster (Coliforms)
- o MRCP
  - – Helpful in delineating biliary tract
  - – Non–superior to CT of the abdomen

➤ Treatment

- o IV antibiotics, as appropriate from microbiological culture
- o Percutaneous drainage

Hydatid cysts

➤ Microbiology

- o *Echinococcus granulosus* or *E. multilocularis*
- o Zoonotic infections with dogs bring to definitive host and humans are intermediate hosts

➤ Clinical

- o Asymptomatic
- o RUQ pain due to mass effect

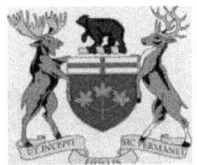

- o Rupture associated with the following:
  - – Biliary colic
  - – Obstructive jaundice
  - – Pancreatitis
  - – Cholangitis

- o Interperitoneal leakage
  - – Peritonitis

- o Systemic leakage
  - – Anaphylactic reaction

➢ Laboratory

- o Serology by ELISA
  - – Positive in 70%
  - – May remain positive for years after surgical removal

➢ Diagnostic imaging

- o U/S of the abdomen shows
  - – Infoldings of the inner cyst wall
  - – Separation of the hydatid membrane from the wall of the cyst
  - – Hydatid sand

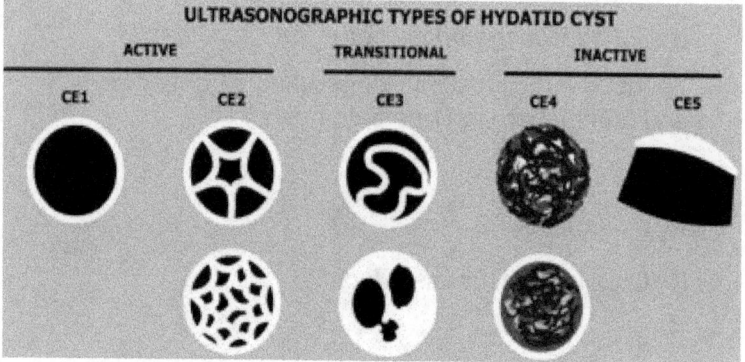

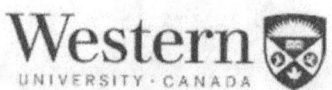

> Treatment
>   o Depends on the size and stage, as shown by one or combination of these diagnostic imaging modalities:
>   – Medical: albendazole
>   – PAIR (Puncture, Aspiration, Installation of scolicidal agent and Reaspiration)
>   – Surgery
>   – Observation

WHO Classification of cystic echinococcus (CE) and treatment stratified by cyst stage

WHO stage	Description	Stage	Size	Preferred treatment	Alternate treatment
CE1	Unilocular unechoic cystic lesion with double line sign	Active	<5 cm	Albendazole alone	PAIR
			>5 cm	Albendazole + PAIR	PAIR
CE2	Multiseptated, "rosette-like" "honeycomb" cyst	Active	Any	Albendazole + either modified catheterization or surgery	Modified catheterization
CE3a	Cyst with detached membranes (water-lily-sign)	Transitional	<5 cm	Albendazole alone	PAIR
			>5 cm	Albendazole + PAIR	PAIR

Amebic Liver Abscess

> Microbiology
>   o Ingestion of *Entamoeba histolytica* cysts
>   o Cysts invade the colonic mucosa
>   o Migrate though the mesenteric venules to the liver

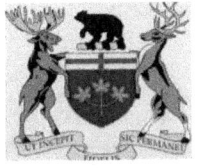

➢ Clinical

    o Recent travel to endemic areas (tropical areas) within the last 8 – 20 weeks

    o Abrupt onset of fever and RUQ pain

    o Preceded by or associated with dysentery

➢ Diagnostic imaging

    o Ultrasound or CT

    o Low density mass with peripherally enhancing ring

    o Serology plus U/S
        – Sensitivity and specificity is > 95%

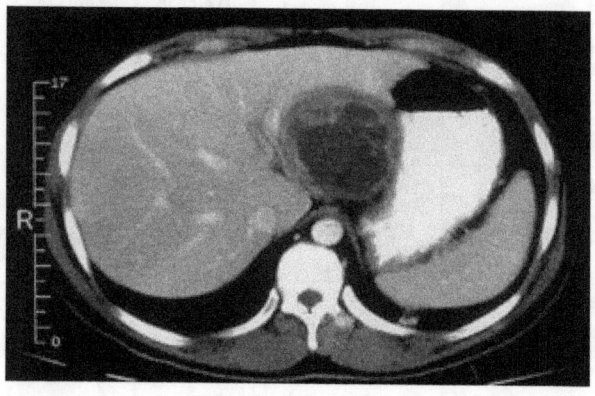

➢ Laboratory

    o Serologic testing (ELISA) specificity and sensitivity > 95% combined with imaging studies

➢ Treatment

    o Uncomplicated
        – Metronidazole 500 – 750 mg *tid po* for 7 – 10 days

    o Complicated

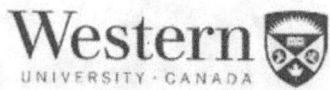

Liver Physiology and Metabolism

David Yik

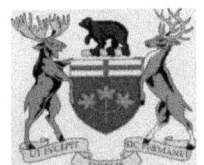

➢ Outline

  o Liver cell types and organization

  o Integration of the functions of the different cell types

  o Regeneration and apoptosis of liver cells

  o Protein synthesis and degradation in the liver

  o Hepatic nutrient metabolism

➢ Anatomy

  o Parenchymal cells
    - Hepatocytes
    - Cholangiocytes (bile duct epithelial cells)

  o Sinusoidal nonparenchymal cells
    - Hepatic sinusoidal endothelial cells
    - Kupffer cells

  o Perisinusoidal non–parenchymal cells
    - Hepatic stellate cells
    - Pit cells

Hepatocytes

  o Large polyhedral cells, ~ 20 – 30 micrometers diameter

  o Composed organelles for synthetic and metabolic activities

  o 30% are binucleate

  o Polarized epithelial cells

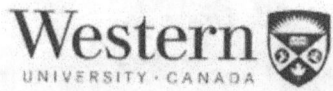

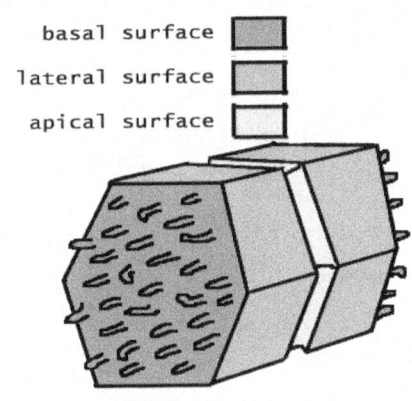

- basal surface
- lateral surface
- apical surface

- o 3 domains:
  - – Sinusoidal surface (basolateral)
  - – Canalicular surface (apical)
  - – Contiguous surface (lateral)

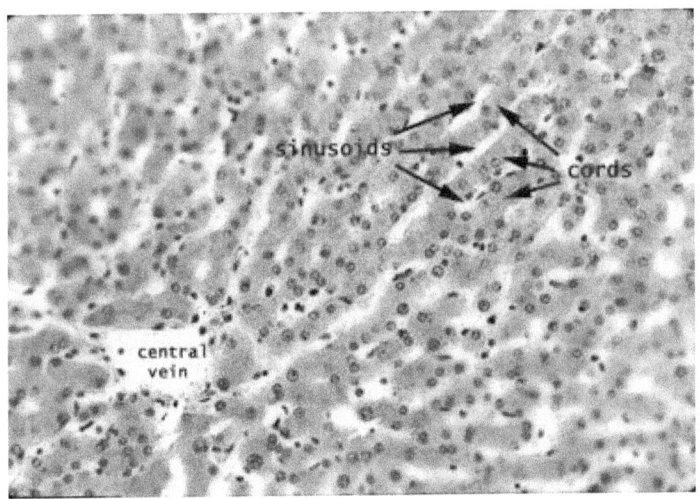

sinusoids

cords

central vein

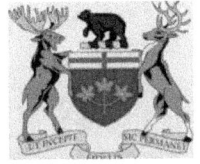

Space of Disse

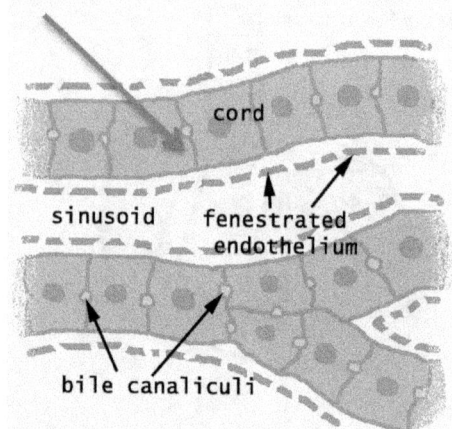

Junctions in plasma membrane

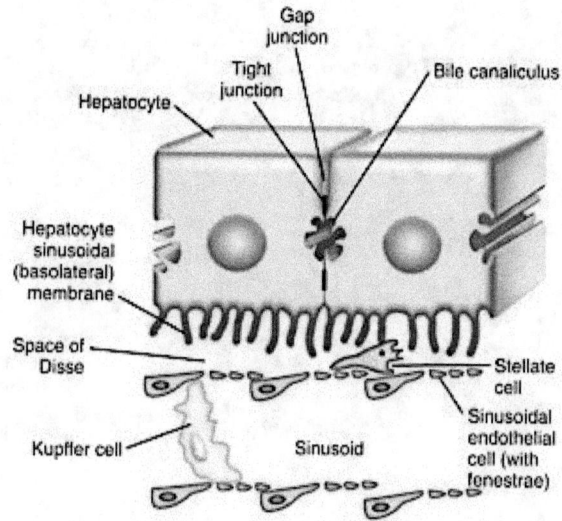

Source: Roy-Chowdawry, N. and Roy-Chowdawry, J. *Sleisenger and Fordtran's Gastrointestinal and Liver Disease*. 10th Edition. 2016. Figure 72-1, page 1224.

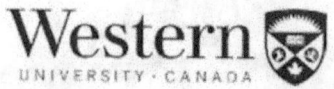

- o Tight junctions (desmosomes)
    - – Seals bile canaliculi, permits concentration difference of solutes between cytoplasm and bile canaliculus
- o Gap junctions
    - – Subdomains of contiguous domains
    - – Composed of bundles of particles that form symmetrical cylinder that opens or closes the central channel
    - – Allows communications between cells (nutrient exchange, electrical conduction, etc.)

- ➢ Cytoskeleton
    - o Supports organization of organelles, cell polarity, intracellular movement of vesicles and molecular transport
    - o Intermediate filaments – polymers of fibrous polypeptides, provide mechanical support to cells
    - o Microtubules – hollow tubular structures serves and tracks for the movement of vesicles mediated by ATPase–powered motor proteins
    - o Microfilaments – composed of actin strands function to maintain cell matrix integrity, facilitate bile canalicular contraction, control tight junction permeability and involved in endocytosis and transport
    - o Collapse of hepatocytes during apoptosis is related to remodeling of the actin cytoskeleton

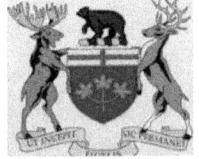

- ➢ Nucleus and Endoplasmic reticulum (ER)
  - o Outer nuclear membrane is continuous with the endoplasmic reticulum membrane
  - o Perinuclear space between 2 nuclear membranes surrounds the nucleus and is continuous with the ER lumen
  - o Endoplasmic reticulum
    - Comprises membranous tubules and flattened sacs (cisternae) enclosing a space that extends throughout the cytoplasm
  - o Rough ER
    - Site of active protein synthesis
  - o Smooth ER
    - No ribosomes
    - Site of lipid biosynthesis, detoxification and Ca regulation

- ➢ Golgi Complex
  - o Many proteins synthesized in the rough ER are transported to the Golgi apparatus in transition vesicles
  - o Golgi complex = stack of cisternae
    - Modifies (glycosylation and phosphorylation), sorts and packages proteins for cell secretion
    - Produces lysosomes
  - o Lysosomes are organelles that contain hydrolytic enzymes
    - Fuse with vacuoles, dispense enzymes, digest vacuole contents in the *cis vs trans* face

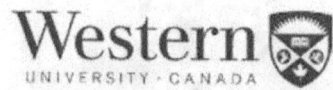

➢ Mitochondria

  o Constitute 20% of cytoplasmic volume

  o Site of cellular respiration

  o Contain enzymes of:
    - Tricarboxylic acid cycle (Krebs)
    - Fatty acid oxidation
    - Oxidative phosphorylation

  o Part of the urea cycle, gluconeogenesis, fatty acid synthesis and heme synthesis

  o Key role in apoptosis

  o Glycolysis + Krebs cycle + oxidative phosphorylation produce 30 ATP molecules per complete breakdown of one glucose molecule

➢ Endocytosis

  o Definitions
    - Pinocytosis: non–selective bulk–phase uptake of extracellular fluid via the engulfment of plasma membrane invagination
    - Phagocytosis: non–specific ingestion of particles, as well as, regions of the cell surface
    - Receptor–mediated endocytosis: uptake of specific molecules and ligands

Cholangiocytes (bile duct epithelial cells)

  o Large and small subpopulations of cells

  o Active role in secretion and absorption of biliary components

  o Regulation of extracellular matrix composition

  o Highly polarized to facilitate excretion and absorption

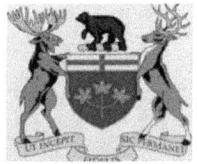

- Na–dependent bile salt transporter (ABAT) on the apical and luminal surface – uptake of conjugated bile acids

- Truncated or spliced ABAT (ASBT) on the basolateral surface – efflux of bile acids in a Na–independent process

- Glucose reabsorption from bile via SGLT1 (Na–dependent) and GLUT1

- Aquaporin–1 at the apical and basolateral surfaces – water excretion into the bile

- Large (not the small) cholangiocytes express secretin + somatostatin receptors, chloride and bicarbonate exchangers, CFTRs – this population may modulate water and electrolyte secretion in response to secretin and somatostatin

Hepatic Sinusoidal Endothelial Cells (HSECs)

- Comprise 20% of total liver cells

- Flat thin extensions that form sieve plates containing *fenestrae*

- Unlike capillary endothelial cells, do not form intracellular junctions

- No junctions, no basement membrane, fenestrae → plasma flows freely into the space of Disse

- Diameters of the fenestrae actively controlled by actin–containing cytoskeleton → *selective barrier depending on hormonal milieu*

- HSECs secrete prostaglandins, IL–1, IL–6, interferon, TNF–α, endothelin

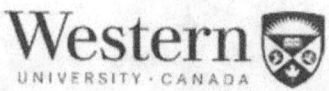

Kupffer Cells

- Specialized tissue macrophages; account for 80-90% of total fixed macrophages in body

- Derived from BM stem cells or monocytes to remove substances from the portal blood

- Features: bristle–coated micropinocytic vesicles, fuzzy–coated vacuoles, lots of lysosomes

- Secrete vasoactive toxic mediators

- Increase in number and activity in response to liver injury

Hepatic Stellate Cells (HSCs; aka, Ito cells)

- 5 – 8% of all liver cells between endothelial lining and hepatocytes

- Sources of paracrine, autocrine, juxtacrine and chemo–attractant factors that maintain homeostasis in the hepatic sinusoid

- Quiescent HSCs have flat cytoplasmic extensions enriched in microfilaments and microtubules, which spread out parallel to the endothelial lining to contact several cells

- After chronic liver injury, HSCs become activated

- *HSC activation is the central event in hepatic fibrosis*

- HSCs transform from slender star–shaped structures to elongated myofibroblasts

- Activation is initiated by paracrine stimulation by HSCs, Kupffer cells, hepatocytes, platelets and leukocytes

- HSCs: produce cellular fibronectin, activates TGF–β

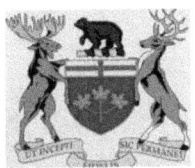

- o Extracellular matrix modulates shape, proliferation, and function of activated HSCs via binding to cell surface *integrins* and changes in cytoskeleton assembly
- o Activation of HSCs perpetuates through behavior change of HSCs: *proliferation*, contractility, over-expression of matrix proteins, release of matrix degradation proteins + cytokines

Pit Cells

- o Natural killer (NK) cells of the liver is located mostly within the sinusoidal lumen, close to Kupffer cells
- o Similar in appearance to large lymphocytes
- o Adherent to the sinusoidal wall that is often anchored with villous extensions
- o Abundant cytoplasm with dense granules, locomotory shape characterized by a uropod (tail–like structure on trailing end)
- o Short–lived, replenished from extrahepatic structures
- o Have tumor–cell killing activity in the liver and thought to remove virus–infected liver cells
- o Possible roles in controlling growth and differentiation of liver cells and liver–graft rejection

Functional Integration of Diverse Liver Cells

- o Occurs through:
  - – Direct cell–cell communication (i.e. via gap junctions)
  - – Paracrine secretion affecting the neighboring cells
  - – Cell signaling
  - – Interaction with extracellular matrix (i.e. HSC activation)

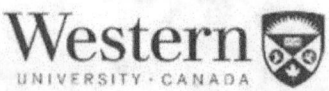

- Integrins: cell surface receptors bind to matrix proteins at specialized attachment sites → changes in cell shape, spreading, migration
- Integrins affect cell proliferation, differentiation, survival, apoptosis and gene expression
- Generalized response to endocrine and metabolic fluxes

Liver Regeneration

o Normal hepatocytes divide infrequently

o But liver has the unique capacity to replace tissue mass after injury or loss of liver mass

o "Restorative hyperplasia" is more accurate since the total liver mass rather than lobulated anatomic configuration is reconstituted

o In rat models
  - Resection of 2/3 liver → proliferation of residual cells and restoration of liver mass in days to weeks
  - 80 – 95% of hepatocytes undergo mitosis
  - Adult hepatocytes (rather than liver progenitor cells) contribute to the regeneration unless inhibited secondary toxic and physical injury

o Liver progenitor cells are thought to give rise to hepatocytes and cholangiocytes

o Liver cells return to quiescent state once liver mass is restored to itsoriginal size (within ~ 10%)

o A balance between mitosis and apoptosis fine–tunes the restoration of hepatic mass

o Strictly self–limited hepatocyte replication suggests the presence of strong regulatory pressures that favor replicative repression

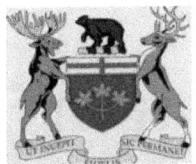

- o Signaling for cessation of replication is less well–understood
- o Immediate early genes
- o Delayed early genes
- o Cell cycle genes

➢ Immediate early genes

- o More than 70 immediate early genes are already identified

- o Activated almost immediately after partial hepatectomy, often without the need for protein synthesis

- o Including proto–oncogenes, i.e. c-*fos*, c-*myc*, and transcription factors

- o In quiescent hepatocytes, nuclear trans–activating factor kappa B (NFκB) remains in the cytosol and inactivated by binding to an inhibitor (IκB)

- o Binding of TNF to the cell surface receptor initiates a signalling cascade → phosphorylation of IκB, releases NFκB that translocates to the nucleus → transcription activation of more than a dozen of genes also involved in the immediate early response, including IL–6

- o *IL–6 is thought to play an important role in regeneration; strong inducer of STAT3 (signal transducer and activator of transcription)*

➢ Delayed early genes

- o Transcribed after the immediate early gene response but before the cell cycle genes reach the maximum level of expression (i.e. G0 → G1 phase)

- o Dependent on protein synthesis

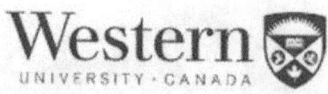

- o Includes anti–apoptotic gene, *bcl-x*
- o Proapoptotic genes (*BAK, BAD, BAX*) are down-regulated initially after partial hepatectomy

➢ Cell cycle genes

- o After priming, progression from G1 through S and M phases, cyclins and cyclin–dependent kinases (cdks) are expressed
- o HGF and TGF–β are crucial until the peak level of cyclin D1 is reached, then cells progress autonomously through cell cycle without the need of futher growth factors

Apoptosis: Programmed Cell Death

- o Provides balance to the fine–tuning and remodeling process in hepatic architecture reconstruction
- o Pathway in removal of damaged, senescent, supernumerary cells without altering the cellular microenvironment (*vs* gross necrosis, for example)
- o *Loss of apoptotic pathways → survival of DNA–damaged cells → several forms of cancer*

➢ Apoptotic signals originate from:

- o Within cells through mechanisms that sense DNA damage or inappropriate proliferative signals
- o Other cells
  - – Immune–mediated cells give apoptotic signals to cells recognized as foreign or pathogenic
  - – Nurturing signals from neighboring cells or matrix is lost, triggering apoptosis
  - – Apoptosis may be triggered by certain growth factors (TGF–β1)

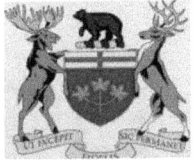

➤ Phases of apoptosis

- o Latent phase
  - – Cell undergoes molecular and biochemical changes and remains morphologically intact

- o Execution phase
  - – Cell death carried out by the activation of specific proteases called caspases, cleave multiple substrates → DNA fragmentation, chromatin condensation, cell shrinkage, membrane blebbing
  - – Cell is phagocytosed or just loses contact with neighboring cells
  - – *No inflammatory reaction* (compare to cell necrosis)

- o Mechanisms of execution
  - – Cell surface death receptors: includes Fas (TNF receptor) – binding of Fas to Fas ligand leads to a cascade–activating caspases
  - – Mitochondrial permeabiilty transition: Various toxic insults cause mitochondria to open its channels and release proteins, i.e. cytochrome C
  - – Cytochrome C triggers events leading to caspase activation; permeabilization also leads to loss of electron transport chain resulting to loss of function (i.e. ATP generation)

Hepatic Protein Synthesis

- o Compared to other organs, liver expresses many genes

- o > 90% of plasma proteins, 15% of total protein mass of body are produced in the liver

- o Gene expression is regulated at multiple levels:
  - – State of chromatin – determines accessibility of specific genes to the transcription machinery and binding of specific transcription factors

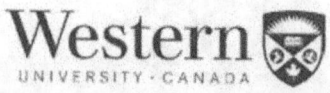

- – Post–transcriptional regulation – differential splicing, protein folding, phosphorylation or other modification
- – Modulation of protein degradation and RNA stability
- o Up–regulation or repression of expression of a particular set of genes are often mediated by nuclear receptors:
    - – Phenobarbital binds to constitutive androstane receptor (CAR) → CAR translocates to the nucleus inducing multiple genes
    - – Bile acids bind to FXR, fibrates to PPAR, thyroid hormones to TR

➤ Hepatic protein folding dependent on chaperones

- o Proteins are translocated to the ER for folding, then to the Golgi

- o ER contains molecular chaperones to promote efficient folding
    - – Different chaperones, different specific functions
    - – "Quality control" via complex series of glycosylation and deglycosylation, prevention of misfolded proteins from being secreted
    - – Misfolded proteins are targeted for degradation through the ubiquitin–proteosome pathway
    - – 50% of polypeptide chains fail the quality control
    - – Percentage failure rises in mutant proteins with AA substitutions
    - – Some chaperones rescue misfolded proteins

➤ Pathways for *protein catabolism*

- o Autophagic–lysosomal pathway
    - – Handles bulk degradation of endogenous proteins and other cellular components (RNA, carbohydrates, lipids)

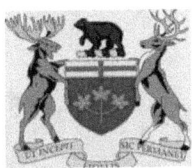

- Regulated by plasma levels of amino acids via binding to cell surface receptors → intracellular signalling

o Ubiquitin–proteosome pathway
  - Principal mechanism is for turnover of normally short–lived proteins
  - Ubiquitin is a small protein covalently links to itself or other proteins
  - Ubiquitin binds to misfolded proteins → directs proteasome–dependent proteolysis
  - Ubiquitin also participates in the following:
    - Protein translocation
    - Cell cycle regulation
    - Directs proteins through endocytotic pathway, including cyclins

Hepatic Nutrient Metabolism

o Hepatic metabolic function regulated by hormones secreted by the pancreas, adrenal gland, thyroid, and neuronal inputs

o Fed (nutrient absorption) state – absorbed nutrients are metabolized, modified for storage in the liver and fatty tissue, or made available to other organs for energy sources

o Fasting (non–absorptive) state – energy supply maintained from the stored fuel and through the synthesis of energy sources
  - Carbohydrate metabolism
  - Lipid metabolism

Carbohydrate Metabolism

o Glucose is the primary energy source of the brain, blood cells, muscle, renal cortex

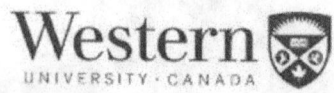

o   After 24 – 48 hours of fasting, brain uses ketones as metabolic fuel, reducing its glucose requirement by 50 – 70%

o   Liver is the principal organ that maintains carbohydrate stores by synthesizing glycogen and generating glucose from precursors

o   Glucose is synthesized from non–oxidative metabolic products of glucose (pyruvate, lactate) that are generated mainly by RBCs; and from amino acid precursors are derived from muscles during starvation and exercise

Glucose Uptake into Hepatocytes

➢   GLUT2 (glucose transpoter–2)

o   Glucose enters into the hepatocytes via glucose transporter–2
   -   Facilitates diffusion across sinusoidal membrane
   -   Functions independently of metabolic conditions, like insulin level
   -   Low affinity, high capacity characteristics of Glut2 means intrahepatic glucose level is determined by plasma glucose level

➢   GLUT1 (glucose transporter–1)
o   High affinity, low capacity
o   Permits glucose uptake by hepatocytes when the circulating plasma glucose level is low
o   During fasting, there is increased expression of Glut1
o   Through various pathways, glucose is converted to amino acids, fatty acids or glycogen

Hepatocyte Metabolism

o   Many possible endpoints and complex pathways are regulated by multiple signals to prevent competing pathways from operating at the same time

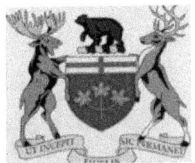

- o 3 major independent metabolic pathways from glucose–6–phosphate (G6P)
  - Glycogen synthesis
  - Anaerobic glycolysis
  - Pentose phosphate shunt

- o Anaerobic glycolysis via Embden–Meyerhof pathway
  - Generates pyruvate or lactate as the substrate for the Krebs cycle

- o Pentose phosphate shunt
  - Generates reducing equivalents necessary for anaerobic glycolysis and fatty acid synthesis
  - Glucose kinase (GK) converts glucose to G6P
  - GK is not inhibited by the reaction product G6P
  - GK activity levels therefore, regulates intrahepatocellular glucose that determines the net uptake of glucose by hepatocytes from the sinusoidal plasma
  - GK is activated by insulin and inhibited by glucagon

- o G6P forms fructose 6–phosphate and fructose–1, 6–diphosphate

- o Starvation decreases GK activity → glucose efflux

- o Mutations in GK gene is associated with some cases of MODY

- o Gl6P is a multi–subunit enzyme, whose active site is located within the ER lumen

- o Inherited deficiency of G6P causes glycogen storage disease, type Ia

- o G6P transport across the ER lumen is mediated by microsomal transport protein → defects in protein → glycogen storage disease, type Ib

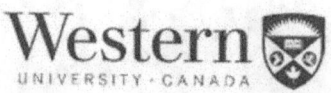

- 6–Fructokinase/Pase produces the regulatory product fructose–2,6–P2
  - Potently activates 6 PF–1–K
  - Potently inhibits fruct–1, 6–P2ase

- During starvation, fructose–2,6–P2 are low and gluconeogenesis is enhanced

- High levels of fructose–2,6–P2 are found during refeeding and insulin administration, promoting glycolysis and fatty acid synthesis

- 4 reactions lead to the formation of PEP with the generation of 8 molecules of ATP

- PK generates another 2 molecules of ATP

- PYR undergo further metabolism in the mitochondria to form acetyl CoA → feeds into the Krebs cycle for aerobic metabolism, ultimately metabolized to water and CO_2

- 15 molecules of ATP are produced per molecule of PYR

- Other PYR pathways lead to precursors of fatty acids (citrate from Krebs) or amino acids, by means of oxaloacetate formation

- PEPCK (phosphoenol pyruvate carboxykinase) converts OAA to the amino acid L–aspartate; inhibited by insulin, up–regulated during fasting

- Other carbohydrates participate in the glycolytic pathway, including galactose and fructose

- Fructose is an abundant sugar in the diet and can be used for gluconeogenesis with glycogen synthesis vs glycolysis

- Fructose provides the glycerol backbone for triacylglycerol and phospholipids

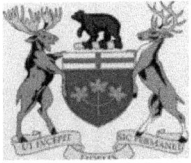

Glycogen Formation and Metabolism

- o Glycogen stored in the liver is the main source of rapidly available glucose for glucose–dependent tissues (RBCs, retina, renal medulla, brain)
- o Hepatic glycogen stores good for 2–day supply of glucose
- o After 2 days, gluconeogenesis occurs, mainly from lactate (end–product of anaerobic glucose metabolism) generated in the muscles, intestine, liver and RBCs
- o Glycogen stored in the muscles is utilized *locally*; cannot be exported out of the cell because muscles lack G6P
- o Glycogen synthase catalyzes the addition of UDP–glucose to the expanding glycogen chain
- o Glycogen phosphorylase catalyzes breakdown of the glycogen subunits
- o Glycogen exists as two distinct populations
  - – Small (proglycogen, MW ~ 4×10^5)
  - – Large (macroglycogen, MW ~ 1×10^7)
- o Two distinct pools of glycogen allows subtle control of glucose levels – this may have clinical contributions to diseases, such as DM

Carbohydrate Metabolism in Cirrhosis

- o Patients with cirrhosis have an increased frequency of hyperglycemia and relative hyperinsulinemia with insulin resistance, similar to that is found in patients with DM and obesity
- o Hyperglycemia secondary to decreased glucose uptake by muscles, and reduced glycogen storage in liver and muscles
  - – Insulin resistance → increased plasma insulin levels

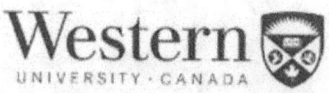

- o Other causes of relative insulin resistance:
    - Increased serum fatty acid levels inhibit glucose uptake by the muscles
    - Altered second messenger activity after insulin binds to its receptors in serum concentrations of cytokines 2° to elevated serum levels of lipopolysaccharides
    - Increased levels of glucagon and catecholamines

Lipid Metabolism Overview

- o Fatty acids are important energy source of the liver
    - Efficient fuel store within and outside the liver
    - Oxidation of fatty acids yields the highest ATP production of any metabolic fuel
    - Most organs use fatty acids
    - Excess glucose is converted to fatty acid and stored in adipose tissue or delivered by lipoproteins to other organs

- o FAs serve as important structural components of cells (cell membrane components, important in cell anchoring)

- o FAs are absorbed directly into the blood via intestinal capillaries; they are also synthesized in hepatocytes

- o Fatty acid synthesis
    - Fatty acid synthesis occurs in the hepatocyte cytosol
    - Regulated by the availability of acetyl–CoA, the basic subunit in developing fatty acid carbon chain
    - Successive malonyl–CoA molecules are used in the fatty acid synthase system to add 2 carbon units at the end of the growing fatty acid chain until a carbon–16 or carbon–18 fatty acid is synthesized
    - Once the fatty acid chain has reached an appropriate length, it is esterified with glycerol to

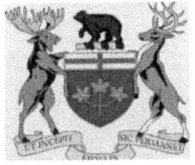

form triglycerides → triglycerides can be transported by lipoproteins → distal sites for storage or use

- Using fatty acids for energy:
    - β–oxidation of fatty acids
    - Important source of energy for many organs, including liver
    - Process occurs in mitochondria and peroxisomes
- Mitochondrial β–oxidation of fatty acids
    - Malonyl–CoA is the basic subunit of fatty acid synthesis and potent <u>inhibitor</u> of CPT1; thus, fatty acid synthesis and β–oxidation never happen concurrently
    - Fatty acids undergo fatty acyl–CoA formation via fatty acyl–CoA synthetases in the mitochondrial outer membrane to form fatty acyl–CoA
    - In the inner membrane, fatty acyl–CoA conjugated with carnitine (via CPT1) → fatty acylcarnitine → mitochondrion in exchange for free carnitine
    - Fatty acyl–CoA is released (via CPT2) and serves as a substrate for β–oxidation
    - Resultant acetyl–CoA can feed into Krebs cycle or enter the 3–hydroxyl methyl glutaryl–CoA cycle to form ketone bodies (only possible in hepatic mitochondria)
- Peroxisomal β–oxidation of fatty acids
    - Peroxisomes have lesser capacity than mitochondria for β–oxidation
- Significant differences:
    - Initial fatty acyl–CoA formation within peroxisome does not require fatty acyl carnitine formation for the entry into the peroxisome
    - In mitochondria, electrons → electron transport system → water and ATP → in peroxisomes ↓ ATP produced per fatty acid chain
    - Less ATP → ↑ peroxisomal fatty acid β–oxidation → ↓ lipid mass and ↓ weight

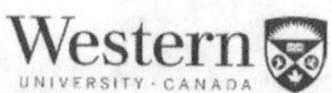

- Peroxisomes proliferate with administration of many hypolipidemic agents, such as *clofibrate*
- Comprised of apolipoproteins, triglycerides, phospholipids, cholesterol and cholesterol esters
  - Mediate transport of lipids from the liver into the plasma and back to liver or to other tissues
- Classification (increasing order of density):
  - Chylomicrons
  - Very low density lipoproteins (VLDLs)
  - Intermediate density lipoproteins (IDLs)
  - Low density lipoproteins (LDLs)
  - High density lipoproteins (HDLs) (density differences reflect differences in components atop)

Different lipid composition of each lipoprotein subtypes

- VLDL, chylomicrons: major component – triglycerides
  - Energy source of peripheral tissues
  - Components of cellular structures
- LDL, HDL: major component – cholesterol
  - Not used as fuel source
  - Used as structural component of membranes
  - Precursor for steroid hormones
- Specific apolipoproteins bind lipids to form lipoproteins
  - Modified by enzymes in plasma and endothelial cells
  - Act as ligands of specific lipoprotein receptors
- Liver expresses cell–surface receptors for circulating lipoproteins, enabling modulation of plasma levels
- Lipid components are in constant dynamic flux because of constant interactions:
  - Delivery of lipids and cholesterol to cells
  - Transfer to other lipoproteins (via lipid transfer proteins)
  - Catalysis by lipolytic enzymes

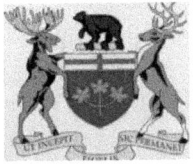

Apolipoproteins

- ➢ ApoA
  - ○ ApoA–I is the major component of HDL
    - – In the lipid-poor state, apoA–I accepts cholesterol from cell membranes
    - – Key activator of lecithin–cholesterol acyltransferase (LCAT)
  - ○ ApoA–II and apoA–IV are minor constitutents of HDL

- ➢ ApoB
  - ○ 2 major apolipoproteins associated with *triglyceride* transport, apoB–100 and apoB–48
    - – ApoB–100 synthesized in liver, apoB-48 in the intestine
    - – In intestinal epithelium, apoB mRNA undergoes post–transcriptional RNA editing → stop codon → form apoB that is 48% length of apoB–100 generated in the liver
    - – Terminal domain is absent in apoB–48 is required to bind LDL receptor
    - – Therefore, VLDL (containing apoB–100) gives rise to LDL
    - – Chylomicron remnants (contain apoB–48) are cleared rapidly from plasma and do not give rise to LDL

- ➢ ApoC
  - ○ ApoC is synthesized mainly in the liver (some intestinal and other)
    - – 3 different gene products inhibit uptake of chylomicron remnants by the liver
    - – ApoC–I: exact function is unknown
    - – ApoC–II: (VLDL, IDL, HDL, chylomicrons) essential activator of lipoprotein lipase (LPL)
    - – ApoC–III: (IDL, HDL, chylomicrons) may be an inhibitor of LDL activity

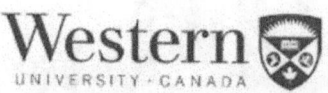

➢ ApoE
- o ApoE is synthesized in the liver and found on all lipoproteins
    - Important for removal of lipoprotein remnants in serum
    - Binds LDL receptors and other membrane proteins
    - Has 3 major alleles: ε2, ε3, ε4 – each has different ability to bind to LDL receptor
    - Absence of apoE → reduced clearance of chylomicron and VLDL remnants and elevated plasma values of these → ↑ *atherosclerosis risk*
    - ApoE is important in lipid transport in the CNS
    - Inheritance of a single ε4 gene only is associated with premature Alzheimer's dementia compared with ε3/ε3

Lipolytic Enzymes

- o Liporotein lipase (LPL) is synthesized in fat and muscles
    - Localized to the *luminal surfaces of the capillary beds of adipose, lungs, muscle tissues*
    - Catalyzes lipolysis of triglycerides in VLDL, chylomicrons, HDL
    - Stimulated by fasting, fatty acids, hormones, catecholamines
    - Patients homozygous for LPL deficiency have severe hypertriglyceridemia in childhood → pancreatitis
    - ApoC–II plays major role in activating LPL

- o Hepatic triglyceride lipase (HTGL) is synthesized in the liver
    - Localized in the *luminal surfaces of hepatic endothelial cells*
    - Catalyzes lipolysis in VLDL, IDL, HDL
    - Major role in LDL formation

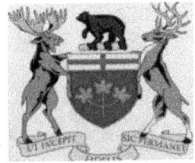

Lipid transport proteins: Crucial to transfer of cholesterol from non–hepatic tissues to liver

- o In the plasma, lipid exchange between particles is facilitated by:
  - LCAT
  - Cholesteryl ester transfer protein (CETP)

- o LCAT (lecithin–cholesterol acetyl transferase) synthesized in the liver
  - ApoA–1 is a cofactor for LCAT activity
  - Converts cholesterol to cholesteryl ester (more hydrophobic)
  - Cholesteryl ester can then be sequestered in the core of lipoprotein

- o CETP (cholesterol ester transfer protein) synthesized mainly in the liver
  - Circulates in association with HDL
  - Exchanges cholesteryl esters from HDL for triglycerides from chylomicrons or VLDL

Intestinal and Hepatic Lipid Transport

- o Liver functions as the hub in receiving fatty acids and cholesterol from *diet* and *peripheral tissues*
  - Packages them into lipoprotein complexes
  - Releases complexes into the circulation

➢ Fatty acid transport from diet

- o Fatty acids and cholesterol absorbed by the intestinal epithelial cells

- o Fatty acids formed into triglycerides

- o Cholesterol is esterified to cholesteryl ester

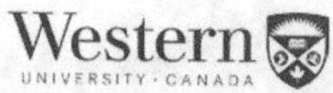

o   These lipids are packaged into nascent chylomicrons, which at this stage:
    - Triglycerides (~ 90%)
    - Phospholipids (6 – 12%)
    - Cholesteryl ester (1 – 3%)
    - Apolipoproteins (1 – 3%): apoB–48, apoA–1, apoA–II, apoA–IV
o   Nascent chylomicrons enter the interstitial space
o   There, they acquire apoC–II, which activates LPL
    - Promotes triglyceride release
o   If apoC–III is acquired, this inhibits LPL activity
o   Release of triglycerides and extraction by peripheral tissues raise the relative concentration of cholesteryl ester in the chylomicron remnant
o   ApoE addition is critical of targeting of the chylomicron remnant, which is identified and taken up by hepatocytes through chylomicron remnant receptors
o   The endocytosed chylomicron remnants are targeted to lysosomes and degraded
o   Atherosclerosis is more likely if chylomicron excretion is impaired
    - Reduced clearance of chylomicron remnants can be due to the following:
      ▪ Inherited mutations of the binding domain of apoE
      ▪ Reduced LPL activity
      ▪ Reduced apoC–II levels
      ▪ Increased VLDL secretion resulting from excess fatty acid absorption (can compete with chylomicron remnant uptake system)
    - With impaired clearance, chylomicron remnants accumulate in the serum
      ▪ Taken up by endothelial cells and macrophages → foamy cells, which are precursors of fatty streaks and atheromas

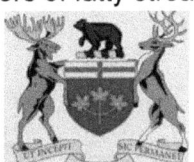

- ➤ Fatty acid transport from adipocytes

    - ○ Fatty acids are released from adipocytes via the intracellular hormone–sensitive lipase
        - – Bind to albumin and are transported to other tissues, including liver
        - – In the liver, they are used for the synthesis of phospholipids, triglycerides and cholesterol (rate–limiting enzyme of cholesterol synthesis is HMG–CoA reductase, target of statins)

    - ○ In the *fasting state*, VLDLs replace chylomicrons as the major transporters of triglycerides and cholesterol → *exported* from the liver

    - ○ The fatty acids released from adipocytes are stored in the hepatocyte cytosol → fatty acid–binding proteins (FABPs) → direct fatty acids to specific subcellular targets (i.e. Smooth ER – VLDL synthesis; peroxisomes – beta oxidation)

- ➤ Lipoprotein transport in the fasting state

    - ○ ApoB–100 is the main transport carrier in VLDL
        - – (apoC–1, apoC–II, apoC–III, apoE arise from other serum lipoproteins)

    - ○ ApoB–100 synthesis and VLDL secretion are regulated by the availability of co–transported lipids and sterols in the smooth ER:
        - – After the synthesis in the smooth ER, apoB–100 interacts with the newly synthesized triglycerides and cholesteryl esters
        - – This apoB–lipid complex is translocated into the lumen, through the Golgi apparatus, secreted into the sinusoidal space as VLDL
        - – If the lipid components are not available, apoB–100 gets *degraded in the ER* (if there are low triglyceride levels, the liver secretes smaller IDL–type particles, even LDL–type particles)

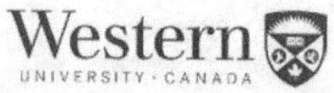

- o In the plasma, LPL and HTGL (the lipolytic enzymes) remove triglycerides from the secreted VLDL
  - The "remnant" becomes smaller and denser IDL and LDL particles
- o Conversion of IDL to LDL requires activity of apoE
- o LDL particles become relatively denser in cholesteryl esters   (via both removal of triglycerides and acquisition of cholesteryl ester from other lipoproteins – mainly HDL, with release of apoC to HDL)
- o LDL is removed from the circulation by LDL receptors in the liver and peripheral tissues – homozygous deficiency in 1:1 million

High Density Liporpoteins (HDL)

- o Protective role against atherosclerosis
- o Nascent HDL formed in the liver (from VLDL) and intestines (from chylomicrons) by lipolysis
- o Initially called HDL_3 – cholesterol–poor molecules
  - LCAT in the plasma converts cholesterol from the peripheral membranes into cholesteryl esters that can move into the core of the lipoprotein
  - Therefore, more available surface of lipoprotein for further cholesterol extraction from cell membranes
- o When complex is large enough to accommodate apoC–II and apoC–III it is called HDL_2
- o CETP removes esterified cholesterol out of HDL in exchange for triglycerides (from chylomicrons or VLDL)
- o Triglycerides are eventually hydrolyzed by HTGL in the liver, regenerating small HDL (HDL_3)

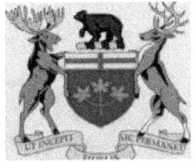

Lipid metabolism is a derangement in chronic liver disease (CLD)

- o Most common lipid abnormality in CLD is hypertriglyceridemia
- o EtOH
  - – Increased fatty acid synthesis and decreased β–oxidation of fatty acids, $2°$ to greater NADH production by EtOH metabolism in viral liver diseases
  - – Moderate EtOH associated with increased HDL_3, therefore the reduce risk of atherosclerosis
- o As cirrhosis advances (Child–Pugh A → C), LDL, HDL and total cholesterol levels decrease, progressively
  - – Prognostic marker in non–cholestatic liver disease

It is wise to keep in mind that, neither success nor failure, is ever final.

Roger Babson

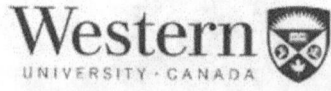

Congenital Liver Diseases

Karim Qumosani

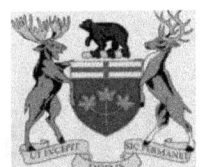

➢ Introduction

- o Membrane transporters–related liver disease
  - – Progressive Familial Intrahepatic Cholestasis (PFIC)
  - – Benign Recurrent Intrahepatic Cholestatsis (BRIC)
  - – Intrahepatic Cholestatsis of Pregnancy
  - – Dubin–Johnson Syndrome

- o Non–membrane transporters–related liver disease
  - – Bile duct present (Abnormal)
  - – Bile duct absent

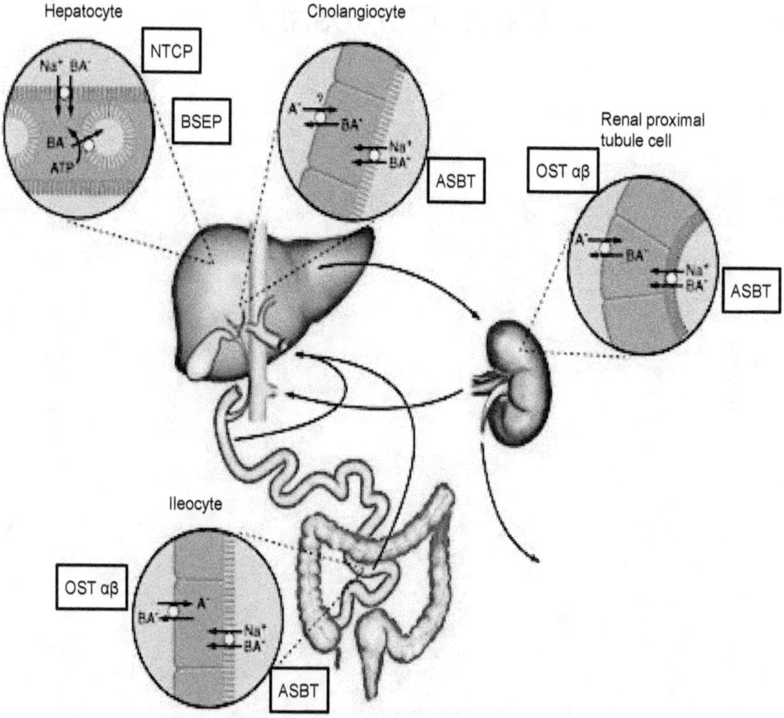

Adapted from: Dowson, P.A. *Sleisenger & Fordtran's Gastrointestinal and Liver Disease.* 10th Ed. Figure 64-3, page 1090.

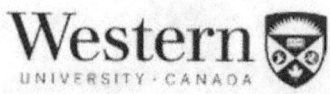

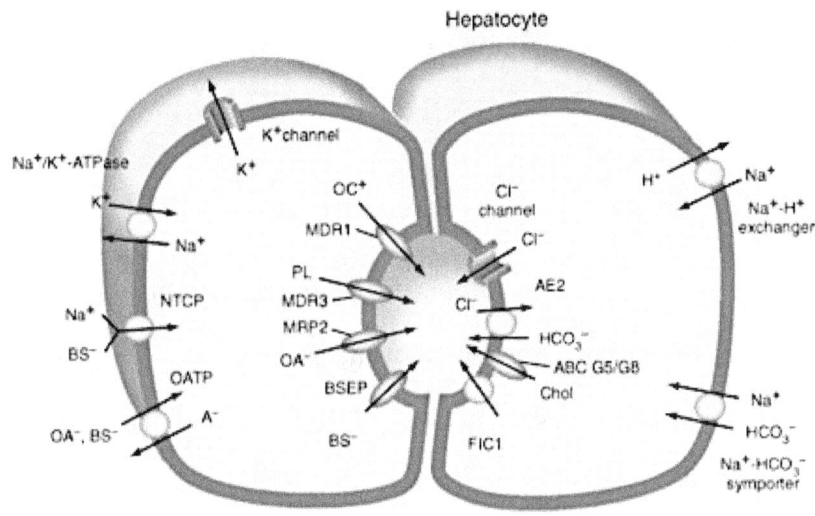

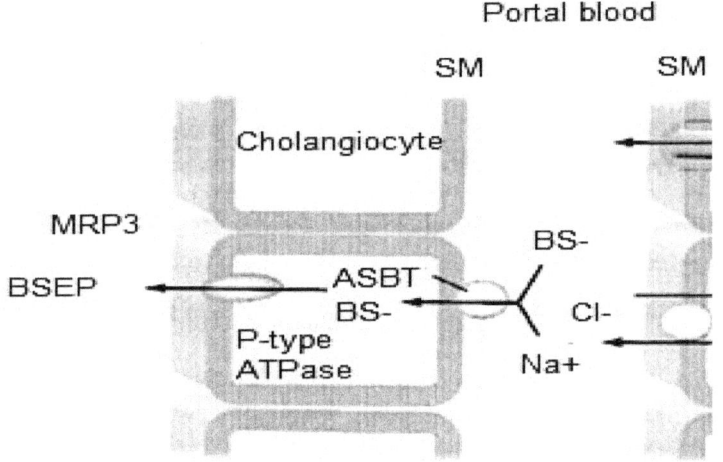

Adapted from: Sherlock and Dooley. 11th Edition. 2002. Figure 64-4, page 1082; Dowson, P.A. *Sleisenger & Fordtran's Gastrointestinal and Liver Disease.* 10th Ed. Figure 64-4, page 1092.

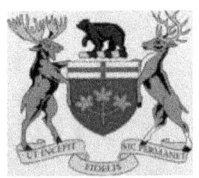

Progressive Familial Intrahepatic Cholestatsis (PFIC)

➢ PFIC Type 1
- o Defect — FIC 1
- o Transport — Aminophospholipids
- o Presentation — Progressive cholestasis, pruritus, pancreatitis, malabsorption

Benign Recurrent Intrahepatic Cholestasis

- o Milder disease phenotype of PFIC

➢ PFIC Type 2
- o Defect — BSEP
- o Transport — Bile acids
- o Presentation — Progressive cholestasis and hepatic fibrosis
  - — ↑ risk of hepatobiliary malignancy

➢ PFIC Type 3
- o Defect — MDR3
- o Transport — Phosphatidylcholine
- o Presentation — Cholestasis and periportal fibrosis

Intrahepatic Cholestatsis of Pregnancy (ICP)

- o Defect — MDR3; BSEP
- o Transport — Phosphatidylcholine, bile acids
- o Presentation — Third trimester cholestasis, fetal loss and prematurity

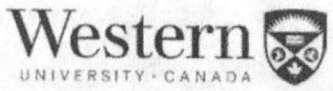

Dubin–Johnson Syndrome (DJS)

- Defect   – MRP2
- Transport   – Conjugated bilirubin (organic anion conjugate)
- Presentation – Asymptomatic direct hyperbilirubinemia with benign prognosis

Rotor Syndrome

- Defect   – MRP2
- Transport   – Organic anion conjugates
- Representation – Simila to DJ5
  - Delayed clearance of bromosulfopthalein, indocyanine green (dyes)

Primary Bile Acid Malabsorption (PBAM)

- Defect   – ASBT
- Transport   – Bile acids
- Representation – Steatorrhea

Sito Sterolemia

- Defect   – ABCG5/8
- Transport   – Cholesterol, phytosteroids
- Representation – Coronary artery disease, xanthoma

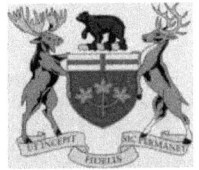

Caroli Disease

- o Congenital disorder characterized by multifocal, segmental dilatation in intrahepatic bile ducts
- o Two variants
  - Caroli disease: less common, only bile duct dilatation (BDD)
  - Caroli syndrome: more common, bile duct dilatation, congenital hepatic fibrosis (CHF) and ARPKD

> CD = BDD
> CS = BDD + CHF + ARPKD

➢ Pathogenesis
  - o Bile Ducts: weakness of the bile duct wall, abnormal proliferation during embryogenesis or congenital Reovirus infection
  - o Liver: arrest or derangement in remodeling of the ductal plate (ductal plate malformation)
  - o Kidney: autosomal recessive PKHD1

➢ Pathology
  - o Bile Ducts: segmental, saccular dilatations of the large intrahepatic bile ducts
  - o Liver: fibrosis and enlargement of portal tracts, dysmophic bile ducts, and hypoplastic portal vein branches
  - o Kidney: multiple cystic lesions

➢ Clinical Manifestations
  - o Bile Ducts: stagnation of bile leading to sludge intraductal lithiasis, cholangitis
  - o Liver: portal hypertension, such as ascites and esophageal varices
  - o Kidney: neonatal kidney disease and hypertension

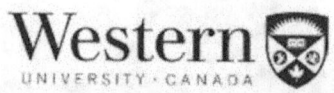

➤ Diagnosis
  o Bile Ducts: imaging with US, CT or MRI showing "**central dot sign**"
  o Liver: fibrosis and enlargement of the portal tracts, dysmophic bile ducts and hypoplastic portal vein branches
  o Bile Ducts
    – Antibiotics
    – Fat soluble vitamin supplements
    – ERCP and ESWL
    – Ursudiol
    – Hepatectomy
  o Liver
    – β–blockers
    – Diuretics
    – Surgical shunt
    – Liver transplant

Paucity of the Interlobular Bile ducts

  o Ratio of the number of interlobular bile ducts to the number of portal tracts is less than 0.5:1

➤ Causes and associations
  o Biliary dysgenesis
  o Intrauterine infection: rubella, CMV
  o Genetic disorder: inborn error of bile metabolism, α–1 antitrypsin

Alagille Syndrome

➤ Definition
  o Autosomal dominant disorder leading to mutations in JAG gene, and leading to disorders in multiple systems, including paucity of the interlobular bile ducts

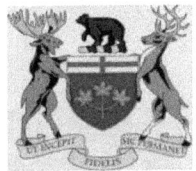

➢ Demographics
  o Most common form of familial intrahepatic cholestasis

➢ Genetics
  o Autosomal dominant with incomplete penetrance
  o Mutations in the JAGGED1 (JAG1) gene on chromosome 20

➢ Clinical
  o CNS
    – Mental retardation
    – Poor coordination and slow speech
  o Eye (> 75% of patients)
  o Dimorphic face
    – Broad forehead
    – Deeply set eyes
    – Small pointed mandible
    – Prominent ears
    – Cleft palate
  o Heart
    – Pulmonary stenosis
  o MSK
    – Butterfly vertebrae
      – Rib anomalies
  o Liver
      – ↓ interlobular bile acids
➢ Treatment
  o Adequate caloric intake
  o Fat soluble vitamin supplements
  o Treat pruritis
  o Liver transplantation
  o Genetic counselling

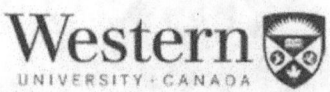

Acute Liver Failure and the ICU

Paul Marotta

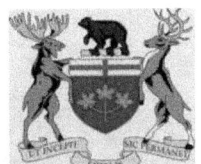

Acute Liver Failure

- ➢ Definition: Evidence of coagulation abnormality (INR ≥ 1.5) and any degree of altered CNS, and ≤ 26weeks (with no known liver disease)

- ➢ Demography
  - o ~ 2,000 cases/year in USA: ~ $4/10^6$ population
  - o 10 – 20 liver transplants annually of ALF in Canada
  - o High mortality rate
  - o Difficult to study due to rarity of cases and variety of etiology and patient demographic

- ➢ Terms
  - o Replace other terms defined by time points
    - – Hyperacute liver failure (< 7days)
    - – Acute liver failure (7 – 21 days)
    - – Subacute liver failure (> 21 days)
    - – Fulminant hepatic failure (within 8 weeks)
  - o Prognosis is based on etiology and not time

Lee, W.M., *et al.* AASLD position paper: The management of acute liver failure: Update 2011. *Hepatology.* 2012; 55(3):965-7.

- ➢ Causes and associations
  - o Etiology is one of the BEST indicators of prognosis
    - – Poor outcomes with AIH, mushroom, Wilson, BCS, Idiosyncratic drug reaction
    - – Better with acetaminophen, pregnancy–related (AFLP/HELLP), ischemic, hepatitis A or E
  - o 20% seen with no discernable cause
    - – 20% acetominophen adducts can be detected

Khandelwal, *et al. Hepatology.* 2011. 53:567-76.

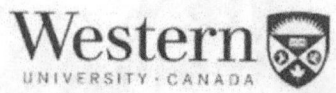

- o Acetaminophen – purposeful, inadvertent, > 10 g (150 mg/kg)
  - – Typically ALT > 4,000, normal BR
  - – Leading cause of ALF, accounts for 20% of indeterminate etiologies
  - – Safe, effective antidote
  - – Give N–acetylcysteine (NAC) promptly and extend up to 72 hours, or until liver profile improves

Mushroom Poisoning

- **Amanita phalloides**
  - o GI distress seen in hours to days after ingestion
  - o Late summer, no lab 'test'
  - o High Mortality
  - o Treatment : Penicillin G (0.5 – 1x10^6 units/kg/day)
  - o Treatment: Silymarin (milk thistle) IV 40mg/kg/day, emergency release

Drug–Induced Liver Injury (DILI)

- ➢ Causes
  - o Guidelines of causality at DILI network
  - o Typically not dose–related (idiosyncratic)
  - o Usually cholestatic with high mortality
  - o Herbals, weight loss, Rx, supplements, illicit drugs

- ➢ Clinical features and complications
  - o Hepatic encephalopathy and cerebral edema
  - o Coagulopathy
  - o Renal dysfunction
  - o Metabolic disturbance
  - o Infection

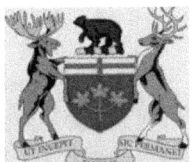

➢ Treatment
  ○ Supportive care
  ○ No corticosteroids, unless with DRESS syndrome

Hepatic Encephalopathy (HE)

➢ Pathogenesis
  ○ Unknown
  ○ Osmotic alterations, loss of autoregulation
  ○ Ammonia
    − Correlates to cerebral edema
    − ArterialAmmonia
      ▪ < 75 ug/dL – rarely develop to HE and ICH
      ▪ > 200 ug/dL – herniation
    − Reduce levels with lactulose (prevents/treatment)
  ○ HE stages 1 – 4
    − Correlates to ICH

➢ Stages
  ○ Stage 1
    − Subtle personality changes, sleep changes, euphoria   Rare ICH
  ○ Stage 2
    − Drowsy, restless, asterixis
  ○ Stage 3   30% ICH
    − Inappropriate, reusable
  ○ Stage 4   >75% ICH
    − Coma

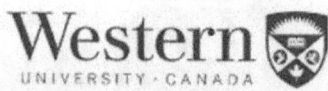

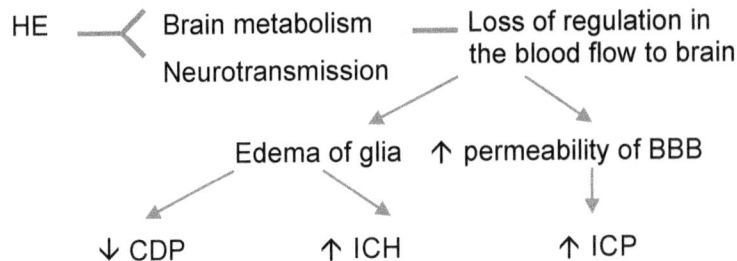

HE — Brain metabolism / Neurotransmission — Loss of regulation in the blood flow to brain

Edema of glia   ↑ permeability of BBB

↓ CDP   ↑ ICH   ↑ ICP

Abbreviations: BBB, blood brain barrier; CPP, cerebral perfusion pressure; HE, hepatic encephalopathy; ICH, intracranial hemorrhage; ICP, intracranial pressure

➤ Initial Assessment
  o History
    – Potential etiology (i.e. viral, drug, immune, pregnancy)
  o Rapid and extensive biochemistry
    – Etiology and severity
  o Progression may be rapid, if there is **any** alteration in the CNS, then the patient admit to ICU
    – Contact transplant center (if appropriate), transport early *vs* late

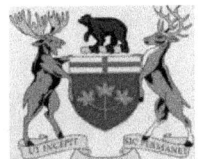

➤ Suggested Initial Investigations

Prothrombin time and INR

- Chemistries
  - Sodium, potassium, chloride, bicarbonate, calcium, magnesium, phosphate, glucose
  - AST, ALT, alkaline phosphatase, GGT, total bilirubin, albumin creatinine, blood urea nitrogen
- Arterial blood gas
- Arterial lactate
- Complete blood count
- Blood type and screen
- Acetaminophen level
- Toxicology screen
- Viral hepatitis serologies
  - Anti–HAV IgM, HBsAg, anti–HBc IgM, anti–HEV, anti–HCV, HCV RNA, HSV1 IgM, VZV
- Ceruloplasmin level
- Pregnancy test (females)
- Ammonia (arterial, if possible)
- Autoimmune markers
- HIV–1, HIV–2
- Amylases and lipases

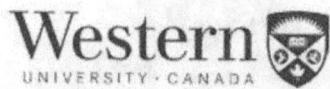

Etiologies of ALF: US ALFSG (1998 – 2008)

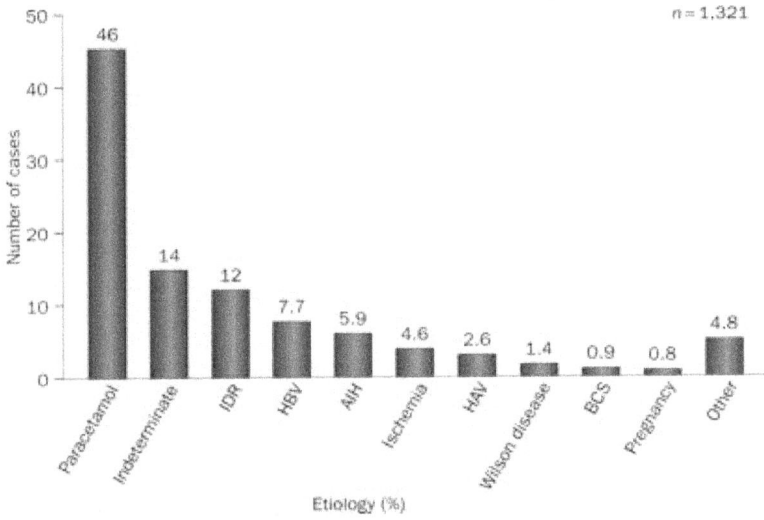

Printed with permission: Stravitz, R.T. and Kramer, D.J. *Nat Rev Gastroenterol Hepatol*. 2009; 6(9):542-53.

ICH Monitoring

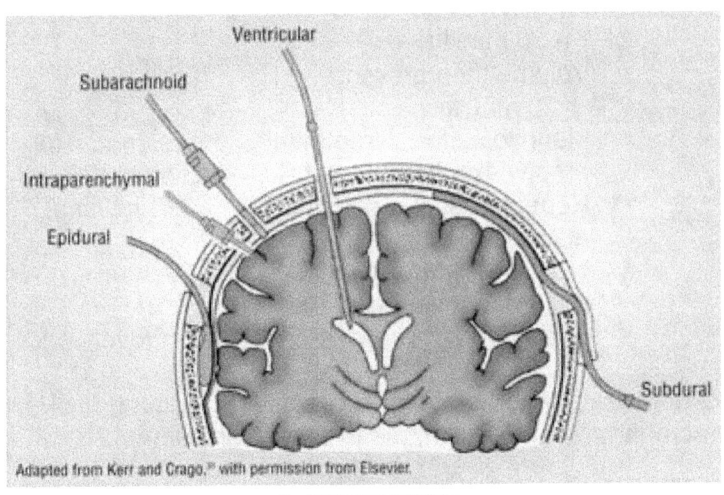

Adapted from Kerr and Crago,[1] with permission from Elsevier.

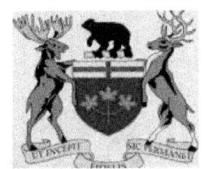

- ○ Hepatic Encephalopathy
    - – I: frequent clinical monitoring, no sedation, lactulose
    - – II: move to ICU
    - – III/IV: hook to ETT or vent, HOB 30°, propofol is useful, monitor pupillary size and reaction, posture
- ○ ICP Monitoring
    - – 50% programs continue to invasive monitoring
    - – PROs: early recognition of ICP, signs in CT are late
    - – CONs: risk of bleeding, 5%; death, 1%
- ○ CPP=MAP-ICP
    - – Keep CPP > 50 – 60 (70*) mmHg
    - – Keep ICP < 20 – 25 mmHg
- ○ Why monitor ICP?
    - – Decerebrate posture ICP = 16 – 20 mmHg
    - – Brain damage ICP = 25 mmHg
    - – SHT, pupil changes ICP = 30 mmHg
- ○ Transcranial Doppler is an alternative

ICP Treatment

- ○ CPP=MAP-ICP
    - – CPP > 60 mmHg
        - ▪ Volume then pressors
    - – ICP < 20 mmHg
        - ▪ Mannitol for treatment only, not for prophylaxis (transient, mild reduction in ICP)
        - ▪ Repeat dosing if s–osmolality < 320 mOsm/L, may require dialysis
        - ▪ Hyperventilation (PaCO$_2$ 25 – 30 mmHg) – not recommended
        - ▪ Hypothermia – core 33 – 34°C (controversial)

Abbreviations: CPP, cerebral perfusion pressure; ICP, intracranial pressure; MAP, mean arterial pressure

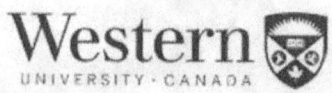

Coagulopathy
- o Best prognostic feature – INR
- o Poor hepatic synthetic function – factors I, II, V, VII, IX, X (INR); factor V has the shortest half life (T1/2), thus has prognostic value
- o Preserve INR
  - – In the absence of bleeding, do NOT correct INR
  - – With elevated INR, overall hemostasis (thromboelastography) is preserved
  - – Treat only if with bleeding, invasive procedure

Hot topics in ALF
- o Predicting need for liver transplantation
  - – Clinical Predictors
  - – Prognostic Models
- o Liver Support Systems
- o Liver transplantation

➤ Prognosis
- o Very difficult to determine who will survive without the need for liver transplantation
- o Etiology is key prognostic variable
  - – Transplant–free survival is > 50%
    - ▪ Acetaminophen, HAV, ischemia, pregnancy–related (AFLP, HELLP syndrome)
  - – Transplant–free survival is < 25%
    - ▪ Wilson disease, Budd–Chiari syndrome, DILI
  - – Best predictors of outcome
    - • Etiology
      - ▪ HE (stage > 3)
      - ▪ INR
      - ▪ Lactate: if arterial lactate > 3.5 mmol/L
      - ▪ Factor V: < 30%, if > 30 years
        - : < 20%, if < 30 years
      - ▪ Liver biopsy (necrosis) > 70%, survival is 10%

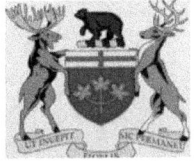

• Prognostic Indicators

Proposed scheme in assessing prognosis and need for orthotopic liver transplantation in patients with ALF

Scheme	Etiology of ALF	Criteria for Liver Transplant
o King's College criteria	APAP	Arterial pH < 7.3; all of the following 1) PT > 100 secs (INR > 6.5) 2) Creatinine > 3.4 mg/dL 3) Grade ¾ encephalopathy
	Non-APAP	PT > 100 secs (INR > 6.5); any 3 of the following: 1) NANB, drugs, halothane etiology 2) Jaundice to encephalopathy > 7 days 3) Age < 10 or > 40 years 4) PT > 50 secs (INR > 3.5) 5) Bilirubin > 17.4 mg/dL
o Factor V	Viral	Age < 30 years: factor V < 20% any age: factor V < 30% and grade ¾ encephalopathy
o Factor VIII / V ratio	APAP	Factor VIII / V ratio is > 30
o Liver biopsy	Mixed	Hepatocyte necrosis in > 70%
o Severity index	HBV, NANB	See reference
o Arterial phosphate	APAP	> 1.2 mmol/L
o Arterial lactate	APAP	> 3.5 mmol/L

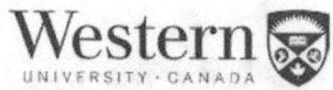

Scheme	Etiology of ALF	Criteria for Liver Transplant
○ Arterial ammonia	Mixed	> 150 – 200 μmol/L
○ APACHE II score	APAP	Score: > 15
○ MELD / Δ MELD score	APAP	MELD: > 33 Δ MELD score: > - 0.4

Abbreviations: ALF, acute liver failure; APACHE, acute physiology and chronic health evaluation; APAP, acetaminophen; HBV, hepatitis B virus; INR, international normalized ratio; MELD, model for end–stage liver disease; NANB, non–A, non–B viral hepatitis; PT, prothrombin time

*Times of data collection vary between studies

Printed with permission: Craig, D.G., *et al. Aliment Pharmacol Ther.* 2010; 31(3):345-58.

Criteria

- ○ King's College Criteria
  - – Based on > 700 ALF
  - – Assumes < 20% survive without LTx
  - – Sensitivity, 70%; Specificity, 85%
  - – PPV: 80 – 100%; NPV: 30 – 95%
  - – AUROC: 0.85
  - – Differentiates ACM from non–ACM

Abbreviations: ACM, acetaminophen; ALF, acute liver failure; LTX, liver transplantation; NPV, negative predictive value; PPV, positive predictive value

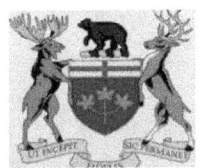

- o ACM
  - – pH < 7.3 or all 3/3
  - – HE stage 3,4
  - – NR > 6.5, * creatinine is > 300

- o Non–ACM
  - – INR > 6.5, or any 3/6 of the following:
    - Age: < 10 – > 40 years
    - Unfavorable etiology: DILI,Wilson, AIH
    - HE: > 7 days from jaundice
    - INR: > 3.5
    - Bilirubin: > 300

Molecular Adsorbent Recirculation System in ALF

- o Reversal of cerebral edema
  - – ↓ ammonia concentration

- o Bridge to the following:
  - – Spontaneous recovery
  - – Liver transplantation

- ➢ MARSTM: 3 compartments

- o Blood circuit
  - – Blood dialyzed across albumin–impregnated high–flux polysulfone dialysis membrane
  - – Pore size cut off:
    - < 50 kDA: ammonia, aromatic amino acids, cytokines
    - > 50 kDa: albumin, immunoglobulins, hormones, growth factors

- o Albumin circuit (dialysate)
  - – 400 cc of 25% human albumin acts as dialysate
  - – Charcoal or anion exchange columns; Dialysate is regenerated

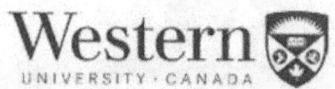

- o Renal Circuit
    - – Hemodialysis or hemofiltration (CRRT)
    - – Can run on pre–existing machines

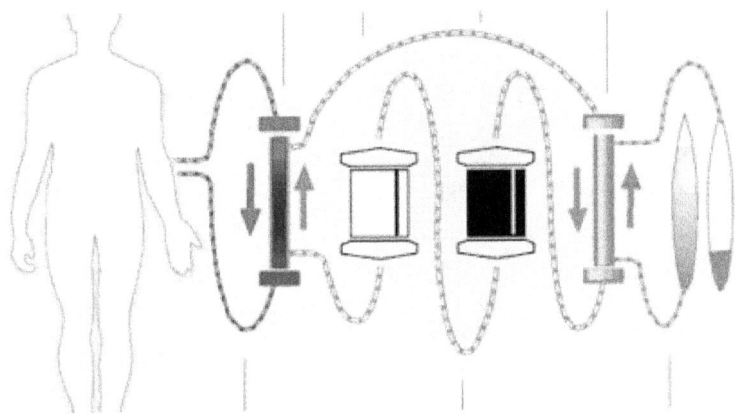

- Phase I–II clinical studies

    - o MARS decreases portal hypertension (Catalina, 2002; Sen, 2005.)

    - o MARS improves hemodynamics (Heeman, 2002; Catalina, 2002; Laleman, 2006; Dona, 2007.)

    - o MARS improves hepatic encephalopathy (Heeman, 2002; Schmidt, 2002; Novelli, 2003; Ding, 2004; DaCostal, 2004; Isoniemi, 2008.)

    - o MARS stabilize renal function (Some cohort studies)

    - o 13 patients (patients) with hyper–acute liver failure"
        - – 8 patients assigned to ONE 6–hour MARS run"
        - – 5 patients to SMT (including CRRT)"

    - o Improvement in hemodynamics in the MARS group"
        - – ↑ SVRI by 46% *vs* 6% (P < 0.0001)"
        - – ↑ MAP (+11 mmHg) *vs* no change (P < 0001)
            - ▪ ↓ CIby 20% (4.6 to 3.7) *vs* 7% (P=.0007)
            - ▪ ↓ HR (105 to 85) *vs* no change (P <.0001)
        - – Arterial lactate and pH levels were unchanged"

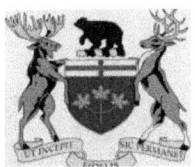

- No mortality difference (62.5vs.60%)" (Schmidt LE, et al., Liv Trans 2003)

➢ FULMAR: Phase 2a / France

- Total 102 patients
- Main etiology of ALF due to Acetaminophen (38%)
  - SMT *vs* MARS+SMT

ITT analysis at 6 months	Causes of ALF	CONV	MARS
Patient survival	- Acetaminophen	85	69
	- Non–acetaminophen	85	82
Transplant–free	- Acetaminohen	85	69
	- Non–acetaminophen	60	60

None of the differences between CONV and MARS was statistically significant.

Faouzi, Saliba., *et al.* AASLD. 2008.

- Possible roles
  - Acetaminophen (LT or non–LT candidate)
    - Bridge to hepatic regeneration and recovery
  - ALF (other etiologies)
    - Bridge to transplant
  - Acute attack in chronic liver disease

Liver Transplantation

- Medical and social criteria
- Transplantation for ALF: ~ 3% Canadian transplant activity (12 cases/year)
- Urgent status: 3F/4F
  - Median wait time is 24 hours (1 hour – 7 days)

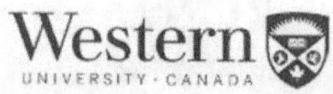

- o Most deaths in the first 1 – 3 years
  - – 1–year survival rate, 60% (poor)
  - – But after 1st year, the 5 – 10–year survival rate is 90%
- o Once listed, 30% recover without LTx and 20% who are transplanted recover
- o Death while listed is 10 – 40%, very dynamic, stressful period

➤ Summary
- o ALF is rare, hence large controlled trials are unlikely
- o Management is based on experience and expert consensus
- o Etiology of ALF is the key of its prognosis
- o Prompt diagnosis is important
  - – Viral, AIH, drugs, ACM (adducts)
- o Management: Position Paper in 2012
  - – Arterial ammonia
    - ▪ < 75 ug/dL is rare in ICH
    - ▪ > 150 ug/dL predicts ICH
    - ▪ > 200 ug/dL suggests impending herniation of brainstem
  - – Hypothermia protocol (32 – 34°C)
  - – MAP > 75, CPP > 60 – 80 mmHg (volume then give norepinephrine)
  - – INR key is variable, no correction needed
  - – Prognosis remains difficult to predict
    - ▪ Kings CC useful, not fully rely on (AUROC)
  - – No good evidence that liver support systems alter morbidity or mortality
  - – Liver transplant is the definitive treatment with excellent long term results

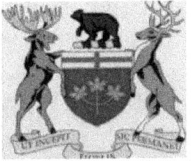

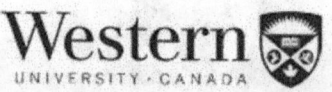

Managing High Risk Individuals for Pancreatic Ductal Adenocarcinoma (PDAC)

Nadeem Hussain

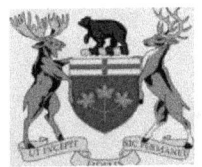

➢ Epidemiology

- o 2nd most common GI malignancy
- o 4th leading cause of cancer–related mortality in both men and women
- o Disease is uncommon before the age of < 45 years
- o General population risk is 1.3 – 1.5%
- o 10 – 20% in patients are operative candidates
- o Median survival is 6 months
- o Dismal 5–year survival rate is 5%
- o Early diagnosis remains the most important challenge in improving prognosis

Jamal, *et al. Cancer Statistics.* 2004. *CA Cancer J Clin.* 54:8, 2004.; Ries, *et al. Seer Cancer Statistics Review.* 1973-1996.; Bethesda, M.D., National Cancer Institute. 2000.

➢ Pathology

- o Pancreatic cells
  - – Acinar, 80% volume of glands
  - – Ductal, 10 – 15% volume of glands
  - – Endocrine, 1 – 2% volume of glands
- o 90% of cancer arises from exocrine component of glands (acinar or ductal) and majority are ductal adenocarcinomas
- o 1 – 2% arise with endocrine component
- o 10% of all pancreatic masses are metastatic
  - – Breast, lung, renal, GI, prostate, melanoma, osteosarcoma (described up to 17 years after diagnosis of renal cell cancer)
- o 60 – 70% are located in the HOP
- o 5 – 10% located in the BOP
- o 10 – 15% located in TOP

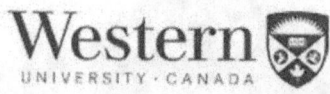

- o Average size
  - – HOP: 2.5 – 3.5 cm
  - – Other: 5 – 7 cm
- o Desmoplasia is common
- o Precursors: PanIN, IPMN, MCN

➢ Precursors
  - o 1999 National Cancer Institute – adopted the "PanIN" nomenclature as a tumor progression model similar to cervical, prostrate and breast cancer
  - o Microscopic
    - – PanIN1
    - – PanIN2; PanIN3
  - o Macroscopic
    - – Cysts
      - ▪ IPMN
    - – MCN

PanIN

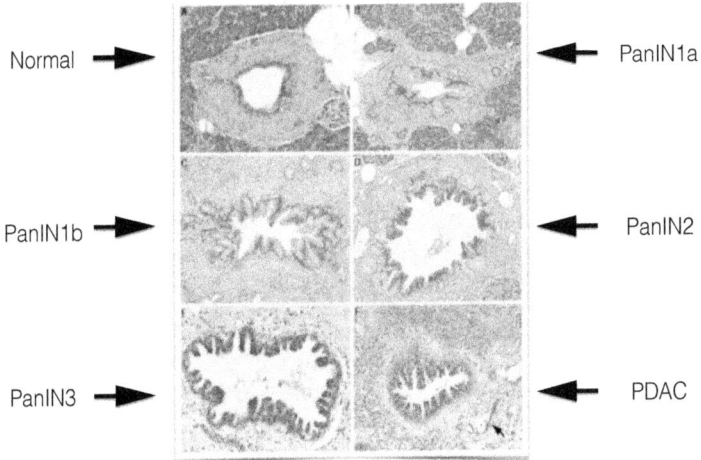

Normal ➡   ⬅ PanIN1a

PanIN1b ➡   ⬅ PanIN2

PanIN3 ➡   ⬅ PDAC

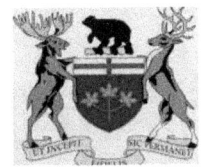

Evidences that PanIN are Precursors

- o Autopsy
  - – Frequent findings of PanIN lesions seen in patients with PDAC
- o Animal models
  - – PanIN1 → PanIN3 → PDAC develop the following exposure to carcinogenic materials
- o Resection margins with PanIN3 shows recurrence of PAC at the margin
- o Prevalence of genetic alterations in cells increases with increasing grades of PanINs

➢ Genetics

- o Molecular Alterations in PanINs

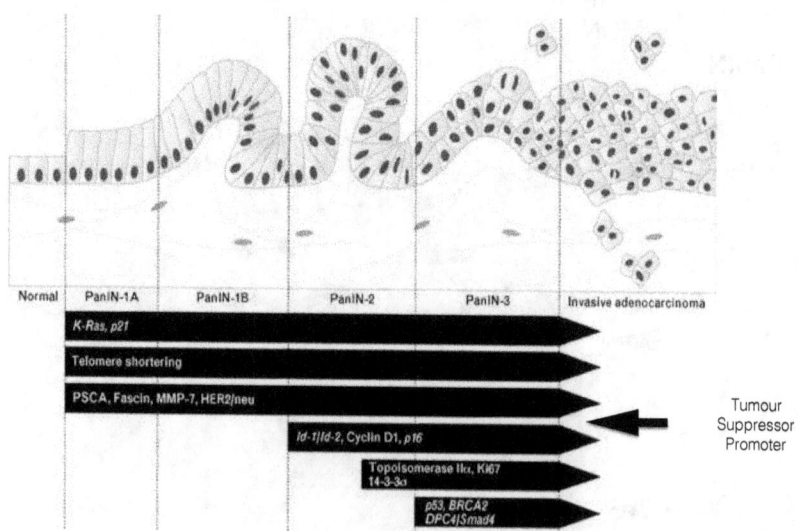

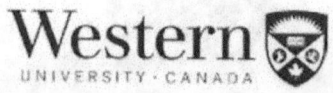

Intraductal Papillary Mucinous Neoplasia (IPMN)

- o   Discovered in 1980s by Japanese investigators

- o   Now accounts for 3 – 5% of all pancreatic neoplasia and 20% of all cystic diseases of pancreas

- o   WHO 2000
  - –   Grossly visible mucin–producing neoplasm that originates from the MPD or side Br with (not always) papillary projections

- o   Diagnosis relies on endoscopy, MRI/MRCP, EUS

- o   Mucin or adenoma → neoplasia produced render patients symptomatic

Abbreviations: Br, branch; MPD, main pancreatic duct

➢   Pathology

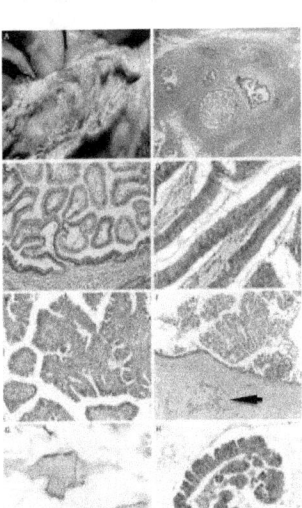

Dilated MPD grossly

Dilated Side Br ducts

Dilated Side Br ducts
Microscopic view LGD
Gastric subtype

Intestinal subtype 35%
most common with LGD

HGD in Pancreaticobiliary type
20% more aggressive

Pancreaticobiliary subtype
with invasive PDAC

Mucin with EUS FNA

EUS FNA with Moderate dysplasia

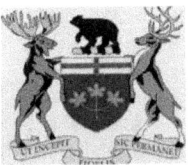

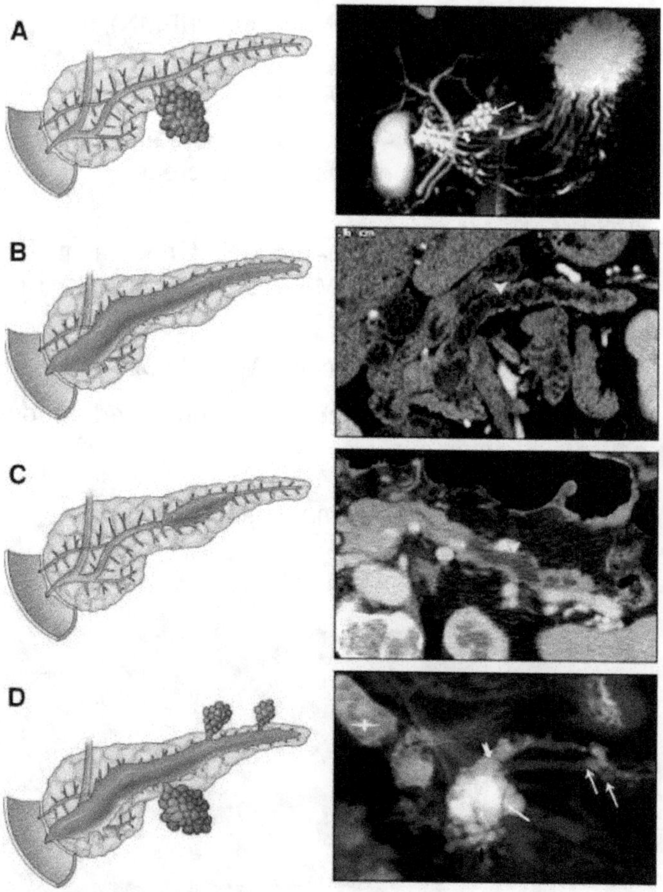

A

B

C

D

Subtypes of IPMN and risk of neoplasm
- ○ MPD/Mixed
  - – Lifetime cancer risk is 60 – 80%
- ○ Side branches
  - – Lifetime cancer risk is10 – 20%
- ○ Resected non–invasive IPMN
  - – 5–year survival: 77 – 96%
- ○ Resected invasive IPMN
  - – 5–yr survival: 34 – 74%

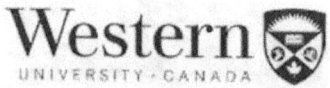

Mucinous Cystic Neoplasm (MCN)

- o 2 – 5% of all pancreatic tumors
- o Exclusively seen in females (over 95%) in BOP/TOP (95%) almost always unifocal (unlike IPMN)
- o No communication with MPD (compared with IPMN)
- o Differentiated from IPMN: supported by ovarian–type stroma

➤ Pathology

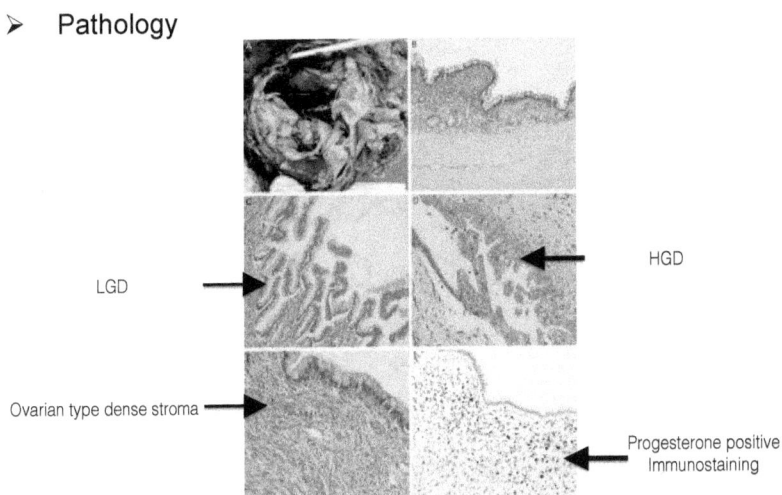

LGD

HGD

Ovarian type dense stroma

Progesterone positive Immunostaining

Pancreatic Ductal Adenocarcinoma

➤ Clinical presentation

- o < 20% present with resectable disease
- o Local extension is common:
    - Duodenum, CBD, PD, PV, SMV, CA, SMA
    - Stomach, spleen, L adrenal gland
- o Metastatic diseases
    - Liver, peritoneum
    - Lung, pleura and bony mets are uncommon

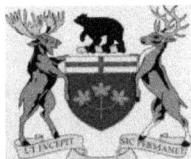

- o Pain (abdominal, back) invasion of celiac or superior mesenteric arterial plexus
- o Fatigue, weight loss and anorexia, depression
- o Obstruction: CBD, PD (acute and chronic pancreatitis), duodenal
- o Idiopathic acute pancreatitis (2 – 3x RR)
- o New onset of DM within 2 years
- o DVT
- o Courvoisier gallbladder – enlarged gallbladder secondary to obstructed CBD

Abbreviations: CA, celiac axis; CBD, common bile duct; DM, diabetes mellitus; DVT, deep venous thrombosis; PD, pancreatic duct; PV, portal vein; RR, relative risk; SMA, superior mesenteric artery; SMV, superior mesenteric artery

➢ Staging (AJCC, 2010)

Primary tumor (T)

TX	Primary tumor cannot be assessed Surgery
T0	No evidence of primary tumor
Tis	Carcinoma *in situ*
T1	Tumor < 2cm in size and limited to the pancreas
T2	Tumor > 2cm in size and limited to the pancreas

T3*	Tumou extends beyond the pancreas but <u>spares</u> the *celiac axis* or *SMA*

T4*	Tumor *involves the celiac axis or SMA* Palliative
N1	Locoregional LN
M1	Disease becomes palliative therapy

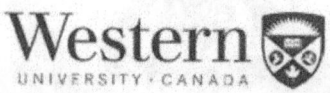

- ➢ Diagnosis and Staging
  - ○ Since majority of patients present with HOP mass, primary modality of presentation is jaundice with local extension into the CBD
  - ○ Abdominal U/S is usually used to differentiate between obstructive and non–obstructive jaundice
  - ○ However, limitation with air limit it's use for imaging of the pancreas
  - ○ A dilated CBD is usually followed by CT of the abdomen

Abbreviations: CBD, common bile duct; HOP, head of pancreas

Pancreas Protocol CT (ppCT)

- ○ Oral contrast given to differentiate between pancreas and duodenum
- ○ No differences between different generation of hCT scanners (4,8,16, and 64–row)
- ○ Mass tends to be hypoattenuating from pancreatic parenchyma (hypovascular)
- ○ Post–processing (multi–planar reformation in coronal and sagital images improves performance) is helpful when looking for vascular invasion

CT objectives

- ○ Maximize attenuation between abnormal hypoattenuating mass and pancreatic normal parenchyma
- ○ Adequately opacify vessels to allow proper staging
- ○ Optimize enhancement of the liver to rule out liver metastases

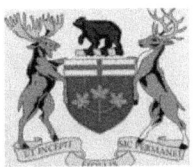

Understand the Vascular Supply of Liver and Pancreas

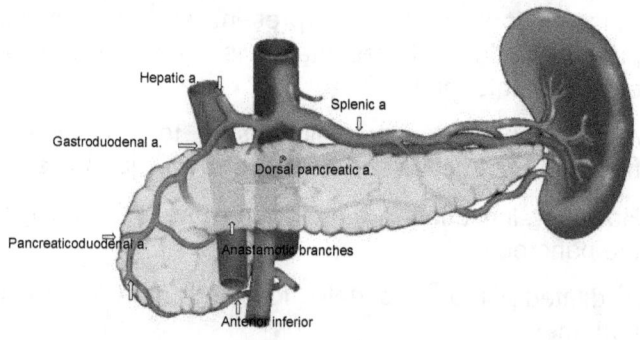

Pancreaticoduodenal a.

Understanding Timing CT Contrast
- o Pancreas supplied by splanchnic arteries
- o Liver is supplied by portal vein (majority – minority by HA)
- o Peak pancreatic enhancement occurs after enhancement of the aorta and before peak enhancement of the liver (portal)
- o Perfect time to visualize the pancreatic mass is between those
- o Still allowing enhancement of the important pancreatic vessels (arteries and veins)
- o Hepatic phase enhancement to visualize hypovascular hepatic metastases
- o Need minimal dual–phase CT

Operating Parameters hCT
- o Most patients with pancreatic cancer have already had a CT of teh abdomen (if at least dual–phase enhancement is not done, then it should be repeated)
- o CT or EUS should be done before biliary stenting is done as the inflammatory reaction occur secondary to stent could interfere with imaging

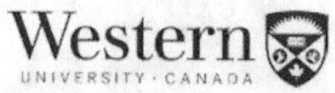

Detecting a Pancreatic Mass

- o The larger the mass the more likely you will find it on your CT

- o Masses < 2 cm in size (best prognosis is 12 – 20% in 5–y survival) are not well–visualized by CT (sen is 65 – 75%) *vs* EUS (sen is 98%)

- o If pretest likelihood of the disease is high with a negative CT should go to EUS

- o 11% of pancreatic cancers are isoattenuating (pathology by local effect)

- o Indirect signs on CT: dilated PD, CBD, double duct sign, mass effect, pancreatic atrophy, pancreatic contour is abnormal

Assessment of Vascular Invasion

Category	Description	Comment
Grade 0	No contiguity of tumour with a vessel	0% invasion
Grade 1	Tumor contiguous with < 25% of the circumference of a vessel	0% invasion
Grade 2	Tumor contiguous with 25-50% of the circumference of a vessel	57% invasion
Grade 3	Tumor contiguous with 50-75% of the circumference of a vessel	88% invasion
Grade 4	Tumou contiguous with >75% of the circumference of a vessel	100% invasion

Lu, *et al.* AJR. 1997; 16:1439-144.; O'Malley, *et al.* AJR. 1999; 173:1513-1518.

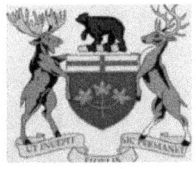

Presence of Metastases

- o Precludes surgery
  - Ascites
  - Hepatic metastases
  - Peritoneal nodules
  - Omental caking
  - Celiac axis metastases

- o CT pitfall
  - Small lesions are difficult to characterize hypodense lesions (< 10 mm) with ~ 12% represent metastases[*] follow–up *vs* MRI *vs* Bx

- o Unexpected hepatic metastases are responsible for 40 – 60% of aborted resections of pancreatic cancer

- o 34% of patients without CT showing distant metastases were found to have metastatic disease on laparotomy[^]; many surgeons perform laparoscopy before

[*]Schwartz, *et al. Radiology.* 1999; 210:71-74.; [^]Liu, *et al. Surg Endosc.* 19:638-642.

MRI

- o MRI is worse than CT in staging PDAC (sens, 84% *vs* 91%) in meta–analysis[*]

- o MRI is helpful with CT lesion < 10 mm with 92% accuracy (for benign cyst, hemangioma *vs* malignant lesion)[^]

[*]Bipat, *et al. J comput Assist Tomogr.* 2005; 29:438-445.
[^]Holakere, *et al. J comput Assist Tomogr.* 2006; 30:591-596.

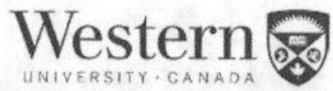

Pancreas

- o A organ, which is difficult to image
- o Close proximity to stomach allows ease of imaging with EUS
- o CLA introduction allows for FNA and FNI
- o Best role in staging, sampling and providing palliative therapy in pancreatic disease

What is EUS?

- o EUS
  - Imaging beyond the lumen
- o Combining endoscope with US with transducer at the tip
- o Bypass
  - Gas
  - Soft tissue
  - Bone
- o Advantage
  - Allows use of higher frequency with resultant better image resolution
  - Allows tissue sampling and therapy

Why bother with EUS?

- o The "appreciated value" of technology is conditional on its use and experience
- o Akin to:
  - EGD and colonoscopy
  - ERCP
  - CT
  - MRI
  - PET

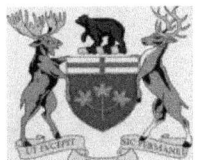

What is EUS used for?

- Mediastinal:
  - Esophageal cancer
  - Lung cancer
  - Mediastinal LN, Mass
  - ENT tumors (thyroid, mets to mediastinum)
- Colonic:
  - Rectal cancer staging
  - Anal sphincter complex
  - Perianal Fistula
- Retroperitoneal:
  - Pancreatic cancer staging
  - Pancreatic mass FNA
  - Pancreatic cystic lesion
  - Chronic pancreatitis
  - Celiac plexus Neurolysis and block
- SMT
- Biliary stones
- Other - interventional

When do the author order an EUS?

- High likelihood of pancreatic carcinoma with negative CT
- CT reveals unresectable disease and you need tissue for palliative care
- Failed CT–guided Bx does not impact tissue diagnosis by EUS
- Suspect the following:
  - Disease is metastatic to pancreas
  - Lymphoma (alters Rx)
  - NET pancreas (alters Rx)
  - Infectious disease (TB)
  - Inflammatory disease (AIP)
- Pain control
  - CPN

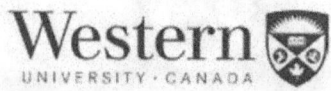

Different Perspectives

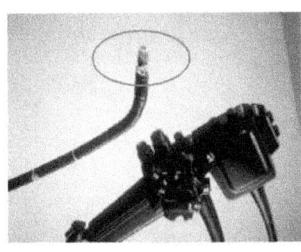
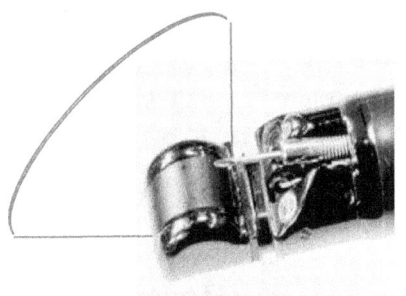

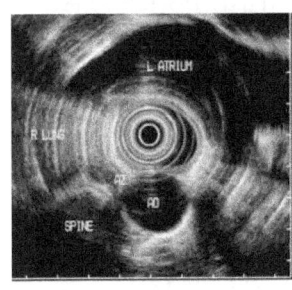
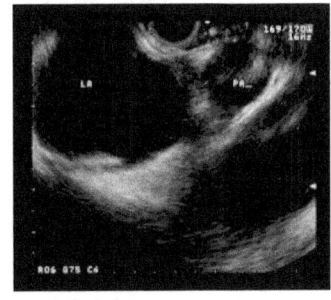

Image Orientation

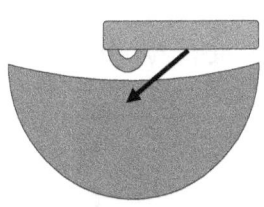
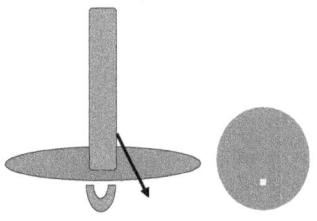

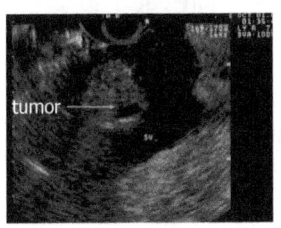
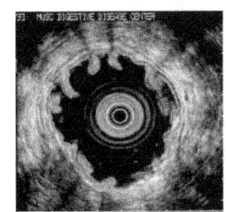

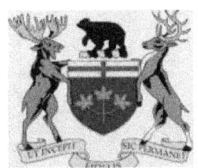

Screening for Pancreatic Cancer

International Cancer of Pancreas Screening (CAPS): Consortium summit in the management of patients with increased risk of familial pancreatic Cancer

Canto, M.I., *et al. Gut.* 2013 ;62(3):339-47.

- ➢ Questions
  - ○ Who should be screened?
  - ○ How should high-risk individuals (HRI) be screened and followed–up?
  - ○ When should surgery be performed?
  - ○ What are the goals of screening and should be considered a success?

- ➢ Yields
  - ○ Theoretically:
    - – PPV =

$$PPV = \frac{\text{sensitivity} \times \text{prevalence}}{\text{sensitivity} \times \text{prevalence} + (1\text{-specificity}) \times (1\text{-prevalence})}$$

    - – General population has risk of 1.3%
    - – Test with 90% sensitivity and specificity
    - – PPV = 12%
    - – 9/10 patients found would be incorrect and would be subject to further unnecessary testing and stress
    - – If Sensitivity/Specificity of test increased to 95%, then PPV = 22%

  - ○ Increasing yields
    - – By either increasing sensitivity or prevalence of the underlying disease, one can increase PPV (yields)
    - – Increasing prevalence of disease
      - ▪ Identify patients at higher risk of PDAC

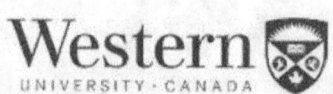

➢ Who should be screened?
- General population risk is 1.3%
- Individuals with risk of > 5% have lifetime risk of 5x RR
- Individuals with known genetic susceptibility identified by gene testing or those with increased risk but no known gene (familial pancreatic cancer)

Modifiable Risk Factors

Risk	Increased PDAC risk
o Current cigarette use	1.7 – 2.2
o Current pipe or cigar use	1.5
o > 3 alcoholic drinks per day	1.2 – 1.4
o Chronic pancreatitis	13.3
o BMI > 40 kg/m^2 male	1.5
o BMI > 40 kg/m^2 female	2.8
o Diabetes mellitus, type 1	2.0
o Diabetes mellitus, type 2	1.8
o Cholecystectomy	1.2
o Gastrectomy	1.5
o *Helicobacter pylori* infection	1.4

Familial Pancreatic Cancer (FPC)
- Based on RR of PDAC, rather than proven efficacy
  - ≥ 2 FDR with PDAC
  - FDR plus ≥ blood relatives with PDAC

Abbreviations: FDR, first degree relative; PDAC, pancreatic duct adenocarcinoma; RR, relative risk

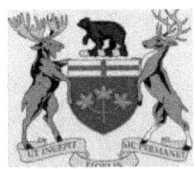

Mutational Carriers

Risk factors	Genes	Increased PDAC risk	Other associated cancers
Hereditary breast and ovarian cancer syndrome	BRCA1, BRCA2, PALB2	2 – 3.5	- Breast, ovarian, prostate
Lynch syndrome (hereditary non-polyposis colorectal cancer)	MLH1, MSH2, MSH6, PMS2, EPCAM	8.6	- Colon, endometrium, ovary, stomach, small intestine, urinary tract, brain, cutaneous sebaceous glands
Familial adenomatous polyposis	APC	4.5 – 6	- Colon, desmoid, duodenum, thyroid, brain, ampullary, hepatoblastoma
Peutz-Jeghers syndrome	STKI1 / LKB1	132	- Esophagus, stomach, small intestine, colon, lungs, breast, uterus, ovary
Familial atypical multiple mole melanoma pancreatic carcinoma syndrome	P16NK4A, CDKN2A	47	Melanoma

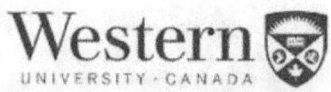

Risk factors	Genes	Increased PDAC risk	Other associated cancers
o Hereditary pancreatitis	PRSS1, SPINK1	69	
o Cystic fibrosis	CFTR	3.5	
o Ataxia-telangiectasia	ATM	Increased	– Leukemia, lymphoma
o Non-O blood group		13	
o Familial pancreatic cancer	Unknown	9(1FDR) 32(3FDRs)	

Becker, A.E., *et al. World J Gastroenterol.* 2014; 20(32):11182-98.

Mutational carriers

- o BRCA2 (HBOCS) with 1 FDR or 2 family members with PDAC
- o MSI (HNPCC) with 1 FDR with PDAC
- o p16 (FAMMM) with 1 FDR with PDAC
- o PALB2 (FPC) with 1 FDR with PDAC
- o PRSS1 (HP)
- o STK11 (PJS)

Abbreviations: FDR, first degree relative; FPC, familial pancreatic cancer; HP, hereditary pancreatitis; PDAC, pancreatic duct adenocarcinoma; PJS, Peutz Jegher syndrome

The Dilemmas of Screening

- o Wide variation of diagnostic yield in various screening programs

- o Unknown at what age to start screening or to stop surveillance

- Give the ideal test features in screening for PDAC.
  - o High sensitivity and specificity
  - o Non–ionizing radiation
  - o Non–invasive
  - o Low complication rate
  - o Eliminates CT or ERCP as test of choice
  - o Presently EUS/MRI; MRCP quality

What test to use?

➢ Laboratory: CA19–9

- o CA19–9 is the only marker available and approved by FDA
  - – Appears to be informative as a predictor of disease recurrence post–resection

- o In low prevalence populations:
  - – Sensitivity, 70%
  - – Specificity, 87%
  - – PPV, 59%
  - – NPV, 92%

➢ Diagnostic imaging: CAPS 3 study

- o Few studies compare CT/MRI/EUS in HRI for PDAC
- o CAPS 3 studied asymptomatic 225 HRI (PJS/HBOS + 1FDR or 1SDR with PDAC/ FPC + 1FDR with PDAC)
- o 92/225 (40%) found to have abnormal (84 cysts; 3 solid; 5 dilated MPD) findings
- o CT detected, 11%; MRI, 33%; EUS, 42.6%

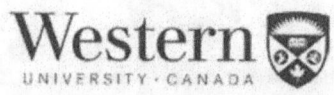

Surveillance
- o A negative test
  - – Followed by repeat imaging in 1 year
- o Positive test by repeat imaging in 3 months
  - – Followed if quick surgical therapy is not possible
- o Low risk lesion found: cystic or solid (LN/NET) < 1 cm in size
  - – Repeat imaging in 3 months

When to consult PB surgeon?
- o Screen only those who are eligible for surgery
- o Solid lesions have > 1 cm seen by multiple modalities should be resected
- o Majority of lesions found are cystic in nature IPMN–BD and should follow the recommendation for IPMN management with lower thresholds for HRI

IPMN–BD Sendai International Guidelines
- o For high risk IPMN–BD:
  - – Cysts > 3 cm (> 2 cm in HRI)
  - – Mural nodularity
  - – Symptomatic
  - – Abnormal cytology

Defining Success
- o CAPS consortium defined success as:
  - – Finding PanIN3
  - – IPMN–BD with HGD
  - – Mucinous cystic neoplasm (adenoma or carcinoma)
  - – Small Invasive resectable PDAC (T1N0M0)

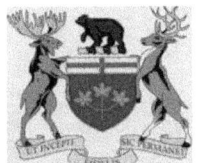

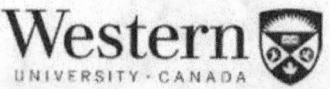

Disease of Excess Fat in the Liver: Non–Alcoholic Fatty Liver Disease

Melanie Beaton

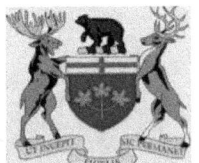

CanMeds – Health Advocate

1. Respond to individual patient health needs and issues as part of patient care
2. Respond to health needs of the communities that they serve
3. Identify the determinants of health of the populations that they serve
4. Promote the health of individual patients, communities and populations

RCPSC, 2006

➢ Objectives

- Advocate for individual patients, populations and communities
- Health promotion and disease prevention
- Fiduciary duty to care
- Medical profession's role in society
- Mobilizing resources as needed
- Patient Safety
- Adapting practice, management and education to the needs of individual patient
- Principles of health policy and its implication
- Community recognition of problem in obesity and its complications
  - Food policies
  - Healthy eating programs
  - Exercise programs
  - Increased access to dietician services
  - Funding for research in metabolic disease
- Encourage and provide information on alcohol cessation programs, healthy diet and lifestyle

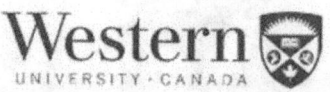

- o Advocate for resources to support patients on these paths
  - As MDs we have a unique voice and ability to mobilize resources

- o Controversies surrounding transplantation
  - Alcoholics
  - Obesity

- o Ensure patient and community are kept "safe"
  - Drivers license
  - SW, Community supports for patient/family (AA, Al-anon...)

- o "As *Health Advocates*, physicians responsibly use their expertise and influence to advance the health and well-being of individual patients, communities, and populations".

- **Non–alcoholic Steatohepatitis** (NASH)

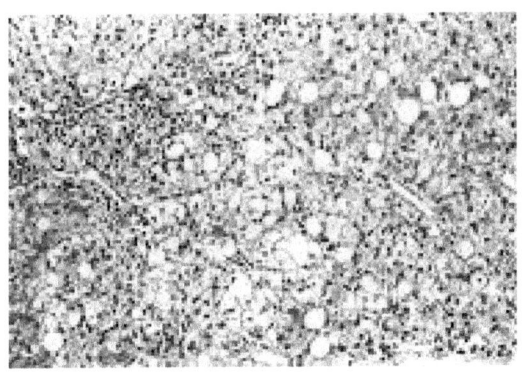

- o 3 – 5% in the general population[1,2]

- o High Risk Groups[3]
  - Type II DM: 10-25%
  - Obesity: up to 50%
  - Hyperlipidemia
  - Metabolic syndrome

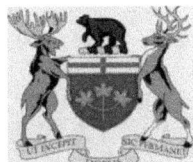

- Male sex
- Hispanic ethnicity
- Aboriginal Canadians

[1]Wanless, I.R. and Lentz, J.S. *Hepatology.* 1990; 12(5):1106-10.

[2]Vernon, G., *et al. Aliment Pharmacol Ther.* 2011; 34(3):274-85.

[3] Williams, C.D., *et al. Gastroenterology.* 2011; 140(1):124-31.

➢ Demography

"Home Sweet Home" Self–reported Overweight and Obesity

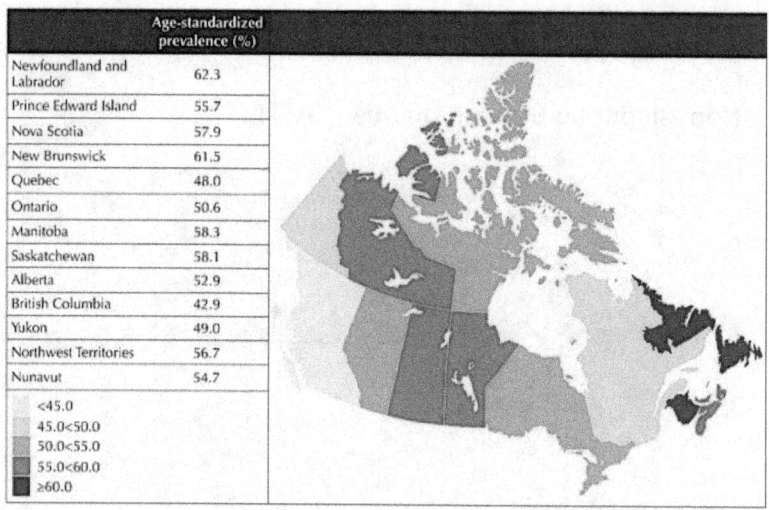

	Age-standardized prevalence (%)
Newfoundland and Labrador	62.3
Prince Edward Island	55.7
Nova Scotia	57.9
New Brunswick	61.5
Quebec	48.0
Ontario	50.6
Manitoba	58.3
Saskatchewan	58.1
Alberta	52.9
British Columbia	42.9
Yukon	49.0
Northwest Territories	56.7
Nunavut	54.7

- <45.0
- 45.0<50.0
- 50.0<55.0
- 55.0<60.0
- ≥60.0

www.publichealth.gc.ca. 2011.

- o A Global Epidemic
  - 1.4 billion people worldwide are overweight
  - 500 million are obese
  - 65% live in countries where being overweight causes more deaths than being underweight

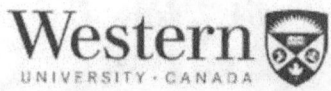

Caution

- o Obesity is now a greater global health threat than malnutrition.

WHO, May 2012

- **Non–Alcoholic Fatty Liver Disease** (NAFLD)
  - o NAFLD is common because obesity is common
    - Hepatic steatosis
      - 20 – 30% of adult population
      - 80 – 90% of obese individuals

  - o Prevalence
    - NHANES III (N=15,700)[1]
      - Assessed NAFLD with aminotransferases
        - *General prevalence: 5.5%*

        } 3 – 10x > prevalence than HCV (1.8% population)

    - Dallas Heart Study (N=2,349)[2]
      - Assessed with liver imaging
        - *General prevalence: 33.6%*

[1]Liangpunsakul, S. and Chalasani, N. *Am J Med Sci.* 2005; 329(3):111-6.
[2]Szczepaniak. L.S., *et al. Am J Physiol Endocrinol Metab.* 2005; 288(2):E462-8.

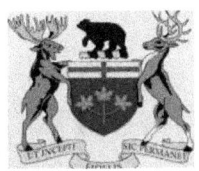

- #1 cause of liver disease in industrialized countries
    - 40% newly diagnosed chronic liver disease[1]
    - ≈ 90% of asymptomatic transaminase elevation when other causes are excluded[2]
- Laboratory alert: up to 80% of patients with NAFLD have normal transaminases[3]

[1]Weston, S.R., *et al. Hepatology.* 2005 Feb; 41(2):372-9.
[2]Angulo, P. *N Engl J Med.* 2002; 346:1221-1231.
[3]Browning, J.D. *Hepatology.* 2006; 44(2):466-71.

➢ Natural History

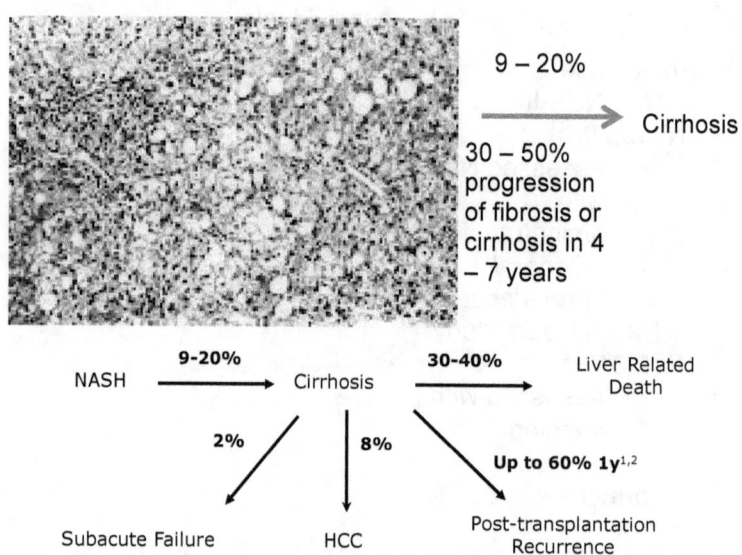

9 – 20%

Cirrhosis

30 – 50% progression of fibrosis or cirrhosis in 4 – 7 years

NASH	→(9-20%)	Cirrhosis	→(30-40%) Liver Related Death

2% / 8%

Up to 60% 1y[1,2]

Subacute Failure   HCC   Post-transplantation Recurrence

[1]Dureja, P., et al. Transplantation. 2011; 91(6):684-9.
[2]Patil, D.T. and Yerian, L.M. *Liver Transpl.* 2012; 18(10):1147-53.

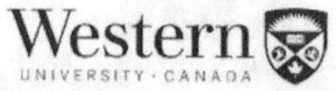

- o NAFLD
    - – ↑ all cause mortality

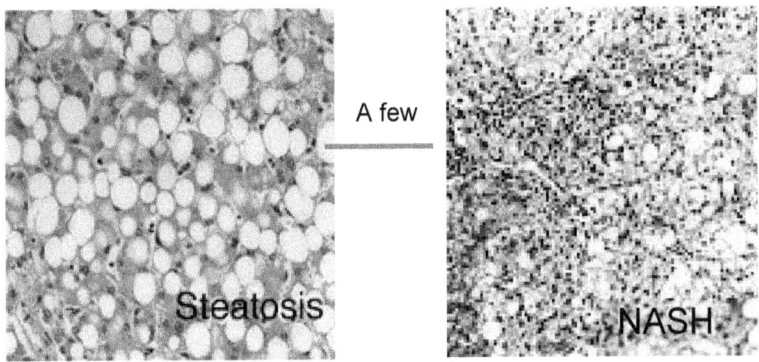

A few

Steatosis   NASH

- o NASH
    - – ↑ liver–related mortality
    - – #3 vs #13 general population
- o #1 cause of death = cardiovascular disease
    - – 25% mortality[1]
    - – > general population
- o NASH
    - – Associated cirrhosis has similar survival to other forms of chronic liver diseases with cirrhosis[2,3]

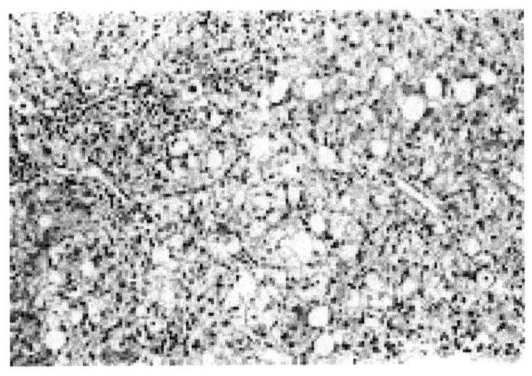

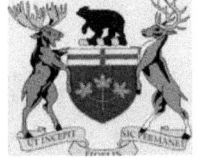

[1]Adams, L.A. and Angulo, P. *Diabet Med.* 2005; 22(9):1129-33.

[2]Sanyal, A.J., *et al. Hepatology.* 2006 Apr; 43(4):682-9.

[3]Yatsuji, S., *et al. J Gastroenterol Hepatol.* 2009; 24(2):248-54.

➢ Other causes and comorbidities of NAFLD

- o Nutrition
  - EtOH, EtOH, EtOH!
  - Rapid weight loss
  - TPN
    - Can occur rapidly
    - Typically reversible

- o Surgery
  - J–I bypass
  - Gastroplasty
  - Extensive SB resection

- o Infection
  - Small intestinal bacterial overgrowth (SIBO)
  - HCV
  - HIV

- o Metabolic disorders
  - Obesity
  - Metabolic syndrome*
  - Diabetes, type 2*
  - Dyslipidemia*
  - Hypo– or Abetalipoprotenemia
  - Lipodystrophies
  - Wilson Disease
  - Glycogen storage disease
  - Hypothyroidism
  - Hypopituitariasm
  - Polycystic ovarian syndrome (POS)

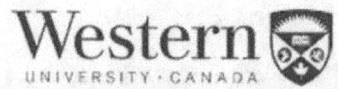

o Drugs
  - Amiodarone
  - Antiretrovirals
  - Corticosteroids
  - Methotrexate
  - Tamoxifen
  - Valproate

o Obstructive sleep apnea (OSA)

*Established comorbidities

Vuppalanchi, *et al. Hepatology.* 2009; 49:306-17.

Advanced Fibrosis in Non–Alcoholic Fatty Liver Disease: Non–Invasive Assessment with MR Elastography

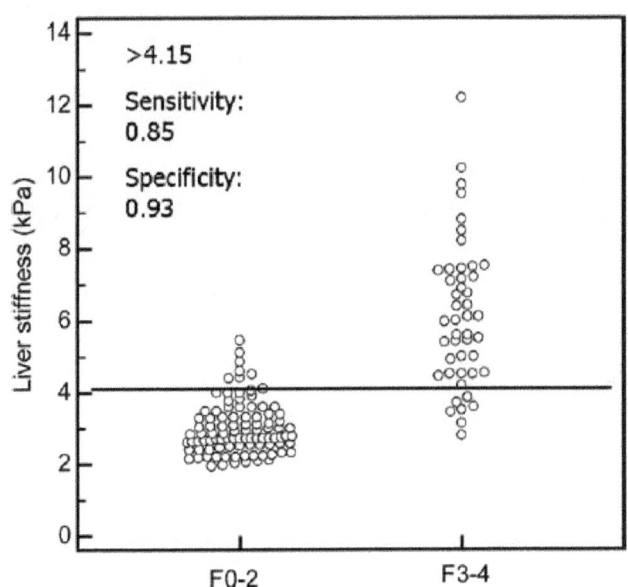

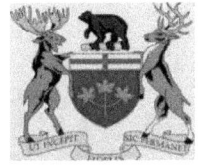

- o 142 NASH subjects with MRE and biopsy
- o Graph shows liver stiffness measured at MR elastography for early (F0–F2) *vs* fibrosis
- o Associated with a sensitivity and specificity of MR elastography in detecting advanced fibrosis of 85% and 92.9%

Kim, D., *et al. Radiology.* 2013; 268(2):411-9.

MR Elastography

NAFLD without fibrosis

NAFLD with advanced fibrosis

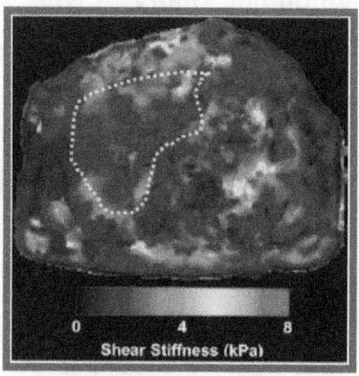 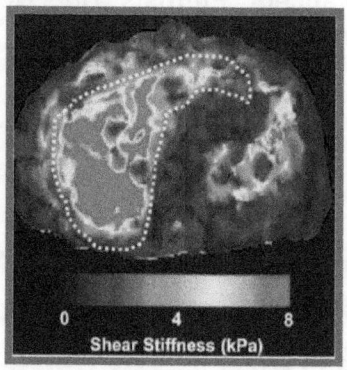

- o Performance characteristics of advanced cirrhosis
- o The best discriminating cut–off of liver stiffness to diagnose advanced fibrosis (F3–F4) from early fibrosis (F0–F2) of 4.15 kPa
  - – Sensitivity, 85%
  - – Specificity, 93%

Kim, D., *et al. Radiology.* 2013; 268(2):411-9.

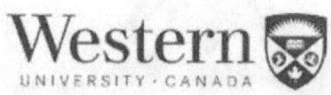

- o Fibroscan and MR elastography
  - – Both good for fibrosis
  - – MRE may be better at distinguishing between grades of fibrosis

- ➢ Diagnosis

  - o Blood tests
    - – Transaminase
      - ▪ If not reliable, assess for steatohepatitis and fibrosis
    - – Radiology
  - o Liver biopsy
    - – Invasive
      - ▪ Associated risks
    - – Current gold standard but somewhat *"tarnished"*
    - – Samples have small portion of the liver
      - ▪ $1/50,000^{th}$ or 0.002%
    - – Sampling variability
      - ▪ K = 0.64 for consecutive biopsies

Non–invasive tests for NAFLD, NASH and advanced fibrosis

- • Laboratory

NAFLD *vs* Non-NAFLD	NASH *vs* Not NASH	No to Minimal Fibrosis *vs* Advanced Fibrosis
Fatty Liver Index (FLI)	CK-18	FIB 4
	FGF 21	AST/ALT Ratio
	NASH Test	NAFLD Fibrosis Score

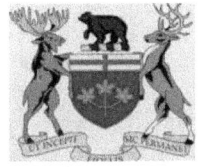

- Diagnostic imaging

NAFLD vs Non-NAFLD	NASH vs Not NASH	No to Minimal Fibrosis vs Advanced Fibrosis
U/S	possibly MRI	Transient elastography
CT		MR elastography
MR spectroscopy		

Apps available: *www.nafldscore.com*; *www.gihep.com*

- ○ NAFLD Fibrosis Score (NFS), FIB–4, BARD
  - – Use the readily available variables
- ○ Each have NPV of ~ 90% for advanced fibrosis
- ○ Annual change over time shown to correlate with risk of mortality

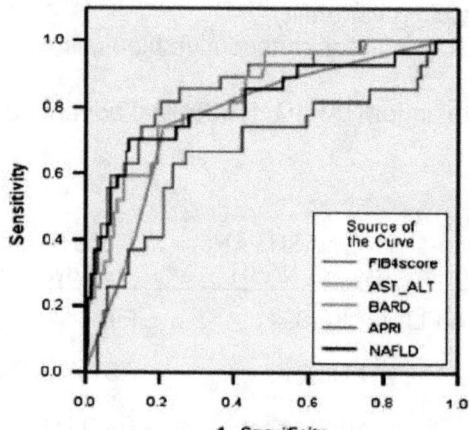

Abbreviation: NPV, negative predictive value

Angulo, P., *et al. Hepatology.* 2007; 45(4):846-54.; McPherson, S., *et al. Gut.* 2010; 59(9):1265-9.; Kim, D., *et al. Radiology.* 2013; 268(2):411-9.; Treeprasertsuk, S., *World J Gastroenterol.* 2013; 19(8):1219-29.

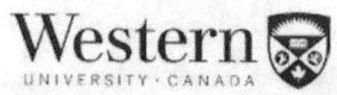

- o Serum Cytokeratin 18 (CK–18)
    - Major intermediate filament protein in liver and substrate of caspase enzymes during apoptosis
    - ↑↑ NASH *vs* NAFLD
    - Performance characteristics
        - Sensitivity, 78%
        - Specificity, 87%
        - AUC, 0.82[1]
    - ↓ post–bariatric surgery and paralleled biopsy changes[2]

[1]Musso, G., *et al. Ann Med.* 2011; 43(8):617-49.
[2]Sutsui, M., *et al. J Clin Gastroenterol.* 2010; 44(6):440-7.

- o PNPLA3 (Patatin–like phospholipase domain containing 3 gene)
    - Meta--analysis
        - Unequivocal evidence of re738409 as a strong modifier of the natural history of NAFLD in different populations around the world
    - N =16 studies, 2,651 subjects with liver biopsy
    - PNPLA3 (*Adiponutrin*) variant associated with:
        - 73% higher fat content
        - 3.2x ↑ risk of the following:
            - Inflammation and ballooning
            - Developing fibrosis

Sookoian, S. and Pirola, C.J. *Hepatology.* 2011; 53:1883-1894.

- ➤ Treatment
    - o Current options
        - Lifestyle modification
            - Intensive intervention appears necessary
                - Treatment arms with basic education about diet, weight loss and exercise have not consistently shown sufficient weight loss to improve liver histology

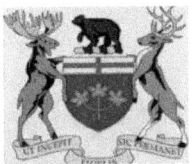

- - Of the 50% of Canadians who are dieting, only 5% are successful
  - Pharmacotherapy
  - Liver transplantation
- ○ Future possibilities
  - Pentoxifylline
  - ARBs
  - Incretin mimetics
  - Probiotics
  - FXR agonists
  - Bariatric surgery
  - Microbiome modification

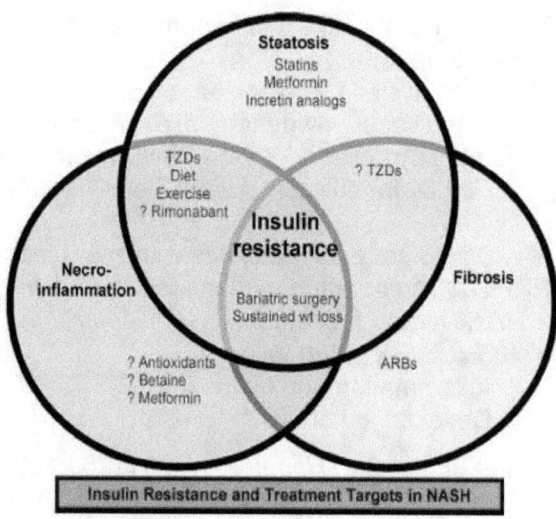

Kashi, M.R., *et al. Semin Liver Dis.* 2008; 28:396-406.

- ○ Basic tenants of treatment
- ○ Lifestyle modifications to ↓ body weight
  - Diet
  - Exercise
- ○ Review medications
  - Hepatotoxins and those associated with steatosis

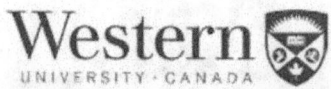

- o Minimize and eliminate EtOH
- o Optimize management of co–morbidities
  - Diabetes
    - Preferably followed by endocrinologist
  - Cardiovascular disease
    - Risk stratification
  - Lipids
    - Statins are safe
  - Consider screening for PCOS, hypothyroidism, OSA

Abbreviations: EtOH, ethanol (alcohol); OSA, obstructive sleep apnea; PCOS, polycystic ovarian syndrome

- o Weight loss
  - #1 cardiovascular disease
  - #2 malignancy
  - Improves transaminases
  - ↓ body weight → ↓ steatosis → ↓ inflammation → ≥ 10% improves fibrosis → ↑ insulin sensitivity

- o Special consideration
  - Dietary fructose

Ligibel, J.A., *et al. J Clin Oncol.* 2014; 32(31):3568-74.

Fructose

- o Monosaccharide

- o Dietary sources
  - Sucrose (disaccharide, glucose + fructose)
  - High–fructose corn syrup, "glucose–fructose"
  - 5x ↑ consumption in the past century and more than doubled in the past 30 years

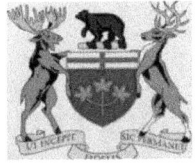

- o Average
  - Consumption of fructose 60 pounds per person–year

- o High Fructose Corn Syrup
  - Daily consumption associated with increased liver fibrosis, inflammation and ballooning
  - "…..a readily modifiable environmental risk factor that may ameliorate disease progression in patients with NAFLD."

Abdelmalek, M.F., *et al. Hepatology.* 2010; 51(6):1961-71.

- o Fructose and liver
  - 1° site of fructose metabolism
  - Fructose differs from glucose metabolism:
    - Insulin independent
      → very rapid hepatic uptake and accumulation
    - Fails to trigger Leptin secretion
      → lacks satiety
    - ↑ *de novo* TG synthesis and ↓ free fatty acid oxidation
      → intrahepatic lipid accumulation
    - ↓ hepatic ATP in obese, DM2 patients[1]
      → hepatocyte injury and fibrosis
- o ≥ 7 servings of fructose per day
  - ↑ severity of fructose in all ages
  - ↑ steatosis, lobular inflammation, hepatocyte, ballooning in patients ≥ 48 years old

Abdelmalek, M.F., *et al. Hepatology.* 2012; 56(3):952-60.

Take Home Facts on Fructose

Reduce daily intake of fructose << 7 servings

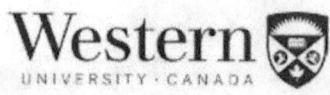

Coffee

- o ↓ weight gain
- o ↓ diabetes
- o ↓ chronic liver disease
- o ↓ Hepatocellular cancer (HCC)

Huxley, R., *et al. Arch Intern Med.* 2009; 169(22):2053-63.; Modi, A.A., *et al. Hepatology.* 2010; 51(1):201-9.; Bravi, F., *et al. Clin Gastroenterol Hepatol.* 2013; 11(11):1413-1421.

- o Further evidence
  - – Moderate coffee consumption may be a benign adjunct to the management of NASH (Molloy, J.W., *et al. Hepatology.* 2012; 55:429-436).
  - – Caffeine is protective in patients with non–alcoholic fatty liver disease (Birerdinc, A., *et al. Aliment Pharmacol Ther.* 2012; 35(1):76-82).
    - ▪ Can daily coffee consumption reduce liver–related mortality?
    - ▪ Is it time to write a prescription for coffee? Coffee and liver disease.
  - – Coffee reduces the risk for hepatocellular carcinoma: An updated meta–analysis
  - – Regular coffee, but not espresso drinking, is protective against fibrosis in a cohort mainly composed of morbidity obese European women with NAFLD undergoing bariatric surgery
  - – > 1000 compounds are potentially responsible
  - – Is it coffee or caffeine?
    - ▪ As yet unanswered
    - ▪ Lower caffeine intake an independent predictor of NAFLD[2]
  - – Espresso or drip?
    - ▪ Regular coffee is protective of fibrosis[1]
    - ▪ Specific to coffee and not in other caffeinated beverages

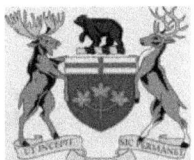

Anty, R., *et al. J Hepatol.* 2012; 57(5):1090-6.; Birerdinc, A., *et al. Aliment Pharmacol Ther.* 2012; 35(1):76-82.

Summary of Lifestyle Modification

- Exercise
  - Aerobic or resistance training 3 – 5x/week for 30 – 60 minutes, at least moderate intensity
- Diet Composition
  - ↓ fructose
  - ↓ carbohydrate benefits in insulin resistance
  - < 10% total energy from saturated fat
  - < 30% total fat
- Coffee
  - Inverse relationship between coffee and NASH fibrosis, fibrosis and HCC
  - Moderate daily unsweetened coffee is a reasonable recommendation

Pharmacotherapy

Agents studied in NASH

Insulin sensitizers / incretin mimetics
- Troglitazone
- Pioglitazone
- Rosiglitazone
- Metformin
- Liraglutide
- Exenatide
- Sitagliptin

Antioxidants
- Vitamin E
- Vitamin C
- Betaine

Cytoprotective agents
- Urso
- Taurine
- Lecithin
- Silymarin
  - Carotene
- Metadoxine

Antihyperlipidemic agents
- Clofibrate
- Gemfibrozil
- Atorvastatin
- Pravastatin
- Probucol
- Omega-3 fatty acids

Antiobesity drugs
- Orlistat
- Sibutramine

Novel treatments
- Losartan
- Probiotics
- Lactulose
- Pentoxifylline
- Oligofructose
- Nateglinide
- Ethyl-eicosa-pentaenoic acid
- Obeticholic acid

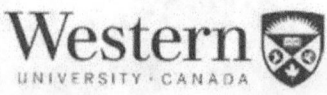

Insulin Sensitizers Metformin

- o Cirrhosis
  - – Not recommended to specifically treat NASH[1]
  - – Benefit of continuing metformin in cirrhotic NASH[2]
    - ▪ Improved survival, 11.8 *vs* 5.6 years
    - ▪ 5–year survival rate
      - Continued metformin, 80%
      - Discontinued metformin, 50%
    - ▪ Regardless of severity of cirrhosis*

[1]Chalasani N, et al. Hepatology. 2012;55(6):2005-23.
[2]Zhang X, et al. Hepatology. 2014;60(6):2008-16.

- o Hepatocellular cancer (HCC)
  - – Background
    - ▪ DM2 confers 3x ↑ risk of HCC
    - ▪ Insulin resistance and hyperinsulinemia influence hepatocarcinogenesis
  - – Proof of principle
    - ▪ Metformin may reduce this risk[1,2]
    - ▪ Activates pathways that inhibit tumor growth
    - ▪ Improves insulin sensitivity
    - ▪ ↑ weight loss
  - – Clinical meta–analysis odds ratio and 95% confidence interval favouring metformin to ↓ risk of HCC 0.502 (0.344 – 0.734)

[1]Miyoshi, H., *et al. Int J Oncol.* 2014; 45(1):322-32.
[2]Singh, S., *et al. Am J Gastroenterol.* 2013; 108(6):881-91.

- o Glucagon–like peptide–1 receptor (GLP–1R) agonists: (Liraglutide and Exenatide)
  - – Cardioprotective, decrease insulin resistance and ↓ BMI
  - – Animal studies and case reports show ↓ steatosis and transaminases
  - – Inconsistent improvement in liver histology[1,2]

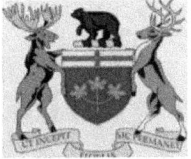

- o Dipeptidyl Peptidase IV (DPP–IV) inhibitors: Sitagliptin (Januvia)
  - – Small studies suggest improved transaminases, histology and weight loss

Kenny, P.R., *et al. Am J Gastroenterol.* 2010; 105(12):2707-9.; Ohki, T., *et al. Scientific World Journal.* 2012; 2012:49(6)453.

- o Lipid lowering agents
  - – Statins, fibrates and ezetimibe are all safe in NASH and improve steatosis and transaminases
  - – Statins presently recommended to treat associated dyslipidemia but not specifically for the treatment of NAFLD
  - – Unclear whether the threshold for treating dyslipidemia in obesity should be reduced
  - – Statins risk of HCC (meta–analysis, odds ratio and 95% confidence interval in favor of statins 0.630 (0.523 – 0.760)

BjorkHem-Bergman, L., *et al. Pharmacoepi Drug Safety.* 2014; 23(10):1101-1106.; Chalasani, N., *et al. Hepatology.* 2012; 55(6):2005-23.; Nseir, W., *et al. Dig Dis Sci.* 2011; 56(12):3439-49.

- o Vitamin E
  - – 0.04% ↑ all–cause mortality
  - – 1% prostate cancer
  - – ↑ hemorrhagic (but ↓ thrombotic stroke) risk
  - – ↑ heart failure
  - – ~ 30% progression to cirrhosis, if high risk
    - Older age
    - Diabetes
    - Obesity
    - NASH + fibrosis

Klein, E.A., *et al. JAMA.* 2011; 306(14):1549-56.

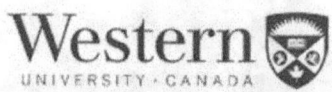

- o Obeticholic acid
  - – Synthetic variant of chenodeoxycholic acid
  - – Potent activator of farnesoid X nuclear receptor
    - ↑insulin sensitivity/ ↓ hepatic gluconeogenesis and TGs
  - – Included were DM and non–DM subjects
  - – 25 mg *po od* given with improved histology (trial stopped early)
    - 45% *vs* 21% placebo
    - However, ↑ TC and LDL, and slight ↓ HDL
    - Pruritis in 23%

Neuschwander-Tetri, *et al. Lancet.* 2015; 385:956-65.

- o Statistically significant

Histopathological improvement	Relative risk (95% CI)
o Resolution of NASH	1.5 (0.9 – 2.6)
o NAFLD activity score	- 0.9 (-1.3 – - 0.5)
o Fibrosis	1.8 (1.1 – 2.7)
o Hepatocyte ballooning	1.5 (1.0 – 2.1)
o Steatosis	1.7 (1.2 – 2.3)
o Lobular inflammation	1.6 (1.1 – 2.2)

- ➤ Bariatric surgery
  - o RCTs being conducted
    - – Safety?
    - – Which surgery is the best?
    - – Longterm efficacy?
  - o Cumulative incidence of type 2 diabetes for 15 years in obese Swedish patients having bariatric surgery hazard ratio, 95% CI 0.22 (0.18 – 0.27), P < 0.001

Carlsson, L.M.S., *et al. N ENgl J Med.* 2012; 367(8):695-704.

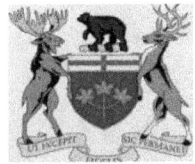

- o   Improvement in liver histology[1]
    - - Maximal benefit seen 1 year post–op
    - - Benefit maintained in 5 years[2]

- o   ↑ satiety hormones

- o   ↑ incretin levels = ↑ insulin sensitivity[3]

[1]Mummadi, R.R., *et al. Clin Gastroenterol Hepatol.* 2008; 6(12):1396-402.
[2]Mathurin, P., *et al. Gastroenterology.* 2009; 137(2):532-40.
[3]Laferrere, B., *et al. J Clin Endocrinol Metab.* 2008; 93(7):2479-85.

➢ Liver transplantation

- o   Outcomes for patients underwent liver transplant for NASH are similar to those with other indications

Microbes

- o   Potential source of hepatotoxic oxidative injury
- o   Dietary intake influences microbiome
- o   NAFLD patients have ↑ gut permeability, which may enhance endotoxin absorption

Wu, G.D., *et al. Science.* 2011; 334(6052):105-8.

- o   Microbiome differs in obese mice *vs* lean
- o   Transfer of microbiota from obsess to lean mice ↑ severity of NAFLD
- o   Infflamasome–mediated   dysbiosis   regulates progression of NAFLD and obesity

Henao-Mejia, J., *et al. Nature.* 482(7384): 179-185.

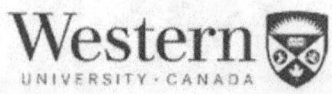

➢ Summary
  o Involves dietician, if resources are available
  o Diet
    – Avoid high fructose foods and beverages
    – Moderate carbohydrate, low fat, low GI foods
    – Portion control, lean protein for satiety
    – Moderate coffee (avoid the "double double")
  o Exercise
    – 30 minutes 3 – 5 days/week, with goal of daily exercise
    – *Note
      ▪ 400 calories/session improves insulin resistance and steatosis, not weight
      ▪ 700 – 800 calories are needed for weight loss

Is this forever?

  o If liver enzymes improve over 12 months
    – Consider liver biopsy to assess histologic improvement
      ▪ Confirm improvement
      ▪ Change and discontinue therapy, if no improvement
  o If no improvement in liver enzymes by 6 months
    – Consider liver biopsy
      ▪ Change and discontinue, if no improvement

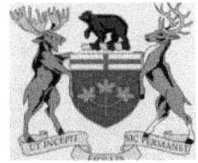

392

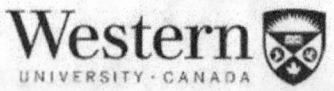

LIVER TRANSPLANTATION

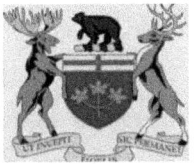

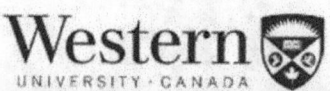

Pulmonary Assessment Pre–Liver Transplantation

Ngoc Han Quang Le

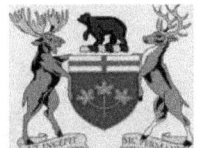

- Demography
  - Incidence
    - 2 – 19%: non–cardiothoracic surgeries

- Impact
  - Equals prevalence and impact on morbidity and mortality, as well as on length of stay (LOS) *vs* cardiac complications
  - Better prediction of long term mortality

- Causes and associations

- Give the potential causes of **increasing dyspnea** in a patient with chronic liver disease.
  - Heart
    - Cardiac failure (cirrhotic cardiomyotomy and tricuspid valve incompetence)
  - Lung
    - Pulmonary hypertension (portopulmonary hypertension syndrome, PPH)
    - Pleural and pericardial effusions
    - Atelectasis is secondary to ascites
    - Pulmonary embolus
    - Aspiration pneumonia
    - Pulmonary infection
    - Pulmonary fibrosis (methotrexate)
    - Interstitial lung disease
  - Metabolic
    - Acidosis
    - Severe anemia

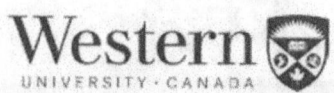

- o Liver disease
  - Liver disease – associated with lung disease
    - Cystic fibrosis
    - α_1–antitrypin deficiency
    - Pulmonary fibrosis from use of methotrexate
  - Pulmonary complications of chronic liver disease
    - Spontaneous bacterial hydrothorax
    - Hepatopulmonary syndrome (HPS)

Adapted from: Kim, Y.K., *et al. Radiographics.* 2009 ;29(3):825-37.

- ➤ Outline
  - o General pulmonary risk assessment pre–LTx (liver transplantation)
  - o Pulmonary complications from underlying chronic liver disease (CLD)
    - Hepatopulmonary syndrome (HPS)
    - Portopulmonay hypertension (PPH)
  - o Impact perioperatively
    - Strategies for optimization of perioperative outcomes

- ➤ Portoperative Pulmonary Complications (PPC)
  - o Definition
    - Atelectasis
    - Infection
      - Bronchitis
      - Pneumonia
    - Respiratory failure
    - Exacerbation of underlying chronic lung disease
    - Others: PE, ARDS, bronchospasm

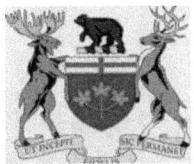

➢ Patient–related risk factors (RF)
- General health and nutritional status
  - Age > 60 years
    - 2nd most commonly validated RF
    - 60 – 69 years old: OR, 2.09
    - 70 – 79 years old: OR, 3.04
  - Weight loss ≥ 10% within the past 6 months
    - Obesity
      - Not a meaningful predictor
      - 6.3 *vs* 7% PPC rate for obese *vs* non–obese patients
  - Functional status
    - Total dependence: OR, 2.51
    - Partial dependence: OR, 1.65

American Society of Anesthesiologist (ASA) classification

		ASA class	Class definition	Rate of PPCs by Class, %
○	Normal	I	Normally healthy patient	1.2
○	Mild	II	Patient with mild systemic disease	5.4
○	Moderate	III	Patient with systemic incapacitating disease	11.4
○	Severe	IV	Patient with an incapacitating systemic disease that is a constant threat of life	10.9
○	Moribund	V	Moribund patient who is not expected to survive for 24 hours with or without operation	NA

Abbreviation: PPCs, post–operative pulmonary complications

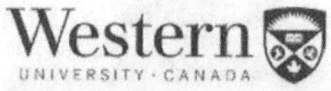

- o Albumin level
  - – Most important predictor of 30–day post–op mortality and morbidity (M&M; usually below 35)
    - Low *vs* normal albumin
  - – 27.6% *vs* 7% PPC

- Respiratory status
  - o Tobacco use
    - – Modest ↑ risk in PPC (OR, 1.26)
      - 2 weeks: risk of respiratory failure
      - 1 year: risk of pneumonia
  - o OSA
    - – ↑ risk of acute hypercapnia and hypoxemia within 24 hours
    - – ICU transfer
      - 24% *vs* 9% in control
  - o Asthma
    - – No effect
  - o COPD
    - – OR, 1.79 (no clear incremental risk even with worsening airflow obstruction [Rybak, D., *et al. Liver Transpl.* 2008; 14(9):1357–65.])
  - o Neurological status (OR, 1.2 – 1.5)
    - – Stroke CVA history
    - – Impaired sensorium
  - o Fluid status
    - – Heart failure (HF)
    - – BUN level > 7.5 mmol/L
  - o Immune status
    - – Diabetes mellitus (DM)
    - – Alcohol abuse
    - – Chronic immunosuppressant

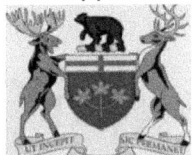

- ➤ Diagnostic Tests
  - o Diagnostic imaging
    - – Chest X–ray (CXR)
      - ▪ Routine pre–op assessment
      - ▪ Findings that alter management: 1 – 4% only
  - o Pulmonary function tests (PFT)
    - – ACP guidelines (1990) recommended PFT in selected patients
    - – Helps establish
      - ▪ Diagnosis, if symptomatic
      - ▪ Baseline for follow–up
    - – Does not translate into effective risk prediction
    - – No established lowest threshold that would prohibit surgery

- ➤ Diagnosis
- • Give the laboratory and radiological tests for the investigation of the pulmonary complications of cirrhosis.

  - o Ascites
    - – Radiolabeled–ascites scan (technetium–labeled scan)
    - – Methylene blue injection followed by tap of pulmonary fluid
  - o CVS
    - – ECG
    - – Echocardiogram with Doppler
    - – Right heart angiogram

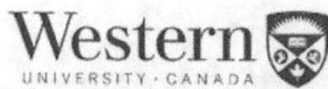

- o Lung
  - – CXR (chest X–ray; normal)
  - – CT chest
  - – ABG in erect and supine positions, for A-a O2 gradient
  - – Hemoglobin concentration, electrolytes
  - – PFTs (pulmonary function tests)
  - – Echo bubble (shunting)
  - – Pleural tap

Adapted from: Kew Michael, C. *Sleisenger & Fordtran's Gastrointestinal and Liver Disease: Pathophysiology/ Diagnosis/Management.* 8th Ed. 2006: page 2009.

> ➢ Risk Index

Arozullah risk class assignment by post–operative pneumonia and respiratory failure risk index score

Risk class	Post–operative Pneumonia Risk Index (point total)	Predicted probability of pneumonia (%)	Respiratory Failure Risk Index (point total)	Predicted probability of respiratory failure (%)
1	0-15	0.2	0-10	0.5
2	16-25	1.2	11-19	2.2
3	26-40	4.0	20-27	5.0
4	41-55	9.4	28-40	11.6
5	> 55	15.3	> 40	30.5

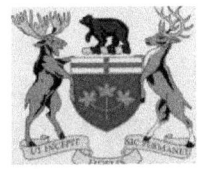

➢ Risk Reduction Strategies

  o Smoking cessation

Time of cessation	PPC
> 10 weeks	Risk similar to non–smokers
> 8 weeks	57% *vs* 14%
2 – 4 weeks	↑ risk

Arozullah, A.M., *et al. Med Clin North Am*. 2003; 87(1):153-73.

  o Lung expansion modalities
     – Incentive spirometry
     – Chest physiotherapy
       ▪ Deep breathing (pain control)
       ▪ Coughing
       ▪ Mobilization
     – Intermittent positive pressure breathing
     – CPAP

Hepatopulmonary Syndrome (HPS)

➢ Definition (diagnostic criteria)
  o Criteria 1
     – Chronic liver disease
  o Criteria 2
     – A–aDO2 ≥ 15 – 20 mmHg
     – ≥ to the age–adjusted value
  o Criteria 3
     – Intrapulmonary vascular dilatation (IPVD)
       ▪ CE-TTE
       ▪ ^{99m}Tc-MAA

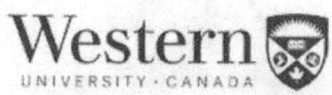

- ➢ Demography
  - o In CLD, ~ 25%
    - Abnormal IPVD in ~ 50% of CLD
  - o In CLD evaluated for LT, 10%

Severity score

Stages	PaO$_2$, mmHg
o Mild	≥ 80
o Moderate	≥ 60 and < 80
o Severe	≥ 50 and < 60
o Very severe	< 50

Aldenkortt, F., *et al. World J Gastroenterol.* 2014; 20(25):8072-81.

- ➢ Clinical
  - o Pulse oximetry
    - SpO2 < 96% predicts PaO2 < 70 mmHg
      - Sensitivity, 100%
      - Specificity, 88%
  - o Arterial blood gases (ABG)
    - P(A–a)O2 gradient ≥ 15 – 20 mmHg (depending on age)
    - PaO2 < 80 mmHg

- • Give the clinical changes seen in patients suggestive of cirrhosis developed to HPS.

  - o Presence of cirrhosis
    - Platypnea (↑ SOB on sitting–up)
    - Cyanosis (especially, distal)
    - Clubbing
    - Permanent telangiectasias of the face (angiomas)
  - o Hypoxemia (PaO2 < 70 mmHg) is usually present, together with cyanosis and clubbing

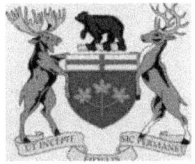

- SOBOE, dyspnea worse when sitting–up (platypnea from orthodeoxia) and better when lying down (result of reduction of intrapulmonary shunting when lying down, with improved oxygenation due to the blood going to both lower and upper parts of the lungs)
- Orthodeoxia (worsening of hypoxemia when patient sits–up or stands) is due to more blood going to the lower lungs when standing, more intrapulmonary shunting and a drop in blood gas arteria PaO_2 decreases by more than 4 mmHg
- Orthodeoxia occurs in HPS, ASD and recurrent pulmonary emboli; oxygen deactivation occur with orthodeoxia during sleep
- Chronic liver disease patients with numerous spider angiomas are more likely to have HPS
- Suspect HPS if alveolar–arterial PaO_2 gradient on room air is > 15 mmHg, and if PaO_2 is < 70 mmHg, or if arterial blood gas PaO_2 falls by more than 4 mmHg on standing
- Seen in 4 – 24% of patients evaluated for liver transplantation

---

SO YOU WANT TO BE A HEPATOLOGIST!

Clubbing is common in patients with liver disease, but when associated with distal cyanosis, HPS is suspected. Neither the presence nor the severity of HPS reflect the severity of the associated liver disease and its dysfunction.

- Differenciate platypnea from orthodeoxia.
    - Platypnea   –   Dyspnea
        - ↑ when upright
        - ↓ when supine
    - Orthodeoxia   –   Hypoxia or hypoxemia
        - ↑ when upright

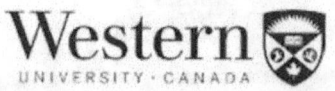

➢ Pathophysiology

SO YOU WANT TO BE A HEPATOLOGIST!

About half of patients with cirrhosis have intrapulmonary vasodilation, but only when severe does HPS occur. The increased production of nitric oxide (NO) and carbon monoxide are important in the pathophysiology of HPS.

• Explain the mechanisms of increased nitric oxide (NO) and carbon monoxide (CO) in cirrhosis complicated by hepatorenal syndrome.

  o NO - ↑ production and release of endothelin–1 → ↑ endothelin–B receptors in pulmonary microvasculature → ↑ eNos (endothelin–1–mediated endothelial NO synthase → ↑ NO

        - ↑ bacterial translocation in gut → ↑ TNF–α → ↑ macrophages adhering to the pulmonary vessels → ↑ iNos (inducible NO synthase) → ↑ NO

  o CO - ↑ adherence of macrophages to pulmonary vessels → ↑ production of CO through heme oxygenase–1

➢ Diagnostic imaging
  o Contrast–enhanced transthoracic echo (CTTE)
    - Most sensitive test
    - Agitated saline injection
    - Differentiates HPS (3 – 6 cycles) *vs* right to left (R → L) shunt (< 3 cycles)

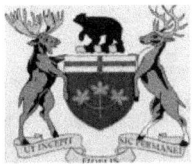

- o Lung perfusion scan: technetium–99m–labelled macroaggregated albumin (MAA) perfusion scanning
  - MAA particles 20 – 50 um in size
  - If shunt MMA particles escape, capillaries and appear in other organs
  - Helpful to rule out other intrinsic lung disease, if shunt fraction is > 6%

➤ Pathogenesis

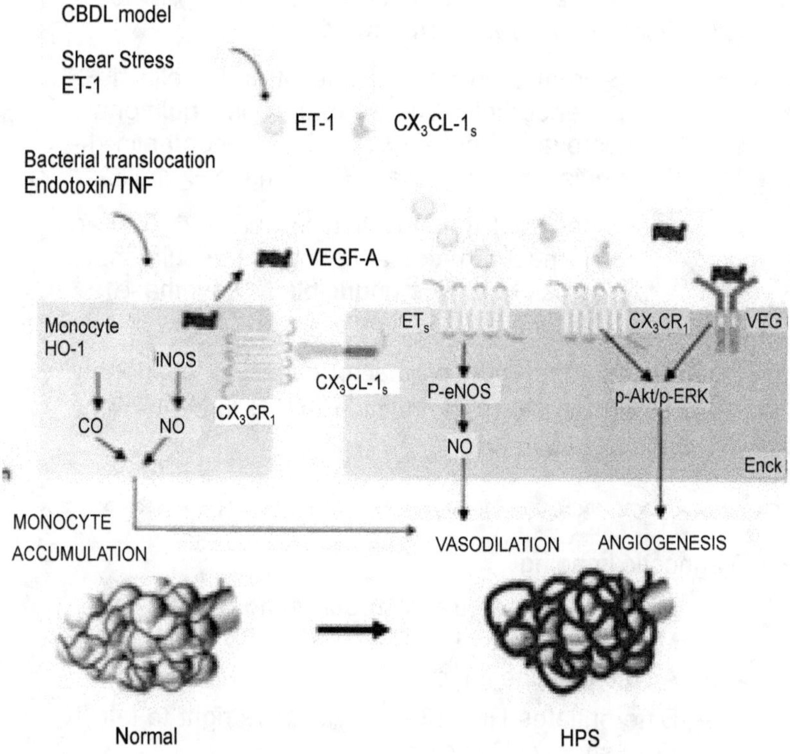

CBDL model

Shear Stress
ET-1

ET-1 CX_3CL-1_s

Bacterial translocation
Endotoxin/TNF

VEGF-A

Monocyte
HO-1

iNOS   ET$_s$ CX_3CR_1 VEG

CX_3CL-1_s

CO   NO CX_3CR_1 P-eNOS   p-Akt/p-ERK

NO

Enck

MONOCYTE
ACCUMULATION   VASODILATION   ANGIOGENESIS

Normal   HPS

Printed with permission: Machicao, V.I., *et al. Hepatology.*
59(4):1627-37.

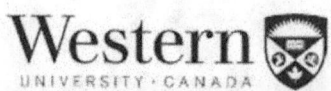

➤ Treatment

Therapies for hepatopulmonary syndrome have only been tested in small and uncontrolled trials.

- o Oxygen therapy
    - Oxygen therapy (0.5 L/min at rest and 2 L/min during exercise) prevents the deleterious consequences of hypoxemia
    - Treatment for 1 year had a beneficial effect on liver function in two patients where their Child–Pugh score markedly improved (Fukushima, *et al.*).

- o Transjugular intrahepatic portosystemic shunt
    - Placement of a transjugular intrahepatic portosystemic shunt (TIPS) to relieve portal hypertension participates in the pathophysiology of HPS has failed to improve patient outcome

- o Cavoplasty and coil emboli
    - In some patients with Budd–Chiari syndrome (BCS), cavoplasty reversed HPS
    - The injection of coil emboli that preferentially distribute to dilated vessels might also decrease hypoxemia by obstructing flow to these areas

- o Pentoxifylline
    - Pentoxifylline inhibits tumor necrosis factor–α overproduction and is effective in attenuating HPS in rats with ligated common bile ducts; the drug has not been tested in patients with HPS

- o Nitric oxide inhibition
    - ↑ production of nitric oxide (NO) causes pulmonary vascular dilatation
    - Therapies that reduce pulmonary NO levels or control its effects have been tested

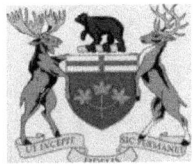

- By blocking the NO–induced activation of guanylate cyclase in smooth muscle cells, methylene blue has been shown to improve pulmonary vascular dilatation and hypoxemia
- Inhalation of the NO synthase inhibitor N^G–nitro–arginine methyl ester, reduces intrapulmonary vascular dilatation, also improved by the PaO_2 and decreases the associated dyspnea in some patients
- It is disputed whether there is any benefit from inhibiting the NO–cyclic guanosine monophosphate pathway (Almeida, *et al.*)

o   Liver transplantation
  - O_2, TIPS, liver transplantation
  - Prolonged post–operative mechanical ventilation may be needed, and mortality rate after liver transplantation is high

Printed with permission: Pastor, C.M. and Schiffer, E. *Nature Clinical Practice Gastroenterology & Hepatology.* 2007; 4(11): page 615.

"To save your world you asked this man to die,

Would this man, could he see you now, ask why?"

W. H. Anden

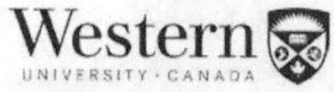

Treatment algorithm

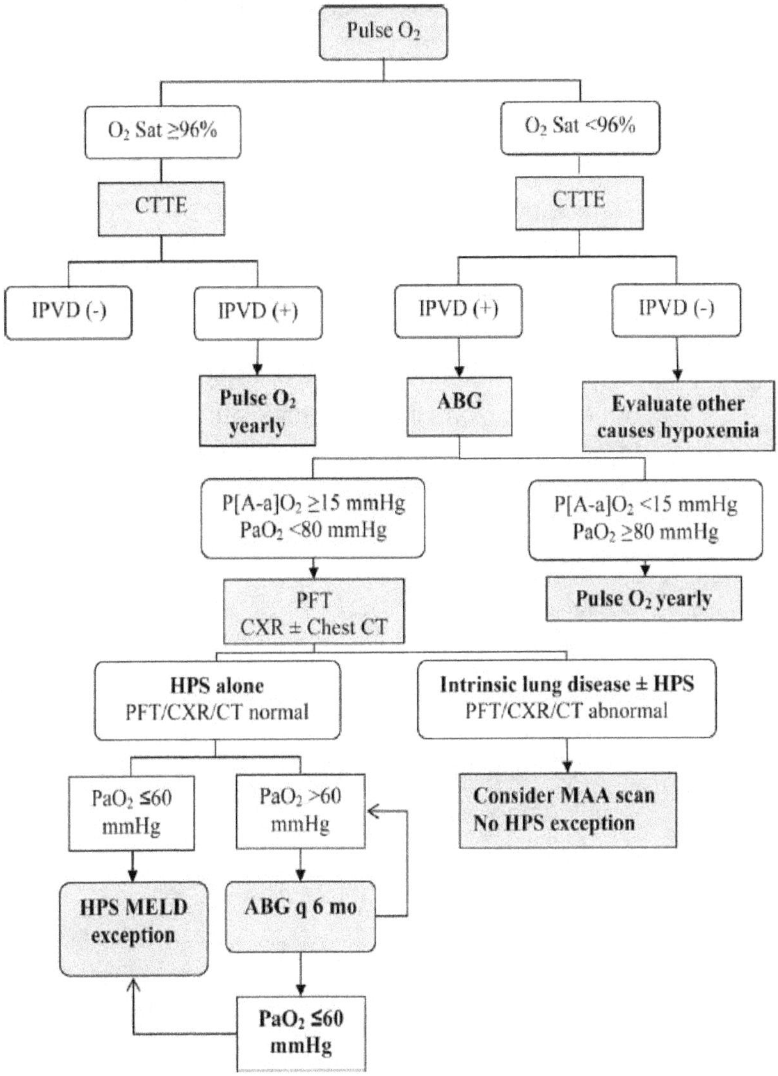

```
                              ┌──────────────┐
                              │   Pulse O₂   │
                              └──────────────┘
                     ┌────────────────┴──────────────────┐
              ┌──────────────┐                    ┌──────────────┐
              │ O₂ Sat ≥96%  │                    │ O₂ Sat <96%  │
              └──────────────┘                    └──────────────┘
              ┌──────────────┐                    ┌──────────────┐
              │     CTTE     │                    │     CTTE     │
              └──────────────┘                    └──────────────┘
          ┌────────┴────────┐              ┌──────────┴──────────┐
   ┌──────────┐      ┌──────────┐   ┌──────────┐         ┌──────────┐
   │ IPVD (-) │      │ IPVD (+) │   │ IPVD (+) │         │ IPVD (-) │
   └──────────┘      └──────────┘   └──────────┘         └──────────┘
                      ┌─────────┐    ┌─────────┐     ┌──────────────────┐
                      │ Pulse O₂│    │   ABG   │     │  Evaluate other  │
                      │  yearly │    └─────────┘     │ causes hypoxemia │
                      └─────────┘                    └──────────────────┘
```

Pulse O₂

- O₂ Sat ≥96% → CTTE
  - IPVD (-)
  - IPVD (+) → **Pulse O₂ yearly**
- O₂ Sat <96% → CTTE
  - IPVD (+) → **ABG**
  - IPVD (-) → **Evaluate other causes hypoxemia**

ABG:
- P[A-a]O₂ ≥15 mmHg / PaO₂ <80 mmHg → **PFT CXR ± Chest CT**
- P[A-a]O₂ <15 mmHg / PaO₂ ≥80 mmHg → **Pulse O₂ yearly**

PFT CXR ± Chest CT:
- **HPS alone** PFT/CXR/CT normal
- **Intrinsic lung disease ± HPS** PFT/CXR/CT abnormal → **Consider MAA scan No HPS exception**

HPS alone:
- PaO₂ ≤60 mmHg → **HPS MELD exception**
- PaO₂ >60 mmHg → **ABG q 6 mo** → PaO₂ ≤60 mmHg → **HPS MELD exception**

Printed with permission: Machicao, V.I., *et al. Hepatology.* 2014; 59(4):1627-37.

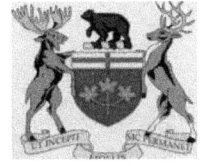

o   Liver transplant
  –   Influence of HRS on outcome of liver transplant

	HPS	No HPS
▪ ↓ survival on LT waiting list	23%	76%

  –   Predictors of poor outcome from HPS
    ▪ PaO_2 < 50 mmHg
    ▪ Shunt fraction, > 20%
  –   ↓ 5–year survival without LT
  –   MELD exception points < PaO_2 < 60 mmHg
  –   Benefit of LT on HPS long term survival related to reversal of HPS
    ▪ Liver transplantation reverses in HPS
      – 6–month, 95%
      – 12–month, 100%
  –   ↓ TNF (no benefit)
    ▪ Pentoxifylline
    ▪ MMF
  –   ↓ bacterial translocation
    ▪ Norfloxacin (no benefit)
  –   ↓ pulmonary angiogenesis
    ▪ Methylene blue
    ▪ No RCT, but repeat use post–LT for weaning
  –   Garlic
    ▪ 18–month RCT
    ▪ ↓ portopulmonary hypertension (POPH) in 2/3

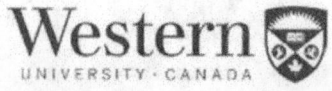

Portopulmonary Hypertension (POPH)

- ➢ Definition
  - o Liver disease (clinical portal hypertension)
  - o MPAP ≥ 25 mmHg
  - o PVR > 240 dyn sec cm^{-5}
  - o PCWP < 15 mmHg

Diagnostic criteria were proposed by the European Respiratory Society and European Society for the Study of the Liver Task Force on Hepatic and Pulmonary Vascular Disorders of POPH

Abbreviations: MPAP, mean pulmonary pressure; PCWP, pulmonary capillary wedge pressure; PVR, pulmonary vascular resistance

Severity of POPH

Severity	MPAP (mmHg)
o Mild	≥ 25 – < 35
o Moderate	35 to < 45
o Severe	≥ 45

- ➢ Demography
  - o Prevalence: 4.5 – 8.5% of transplant candidates
  - o RVSP on TTE
    - – Right ventricular pressure (RVSP) measured on transesophageal echocardiography (TTE) as a surrogate marker for POPH

RVSP	Diagnosis of POPH
> 30 mmHg	59%
> 50 mmHg	65%

Sensitivity, 100%
Specificity, 96%

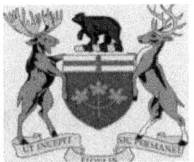

- ➢ Pathogenesis
  - ○ Cirrhosis causes ↑ (pulmonary artery) pressure due to:
    - − Volume overload and ↑ cardiac output (from ↓ systemic vascular resistance and hyperdynamic circulation)
  - ○ ↑ pulmonary vascular resistance in PPH →
    - − ↓ NO plus ↑ endothelin–1 → PA vasoconstriction
    - − Obliteration of pulmonary arterioles may occur from intimal proliferation, adventitial fibrosis, and thrombosis of pulmonary vasculature
    - − ↑ MPAP > 25 mmHg
    - − ↑ PVR > 240 dynes/s/cm^{-5}
    - − ↓ PCWP < 15 mmHg
  - ○ ↑ mPAP (mean pulmonary arterial pressure)
    - − > 25 mmHg, at rest
    - − > 30 mmHg, with exercise
  - ○ ↑ PVR (pulmonary vascular resistance) > 240 dynes/sec/cm^{-5}
  - ○ The presence of
    - − PHT (pulmonary hypertension)
    - − Portosystemic shunts
    - − Hemodynamic abnormalities in portal vein
  - ○ Severity
    - − Mild, mPAP of 25 – 35 mmHg
    - − Moderate, mPAP of 35 – 50 mmHg
    - − Severe, mPAP of > 50 mmHg (prohibitive operative mortality from liver transplantation

Abbreviations: MPAP, mean pulmonary artery pressure; AVR, pulmonary vascular resistance; PCWP, pulmonary capillary wedge pressure

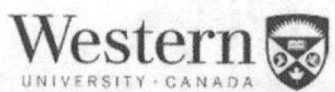

➢ Pathophysiology

   o ↑ CO → ↑ PVR → ↑ mPAP → POPH
                    ↑ PAOP
        – Collateral shunts
        – Vascular remodeling

Abbreviations: CO, cardiac output; mPAP, mean pulmonary artery; PAOP, pulmonary artery pressure; POPH, portopulmonary hypertension; PVR, pulmonary vascular resistance

➢ Clinical

   o Most asymptomatic (60%)

   o Eventual RV dysfunction (↑ RVSP) → syncope, dyspnea

➢ Differential diagnosis

Hemodynamic patterns on right heart catheterization in cirrhosis patients, with elevated RVSP on echocardiogram

Hemodynamic pattern	Mean pulmonary artery pressure (mPAP)	Pulmonary vascular resistance (PVR)	Pulmonary artery occlusion pressure (PAOP)	Cardiac output (CO)
Hyperdynamic circulation	↑	↑	↑	↑
Pulmonary venous hypertension	↑	↔↑	↑	↑
Portopulmonary hypertension	↑	↑	↑	mild ↑ / severe ↓

Printed with permission: Machicao, V.I., *et al. Hepatology.* 2014; 59(4):1627-37.

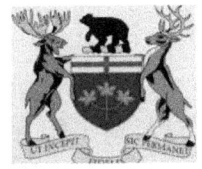

- Distinguish hepatopulmonary syndrome from portopulmonary hypertension.

Clinical	Hepatopulmonary syndrome (HRS: AV shunts)	Portopulmonary hypertension (PPH: constriction of pulmonary vessels)
o Prevalence in cirrhotics evaluated for LT	– ~ 25%	▪ 5%
o Production of NO and CO	– ↑ (iNos, HO-1)	▪ Normal
o ECG findings	– None	▪ RBBB, rightward axis ▪ RV hypertrophy ▪ No to mild hypoxemia
o Symptoms	– Progressive dyspnea – SOB on sitting up (platypnea) – Cyanosis – Finger clubbing – Spider angiomas	▪ Chest pain ▪ SOB on lying down ▪ No cyanosis ▪ RV heave ▪ Pronounced P2 component

o Pathophysiology	– ↑ VEGF → ↑ angiogenesis
	– ↓ gas exchange – hypoxemia
	– Intrapulmonary vasodilation in precapillary and capillary PA circulation due to vasoactive mediators
		▪ Vasoconstriction
		▪ Remodeling of resistance vessels
		▪ ↑ PAP
		  - Medial proliferation and hypertrophy
		  - Arteriopathy
		  - Thrombosis
		  - ↑ endothelin–1

o Arterial blood gas levels	– Moderate to severe hypoxemia	
o Chest radiograph	– Normal	▪ Cardiomegaly ▪ Hilar enlargement

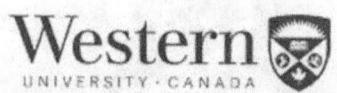

Clinical	Hepatopulmonary syndrome (HRS: AV shunts)	Portopulmonary hypertension (PPH: constriction of pulmonary vessels)
○ 99mTcMAA shunting index ("bubble study")	– Normal/low PVR	▪ < 6% roatrial opacification ▪ Elevated PVR ▪ Normal mPAOP ▪ Large pulmonary arteries
○ CEE	– Tri-regurg; Always positive; left atria opacification for > 3-6 cardiac cycles after – right atrial opacification – > 6%	▪ Usually negative. Positive for <3 cardiac cycles; if arterial septal defect or patent foramen ovale
○ Pulmonary hemodynamics	– Normal/ 'spongy' appearance (type I)	▪ Distal arterial pruning
○ Pulmonary angiography	– Discrete arteriovenous communications (type II) (usually lower lobe)	▪ Only indicated in mild-to-moderate stages
○ OLT	– Always indicated in severe stages	▪ Late contraindication
○ MELD exception points	– Yes	▪ No
○ Role of LT	– Reverses HPS in 80%	▪ Useful when MPAP > 25 and < 35 mmHg

Abbreviations: 99mTcMAA, technetium-99 m-labelled macroaggregated albumin; CEE, contrast enhanced echocardiography; ECG, electrocardiogram; HPS, hepatopulmponary syndrome; MPAP, mean pulmonary artery pressure; OLT, orthotopic liver transplantation; PAOP, mean pulmonary artery occlusion pressure; PAP, pulmonary arterial pressure; PVR, pulmonary vascular resistance; RBBB, r

Printed with permission: Herve, P., et al. Best Practice & Research Clinical Gastroenterology. 2007; 21(1): page 142.

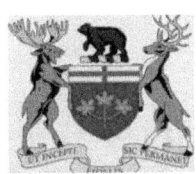

> Treatment algorithm

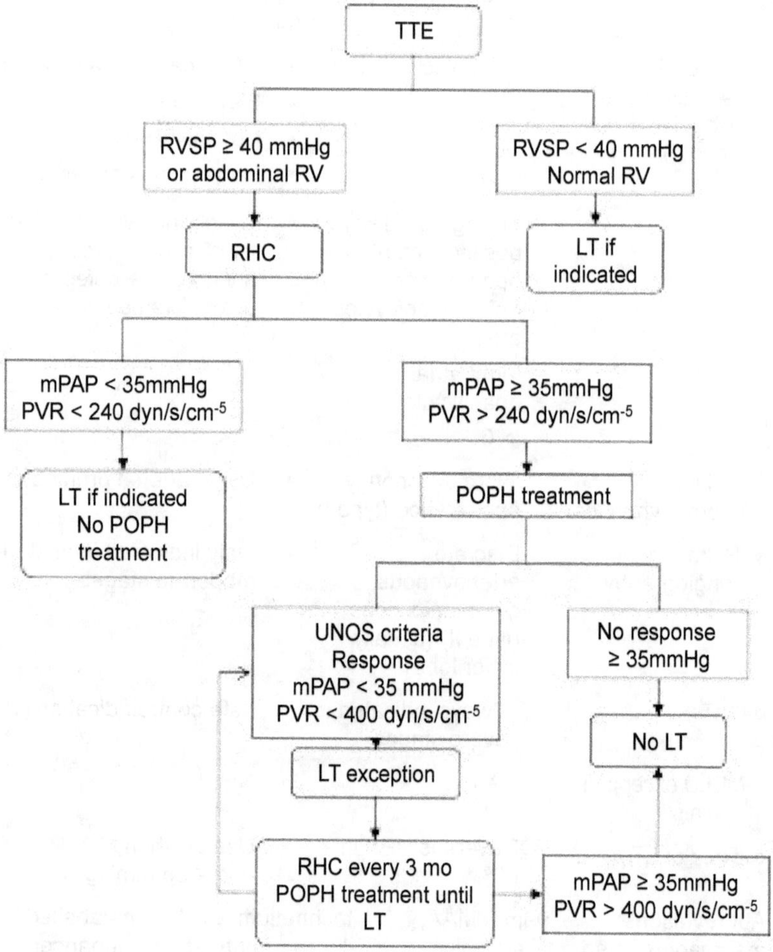

```
                        ┌──────────────────┐
                        │       TTE        │
                        └──────────────────┘
              ┌───────────────────┴───────────────────┐
  ┌──────────────────────┐            ┌──────────────────────┐
  │  RVSP ≥ 40 mmHg       │            │  RVSP < 40 mmHg       │
  │  or abdominal RV      │            │  Normal RV            │
  └──────────────────────┘            └──────────────────────┘
            │                                     │
      ┌──────────┐                         ┌──────────────┐
      │   RHC    │                         │  LT if        │
      └──────────┘                         │  indicated    │
            │                              └──────────────┘
   ┌────────┴─────────────────────────────┐
┌─────────────────────┐        ┌─────────────────────┐
│ mPAP < 35mmHg        │        │  mPAP ≥ 35mmHg       │
│ PVR < 240 dyn/s/cm⁻⁵ │        │  PVR > 240 dyn/s/cm⁻⁵│
└─────────────────────┘        └─────────────────────┘
            │                             │
   ┌─────────────────┐          ┌──────────────────┐
   │ LT if indicated │          │  POPH treatment  │
   │ No POPH         │          └──────────────────┘
   │ treatment       │
   └─────────────────┘
```

mPAP < 35mmHg, PVR < 240 $dyn/s/cm^{-5}$

mPAP ≥ 35mmHg, PVR > 240 $dyn/s/cm^{-5}$

LT if indicated
No POPH treatment

POPH treatment

UNOS criteria
Response
mPAP < 35 mmHg
PVR < 400 $dyn/s/cm^{-5}$

No response
≥ 35mmHg

LT exception

No LT

RHC every 3 mo
POPH treatment until
LT

mPAP ≥ 35mmHg
PVR > 400 $dyn/s/cm^{-5}$

Printed with permission: Machicao, V.I., *et al. Hepatology*. 2014; 59(4) 1627-37.

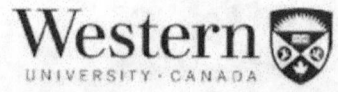

- o Pharmacological agents
    - – PDE–5 inhibitors
    - – Endothelin receptor antagonists
    - – Prostacyclins (EPO, 0.5 – 100 mg/kg/minute IV for 3 – 5 minutes)
        - ▪ Early suggestion of benefit with IV EPO (Khaderi, S., et al. *World J Gastroenterol.* 2014; 20(32):11281-6.)

➢ Prognosis

o Mortality rate (MR)	Years
12%	1
33%	2
60%	5

- o Months of survival
    - – Mean, 15 months
    - – Median, 6 months
- o Liver transplantation
    - – With LT

POPH	mPAP	MR
▪ Mild	< 25	No effect
▪ Moderate	> 35	50%
▪ Severe	> 50	100%

  - – In severe POPH, there is ↓ CO which ↑ 3x after LT reperfusion
  - – If there is non–compliant vascular bed, this sudden ↑ CO acute right ventricular heart failure (RVHF)

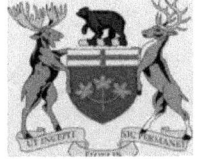

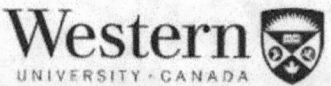

Liver Transplantation and Neuroendocrine Tumor

Gavin Beck

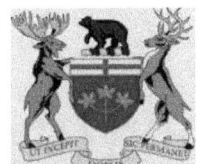

Neuroendocrine tumour

➢ Pathology

- o Tumors arising from the different parts of the widespread neuroendocrine system

- o Majority (85%) from the gastrointestinal tract

- o Majority is sporadic but can be associated with inherited conditions (MEN–1)

- o GI neuroendocrine tumors are often slow growing and majority (40 – 80%) are found in metastatic phase with liver predominant as the site of GI tumor metastasis (40 – 93%) followed by the bones and lungs in 10 – 20%

- o 1st pass portal venous drainage assured from the midgut (duodenum, small bowel, right colon and part of pancreas)

- o Metastasis to the liver also slowly progressive, and untreated individuals have up to 30% 5–year survival

- o Locoregional liver–directed therapies have included hepatic artery embolization, TACE, RFA, cryoablation I^{131}MIBG, along with somatostatin analogues and chemotherapy in effort to reduce tumor bulk and activity in unresectable cases

- o Many lessons learned regarding the biology of NET metastasis to the liver with hepatic resection treatment over the last few decades

➢ Clinical

- o Can be symptomatic both from volume of tumor bulk

- o Clinical syndromes secondary to their hypersecretory activity (hormones include serotonin, insulin, gastrin, glucagon)

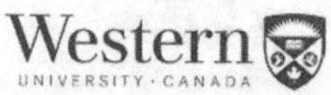

➢ Selection of patients

Criteria for liver transplantation in neuroendocrine patients with hepatic metastasis

1. Confirmed histology of carcinoid tumor (low–grade neuroendocrine tumors) with or without syndrome

2. Primary tumor drained by the portal system (pancreas and intermediate gut: from distal stomach to sigmoid colon) removed with a curative resection (pre–transplant removal of all extrahepatic tumor deposits) through surgical procedure is different and separate from transplantation

3. Metastasis diffusion to liver parenchyma ≤ 50%

4. Good response or stable disease for (6 – 12 months during the pre–transplantation period)

5. Age ≤ 70 years

➢ Treatment

o Up to 90% are multifocal and bilateral

o Only 10 – 25% of liver metastatis can be treated with surgical curative intend (either due to lack of clear margins or multiple foci)

o Even with unilobar disease, high risk recurrence (5–year, 80%) due to R0 resection is rarely achievable

o Role of LT in metastatic neuroendocrine tumor disease should aid in the following:
   - Complete R0 resection
   - Relief of tumor secretory symptoms
   - Reasonable chance of long term cure

Abbreviation: LT, liver transplantation

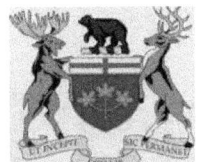

> Prognosis

	Perioperative mortality	Patient survival		Disease free survival
o Resections, all carcinoid	0-6%	5-year	46-79%	16-36%
		10-year	35-59%	19%
o Transplantation		5-year	36-90%	9-24%

Adapted from: Mazzaferro, V., *et al.* *J Hepatol.* 2007; 47:460-8.; Grossman, E.J. and Millis, J.M. *Liver Transpl.* 2010; 16(8):930-42.

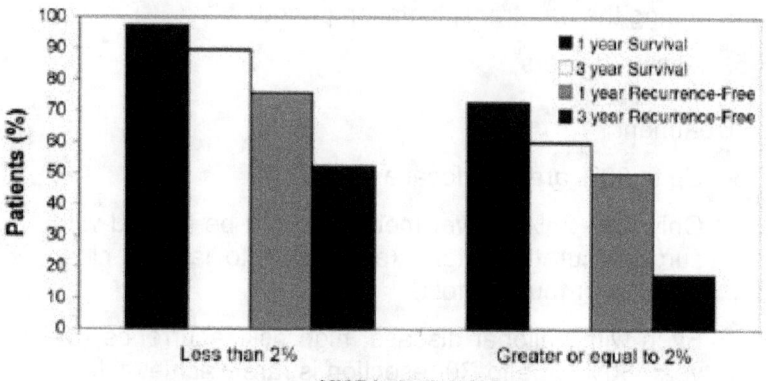

o 55 low risk patients identified (Ki67 < 2%) with 37 having 1–year follow–up and 18 with 3–year follow–up

o 22 high risk identified (Ki67>=2%) with 1–year follow–up and 9 with 3–year follow–up

Printed with permission: Grossman, E.J. and Millis, J.M. *Liver Transpl.* 2010; 16(8):930-42.

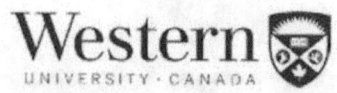

Liver Transplantation for the Treatment of Liver Metastases from Neuroendocrine Tumors: An Analysis of the UNOS Database

Survival of patients with NETs and HCC treated with LT

Tumor types	Survival		
	1–year	3–year	5–year
o Carcinoid NET	71-81%	51-55%	44-47%
o Non–carcinoid	75-82%	62-82%	44-48%
o HCC	79-87%	52-78%	43-58%

Rates of similar patient survival after liver transplantation

Adapted from: Gedaly, R., *et al. Arch Surg.* 2011; 146(8):953-8.

Five–year survival rates in liver transplantation patients for neuroendocrine tumors by quartile of wait time

Wait time, days	5–year survival, mean (SE), %
≤ 22	33(9)
23 – 67	40(12)
68 – 170	52 (11)
≥ 171	74 (9)

Adapted from: Gedaly, R., *et al. Arch Surg.* 2011; 146(8):953-8.

Wait time, days	5–year survival, mean (SE), N = 150)	
	Age ≤ 55 years	Age > 55 years
≤ 67	41 (8)	17 (14)
> 67	63 (8)	62 (14)

Adapted from: Gedaly, R., *et al. Arch Surg.* 2011; 146(8):953-8.

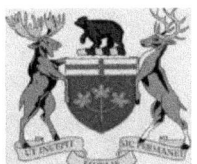

- o Limitations to the UNOS data
    - No information regarding tumor size location, number of metastasis, percent liver parenchyma involved, cell differentiation
    - No histology
    - No characteristics and treatment of primary tumor
    - Large percentage of "unspecified" NET
    - Pre– and post–LT treatment
    - Pretransplant extent of disease

Liver Transplantation for Symptomatic Liver Metastases of Neuroendocrine Tumors

- o Review of literature and our center's experience

- o Selection criteria proposed for liver transplantation and metastatic neuroendocrine tumors

- o Initial assessment investigations
    - Abdominal CT, including liver protocoled CT +/- MRI
    - Ocreotide scan
    - MIBG scan
    - Laboratory tesing, including CBC, Creatinine, Urea, INR, LFT, chromogranin A
    - Pathology reporting Ki67 index

- o All reviewed by multidisciplinary NET board

- o LRCP mNET patients
    - Systemic treatment with 5–FU or oral capecitabine, epirubicin, carboplatin
    - Intrahepatic ^{111}In-ocretate or I^{131}MIBG
    - TACE (doxorubicin/ethiodized oil or cisplatin/^{131}I-ethiodized oil)

- o Post–transplant tumor–specific investigations include chromogranin A and CT of the chest, abdomen, and pelvis q 6 months

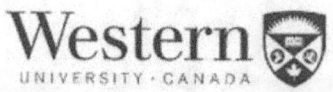

- o Our experience (University Hospital, London, ON, LHSC)
  - 1988
    - 35–year old female, no symptoms or antineoplastic treatment pre–LT; unidentified primary tumor; 9 months post–LT had retroperitoneal lesions and mass in the head of pancreas, resection and debulking enucleation; died 3 years post–LT
  - 1991
    - 61–year old male; liver metastais from GI NET; resection 20 years prior right hemicolectomy; LT complicated by PNF, retreated with POD4, died of sepsis and MOF post–op 1 month
  - 2007
    - 65–year old male, secondary biliary cirrhosis complications from TACE for mNET; diagnosed 7 years with prior resection of terminal ileum and liver mets; Ki67 1%; post–LT had uneventful recovery; recurrence in small bowel mesentery resected in 2010; last follow–up on December 2013 with no evidence of recurrence on CT and was feeling well
  - 2008
    - 34–year old male, carcinoid syndrome, unresectable disease, refractory to octretide; radiation with 7 combined chemotherapy for hepatic artery radionucletide; Ki–67 1%; hepatomegaly from enumerable liver metastasis; cardiac valvular disease is found to be acceptable risk and underwent LT 2008; subsequent recurrence in the abdomen and bone but doing well with stable recurrence; last seen for follow–up on December 2013
  - 2014
    - Mrs FT
  - Currently 1 other NET patient waitlisted for LT at LHSC

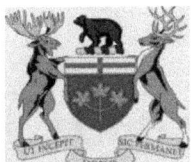

- o Poor prognosis, include the following features
  - – Age > 50 – 55 years
  - – Concomitant radical resection (LT and primary resection at the same time)
  - – Primary pancreatic and duodenal
  - – Hepatomegaly

Selection criteria for liver transplantation for liver metastases of neuroendocrine tumors

Criteria	Center		
	UWO	Mayo	ENETS
o Previous resection of primary disease site	+	+	+
o Unresectable hepatic metastases	+	+	+
o Absence of extrahepatic metastases	+	+	+
o Low-grade tumor with Ki–67 < 2%	+		+[a]
o Duration of stable disease (months) before listing for transplantation[b]	12	6	+
o Trial of therapy for metastatic neuroendocrine tumor	+		+
o Refractory symptomatic disease	+		+
o Otherwise eligible for transplantation			

[a]The suggestion of the ENETS consensus was that Ki–67 should not, as a maximum, exceed 10%.

[b]The UWO calculates its waiting period from the date of the initial consultation for metastatic neuroendocrine tumor. Mayo clinic calculates its waiting period from the date of operation for the primary disease.

Abbreviations: UWO = University of Western Ontario; Mayo = Mayo Clinic; ENETS = European Neuroendocrine Tumor Society

Source: Chan, G., et al. Curr Oncol. 2012; 19(4):217–221.

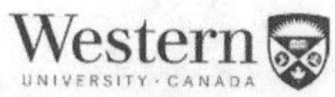

Liver Transplantation for Neuroendocrine Tumors in Europe—Results and Trends in Patient Selection: A 213-Case European Liver Transplant Registry Study

- Published in May 2013
- European registry, 213 LT for NET
- 35 centers over 27 years (1982 – 2009)
- Average 6 of patients/center; 10 centers 1 – 2 patients
- Majority from GI primary, 16 (7.5%) from bronchial tree, 17(8%) had undetected primary

➤ Conclusions

- Although no randomized studies or prospective trials compared to non–transplant management, it is apparent LT has a role in the management of unresectable, confined to the liver, well–differentiated metastatic neuroendocrine tumors
  - Curative intent, symptom management
- Excellent results with Milan criteria compared to very diverse ELTR and UNOS (lack of important data)
- UWO criteria is more stringent than Milan criteria (other inclusion recommendations, i.e. Ki – 67 <10 %)
  - Although, only few patients in comparative analysis are important as our database grows using our selection criteria

Changes in patient characteristics and results over time

	(n=107)	(n=106)	P
Overall 5–year survival from LT	46%	59%	< 0.05
Disease–free 5–year survival from LT	22%	39%	< 0.001
Overall 5–year survival from the diagnosis of LM	62%	84%	< 0.01

Abbreviations: LM, liver metastases; LT, liver transplantation

Adapted from: Le Treut YP, et al. Ann Surg. 2013; 257(5):807-15.

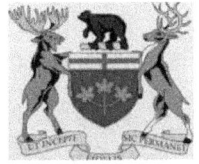

Case series and reviews of the liver transplantation for metastatic neuroendocrine tumors

Reference	Patients (n)			Concurrent resections	Follow-up (years)	OS (%)	RFS (%)
	Overall	OLT	MVT				
Lehnert et al., 1998 [3]	103	103	0	39	5	47	24
Rosenau et al., 2002 [4]	19	19	0	6	5	80	21
Frilling et al., 2006 [5]	15	14	1	2	5	67.2	48.3
van Vilsteren et al., 2006 [6]	19	19	0	1	1	88	80
Olausson et al., 2007 [7]	15	10	5	5	5	90[a]	20
Le Treut et al., 2008 [8]	85	85	0	34	5	47	20
Gedaly et al., 2011 [9]	150	133	13	—	5	49	32
Máthé et al., 2011 [10]	89	89	0	45	5	44	—

[a] Includes only the OLT patients.

OLT = orthotopic liver transplantation; MVT = multi-visceral transplantation; OS = overall survival; RFS = recurrence-free survival.

Source: Chan G, et al. Curr Oncol 2012; 19(4): 217–221.

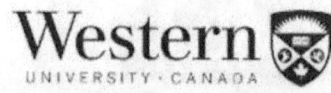

Cardiac Assessment Prior To Liver Transplantation

Amindeep Sandhu

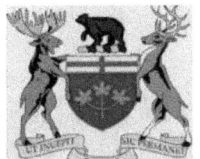

Introduction

o   Liver transplant (LT) candidates are older, have more comorbidities, higher MELDs than before → higher risk profiles

o   Purpose of cardiac evaluation pre–LT
-   Assess peri–operative risk

o   Exclude cardiopulmonary disorders
-   Help ensure good long term outcome

Cardiac Disturbances in ESLD

o   ↑ cardiac output

o   Left ventricular hypertrophy

o   Chamber enlargement

o   Causes "Cirrhotic Cardiomyopathy" (CCM)
-   ↓ contractile response to stress
-   Diastolic dysfunction
-   Electrophysiological abnormalities
    ▪   QT prolongation
    ▪   Heart block

o   Autonomic dysfunction and impaired baroreceptors

o   All in absence of known cardiac disease

o   Mediated by ↓ β–agonist signaling

o   ↑ inflammatory mediators

o   Results to the following:
-   ↓ cardiac functions
-   ↓ SVR
-   Repolarization changes
-   Bradycardia

o   All contribute to CV complications pre– and post–LT

Abbreviation: ESLD, end–stage liver disease

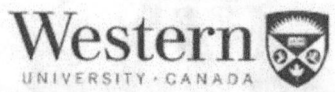

Coronary Artery Disease (CAD)

- o With CAD
    - – 40% mortality 1 year post–LT with > 50% stenosis
- o LT candidates
    - – Angiography → 30% had >/= 50% stenosis
    - – Obstructive CAD is most common in 2+ cardiac RF
    - – Hypertension (HTN)
    - – Dyslipidemia
    - – DM on insulin (40% lower 4–year survival)
- o Difficult dilemma with NASH cirrhosis

Abbreviations: CAD, coronary artery disease; DM, diabetes mellitus; HTN, hypertension; LT, liver transplantation; NASH, non–alcoholic steatohepatitis; RF, risk factors

Liver Transplantation

- o Hemodynamic stress ↑ after reperfusion of transplanted liver
    - – Sudden ↑ in preload
- o ↑ in preload and CCM → abrupt elevations of PCWP → RHF → hepatic congestion in early post–LT
- o Arrhythmias, MI, L–HF can also ensue
- o Pre–cardiac assessment is critical

Abbreviations: LT, liver transplantation; PCWP, pulmonary capillary wedge pressure; RHF, right–sided heart failure

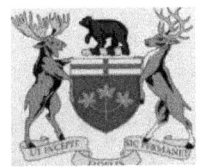

Recommendations – AASLD

- o Pre–LT, ALL patients should get:
  - – Routine history and physical examination to assess for smoking, CAD RF, DM types and control, family history, HF
- o Transthoracic Echo
  - – To assess LV and RV size/function, valve function, PAP + exclude pericardial disease, LVOTO
  - – LVD is not a CI for LT but requires optimization and is a RF for post-LT HF/other complications

Abbreviations: AASLD, American Association for the Study of Liver Disease; CAD RF, coronary artery disease risk factors; CI, contraindicated; DM, diabetes; Echo, echocardiogram; HF, heart failure; LT, liver transplantation; LV, left ventricular; LVD, left ventricular dysfunction; PAP, pulmonary artery pressure

Recommendations: Who to Screen?

- o Routine cardiac Hx and PEx pre–operatively
- o Evaluate for CAD with the following:
  - – Chronic smoker
  - – Personal or family Hx of CAD
  - – Diabetes mellitus
- o First line is Dobutamine Stress Echo (DSE)
  - – NPV 75 – 89% for obstructive CAD

Abbreviations: CAD, coronary artery disease; DSE, dobutamine stress echocardiogram; Hx, history; NPV, negative predictive value

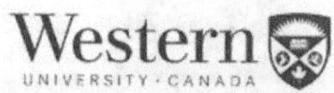

Who gets Coronary Angiography?

- o Known CAD of any kind
- o Diabetes mellitus
- o 2+ cardiovascular RF
- o Moderate or high risk features on dynamic perfusion defects (DSE)
- o Cardiac CT angiography is considered reasonable alternative
- o Obstructive CAD (> 70%) should get revascularized
    - – BMS > DES because of prolonged dual anti–platelet Rx

Abbreviations: BMS, bare metal stent; CAD, coronary artery disease; CT, computed tomography; DES, drug–eluting stents; DSE, dobutamine stress echocardiogram; Rx, treatment (prescription medication)

Heart Failure

- o Pre–DSE LVD/RVD is not contraindicated for LT
- o Volume status and symptoms of CHF should be monitored and optimized prior to LT
- o Aggressive monitoring post–LT is the key with a given high risk of post–LT HF/volume O/L
- o Maintain BB, ACEI or ARB or Aldosterone–blockade peri–operatively unless CI (low BP, AKI/CKD/HRS)

Abbreviations: ACEI, angiotensin converting enzyme inhibitor; AKI, acute kidney injury; ARB, angiotensin receptor blocker; BB, beta–blocker; BP, blood pressure; CI, contraindication; CKD, chronic kidney disease; HF, heart failure; HRS, hepatorenal syndrome; LT, liver transplantation; LVD, left ventricular dysfunction; O/L, overload; RVD, right ventricular dysfunction

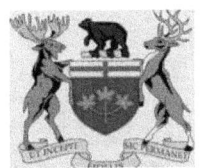

LVH and LVOTO

- o Volume O/L in ESLD leads to a hyperdynamic circulation + LVH = LVOTO

- o Retrospective review of 106 transplant recipients: inducible LVOTO in > 40%, on DSE

- o Exhibits poor tolerance to ESLD and LT

- o Outflow gradient of > 36 mmHg associated with intra–operative hypotension

- o TTE can establish the diagnosis and gradient

- o Requires optimization of volume status pre–op

- o Excessive LVH with LVOTO due to HOCM requires septal ablation if symptomatic, HF that would preclude transplant

- o Careful intra–operative monitoring
  - Avoid tachycardia, limit inotropic agents
  - TEE–guided volume administration

Abbreviations: DSE, dobutamine stress echocardiogram; Dx, diagnosis; ESLD, end-stage liver disease; HOCM, hypertrophic obstructive cardiomyopathy; LVH, left ventricular hypertrophy; LVOTO, left ventricular outflow tract obstruction; pre-op, preoperative; TEE, trans–esophageal echocardiogram; TTE, transthoracic endocardiogram

Pulmonary Heart Disease

- o Hepatopulmonary Syndrome
  - Abnormal intrapulmonary vascular dilation = physiologic shunting + V/Q MM + Hypoxemia

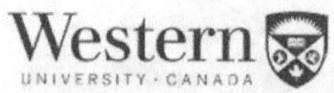

- o Portopulmonary Hypertension (POPH):
  - – mPAP >/= 25 + portal HTN
  - – Pulmonary arterial hypertension + increased PVR (vasoconstriction)
  - – Leads to progressive vascular remodeling
  - – Must have concomitant PHTN, but not correlated with it
  - – Hypoxemia occurs late
  - – LT is contraindicated if untreated

Abbreviations: BP, blood pressure; HPS, hepatopulmonary syndrome; LT, liver transplantation; mPAP, mean pulmonary artery pressure; PHTN, pulmonary hypertension; POPH, portopulmonary hypertension; PVR, pulmonary vascular resistance; V/Q MM, ventricular/perfusion mismatch

Portopulmonary Hypertension (POPH)

- o Present in 8% of all LT candidates
- o Half = moderate to severe: mPAP >/= 35 mmHg
- o Traditionally considered CI to LT
- o Pre–op mPAP > 35 = 50% mortality at 1 year post–LT, 100% if > 50
- o Diagnostic dilemma as Vol O/L and increased CO + LVSD all contribute to higher mPAPs

Abbreviations: CI, contraindicated; CO, cardiac output; LT, liver transplantation; mPAP, mean pulmonary arterial pressure; POPH, portopulmonary hypertension; Vol O/L, volume overload

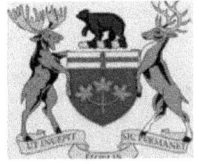

POPH Evaluation

- All LT candidates: evaluate PAPs with TTE
  - Preferably contrast–enhanced
- If elevated (> 25) or RHF → right heart catheterization (RHC)
  - Provides the following:
    - PCWP/RVSP
    - PVR
    - Confirmation of mPAP
- If mPAP > 35 and PCWP > 15 mmHg → diurese and repeat RHC
- If mPAP > 25 persists then PAP is significant
- In the absence of other WHO criteria for PAP, in the setting of ESLD, POPH is confirmed
- Mild: mPAP 25 – 34 mmHg
  - Not CI to LT if RH function preserved, minimal effect on outcome
- Moderate to severe: >/= 35 mmHg
  - Relative CI – depends on the response to pulmonary vasodilators
  - Prostanoids, PDEIs, endothelin–receptor antagonists can lower PAP's enough to facilitate LT
  - Case series have demonstrated successful LT and one-year outcome if response to MM pre–op
    GOAL = PVR < 400, mPAP < 35 persistently → LT safe

Abbreviations: CI, contraindication; LT, liver transplantation; mPAP, mean pulmonary artery pressure; PDEI's, phosphodiesterase inhibitors; PVR, pulmonary vascular resistance; RH, right heart

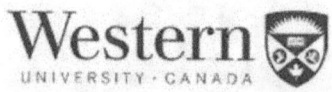

POPH Intraoperative Care

- o TEE to monitor for RV dysfunction
- o Venovenous bypass to prevent sudden RV O/L after reperfusion
- o Inhaled NO to lower PAP
- o Optimize pre–load so ot to cause RV compromise intra–operatively

Abbreviations: NO, nitric oxide; PAP, pulmonary artery pressure; RV O/L, right ventricular overload; RV, right ventricle; TEE, trans–esophageal echocardiogram

Hepatopulmonary Syndrome

- o Seen in 5 – 32% of LT candidates
- o Intrapulmonary shunting demonstrated via contrast echo or [99m]TC macro–aggregated albumin (MAA) lung–brain perfusion scanning
- o HRS almost fully resolves at 6 months post–LT
- o Perioperative risk is high as PaO_2 < 50 mmHg or MAA shunt scan of > 20%
  - Also predicts long term supplemental O_2 and longer recover post–operatively
  - Any degree increases in mortality
- o Work–up, initially includes:
  - PaO_2 < 70 – 80 on RA or A–a gradient >/=15, excluding alternative causes → must screen further
  - CXR, PFTs, CT Chest
  - MAA or pulmonary arteriography if clinical suspicion is warranted – clinches the diagnosis

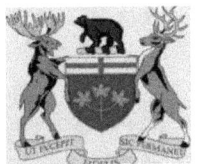

- o No acceptable therapies pre–op, only supplemental O2 and LT (improves mortality)

Abbreviations: A–a, arteriolar–arterial; CT, computed tomography; CXR, chest X–ray; LT, liver transplantation; MAA, macro–aggregated albumin; O_2, oxygen; PaO_2, arterial pressure of oxygen; PFTs, pulmonary function tests; Pre–op, preoperative; RA, room air

Pericardial Effusions

- o Can be associated with Hepatitis C and cryoglobulinemia
- o Hepatohydropericardium = associated with ascites
- o Assessment required for any of the following:
  - – Clinical evidence for tamponade
  - – TTE to confirm the lack of any effusion causing LV outflow compromised

Abbreviations: LV, left ventricle; TTE, transthoracic echocardiogram

QTc prolongation

- o QTc > 440 ms → risk of ventricular arrhythmia
- o Common in ESLD
  - – Retrospective cohort: 50%, n = 600, half of which resolved post–transplant
- o Independent RF:
  - – Age, alcoholic cirrhosis, high Child–Pugh
- o Not contraindication to LT
  - – Search for reversible causes, especially with medications

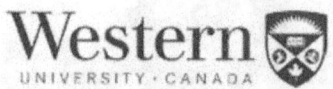

Some reported causes and potentiators of the long QT syndrome
1- Congenital
2- Aquired:
    a. Hypokalemia
    b. Hypmagnesemia
    c. Hypocalcemia
3- Drugs
    a. Amiodarone
    b. Sotalol
    c. Quinidine
    d. Antipsychotic drugs

"Great thoughts speak only to the thoughtful mind, but great actions speak to all mankind."

Emily P. Bissell

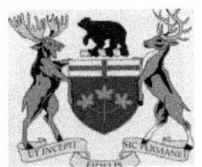

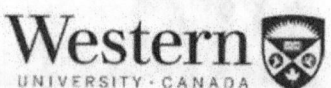

Liver Transplantation for Alcoholic Liver Disease: The Importance of Recidivism

Amindeep Sandhu

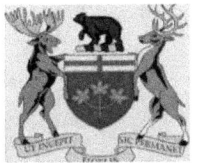

- ➢ Background
  - o Alcoholic liver cirrhosis (ALC) = 2nd most common indication for DDLT in N. America
  - o Offers excellent survival advantage in appropriately selected patients with ALC
  - o Cost–effective
  - o Initial reluctance
    - – Perception of self–infliction
    - – Non–compliance with proven abstinence
    - – Alcohol–mediated damage outside the liver

Abbreviations: ALC, alcoholic liver cirrhosis; DDLT, dead donor liver transplantation

Recidivism Post–LT

- o 10 – 90% is difficult to quantify ("slips", occasional, harmful or addictive drinking)
- o 5 distinct patters of drinking
  - – 80% - no drinking, rare slip
  - – 20% - early harmful use and reduction, gradual increase and reduction, severely harmful
- o Those with "significant" relapse are more likely to be non–compliant with immunosuppression

- ➢ Predictors of Recidivism
  - o Based on meta–analysis of 54 studies:
    - – Poor social support
    - – Family EtOH history
    - – Pre–transplantation abstinence </= 6 months
    - – Pre–LT treatment of psychological condition (not EtOH)
    - – Non–compliance with clinic visits post–LT
    - – Smoking after recidivism

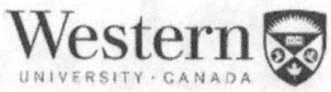

- o Studies are difficult to assess
  - – Wide confidence interval (CI)
  - – Poor quality studies, poor associations overall

- ➤ Patient Selection
  - o Must take into account the history of addiction and alcoholism
  - o 6+ months of abstinence
    - – Widely used in predicting recidivism
    - – 75% of centers in NA adopt this interval
    - – Allows recovery of liver injury
  - o Most require enrollment in an alcohol rehabilitation program
  - o Functional level, employment, social support

Why is 6 months recidivism required?

- o Based on 3 small studies
- o 73 patients, treated for ALC, followed 25 months post–LT compared *vs* age and sex–matched population not LT for alcohol
- o 43% resumed alcohol intake if abstinent is < 6 months *vs* 7%, if > 6 months
- o Other data are similar, smaller, poorly controlled, inconsistent diagnosis of alcoholism
- o Recent studies report recidivism rates of ~ 50% post–LT for ALC, despite of 6 months previous abstinence
  - – Recurrent alcohol consumption and hepatic disease may be mild

Abbreviations: ALC, alcoholic cirrhosis; LT, liver transplantation

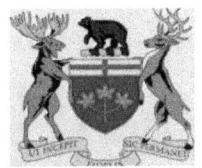

Should an exception be made for 6 months abstinence in severe alcoholic hepatitis?

- o Some studies have refuted the notion that liver transplantation is never indicated in acute alcoholic hepatitis
- o Suggests that attempts be made to identify patients who are at low risk for future recidivism, urgently
- o French study
  - 26 patients with severe alcoholic hepatitis → LT after failing medical management
  - Good social support, contract for abstinence, no prior episodes of known alcoholic liver disease, no active psychological illness
  - Matched with 26 controls with severe alcoholic hepatitis without LT
  - Cumulative 6–month survival is higher in LT group (77 *vs* 23%) and at 2 years (71 *vs* 23%)
  - 3/26 resumed drinking at 2–year follow–up
- o Reproduced in 2 other smaller trials
- o Highly controversial

Reducing Recidivism Pre–LT

- o Many centers in the US require abstinence contract
  - Ongoing attendance to AA post–liver transplantation (LT)
- o Ongoing communication with LT team, social workers, allied health, transplant coordinators
- o Motivational Enhancement Therapy
  - Marginal benefit*

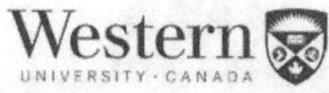

- o Random blood alcohol checks
  - – Ethanol use = less likely with a higher number of random BALs   (P = 0.001)
  - – No patients with pre–existing abstinence of > 24 months had a positive screen
- o Managing addiction (including co–existing) by trained addiction specialist (with special interest in transplant medicine)
  - – Used by many transplant centers in the US

Weinreib, R.M., *et al. Liver Transpl.* 2011; 5:539-47.

Multivariable Analysis for Predictors of Alcohol Use While on Transplant Waiting List

Variables	Risk (hazard) Ratio (95% Confidence interval)	P values
– Abstinence (months)	0.88 (0.83, 0.94)	0.001
– Number of levels drawn	0.63 (0.52, 0.76)	0.001
– Number of times that residential rehab was attended	1.21 (0.81, 1.84)	0.35

Printed with permission: Carbonneau, *et al. Liver Transpl.* 2010; 16(1):91-7.

Increased Risk of Alcohol Use While on Transplant Waiting List with Shorter Duration of Prelisting Abstinence

		Abstinence (Mon)				
		< 6 mon	6-12 mon	12-18 mon	18-24 mon	> 24 mon
EtOH screen	Negative	3 (60%)	53 (79.1%)	16 (76.2%)	16 (88.9%)	23 (100%)
	Positive	2 (40%)	14 (20.9%)	5 (23.8%)	2 (11.1%)	0 (0%)

Abbreviation: EtOH, ethanol

Printed with permission: Carbonneau, *et al. Liver Transpl.* 2010; 16(1):91-7.

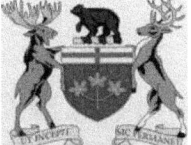

Estimating Future Abstinence Pre–LT

o No single measure is a reliable prognosticator for future relapses in post–LT

o Increased duration of abstinence is associated with reduction of recidivism post–LT

o Liver biopsy = unreliable estimate of recent alcohol use

o Psychosocial assessment determines higher or lower relative but not absolute risk

Post–Liver Transplantation

o Alcohol recidivism rates are difficult to quantify

	Cumulative Abstinence post–LT (mon)		
	12	24	36
o With ALC (recidivism)	82	58	38
o Without ALC (abstinence)	52	38	38

o Post–transplant survival similar to non–ALD

o ALC significantly more likely to have death from CV causes and from *de novo* cancers (abstinent)

Effect of Recidivism

o < 15% of ALD patients heavily drink post–LT

o Heavy drinking post–LT associated with:
  - Rapidly progressive liver injury
  - Allograft failure
  - Fatal alcoholic hepatitis
  - ↓ survival
  - Also associated with:
    - Non follow–up
    - Non–compliance of immunosuppression

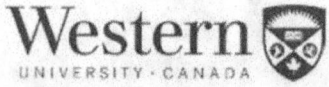

- Alcohol use and long term survival post –LT

	Patient survival (%) years after LT			
	3	5	10	12
o With ALC (recidivism)	95	94	77	52
o Without ALC (abstinence)	95	90	21	21

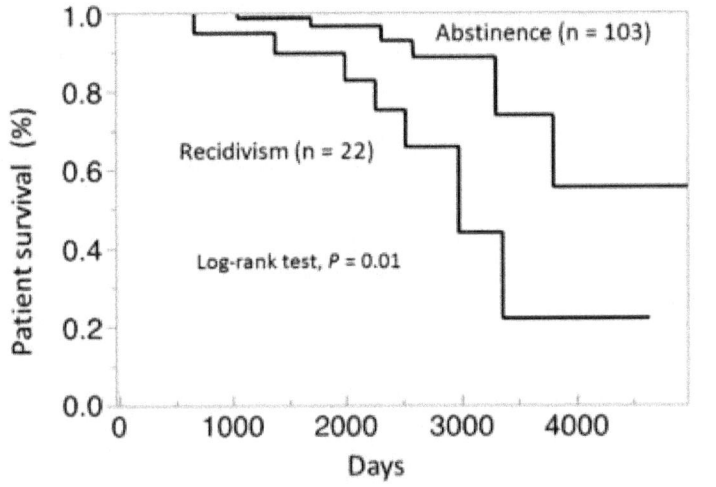

Numbers at risk	0 year	1 year	3 years	5 years	7 years	10 years
Recidivism	22	22	19	14	7	2
Abstinence	103	103	70	42	25	5

- Impact of alcohol relapse on patient survival: comparison of recidivism and abstinence 18 months after transplantation
  - There was a significant difference in survival between the groups (log rank test, P = 0.01)

Printed with permission: Egawa, H., *et al. Liver transpl.* 2014; 20(3):298-310.

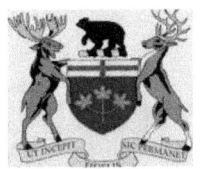

Smoking

- o Smoking remains the critical RF for post–LT morbidity and mortality – independent of relapse
  - – ↑ rate of lung, liver, orophayngeal Ca (*vs* non–ALD post–LT)
  - – DiMartini, *et al.* said 40% of patients who underwent LT for ALD resumed smoking within 6 months
- o Some centers also advocate pre–LT enrollment into smoking cessation programs or removal of smoking
- o 20% of transplant centers in US refuse to list patients, if smoking

Reducing Recidivism Post–LT

- ➤ Summary
  - o Careful and intense follow–up
  - o ↓ in recidivism in 5 years (22% *vs* 44% in matched historical group)
  - o Contract of abstinence
  - o Random blood alcohol sampling
  - o Ongoing psychiatric evaluation or addictions specialist or MET
  - o Ongoing alcohol rehabilitation
  - o Treat co–existing addictions, including smoking

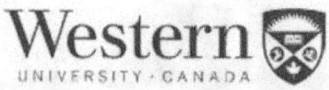

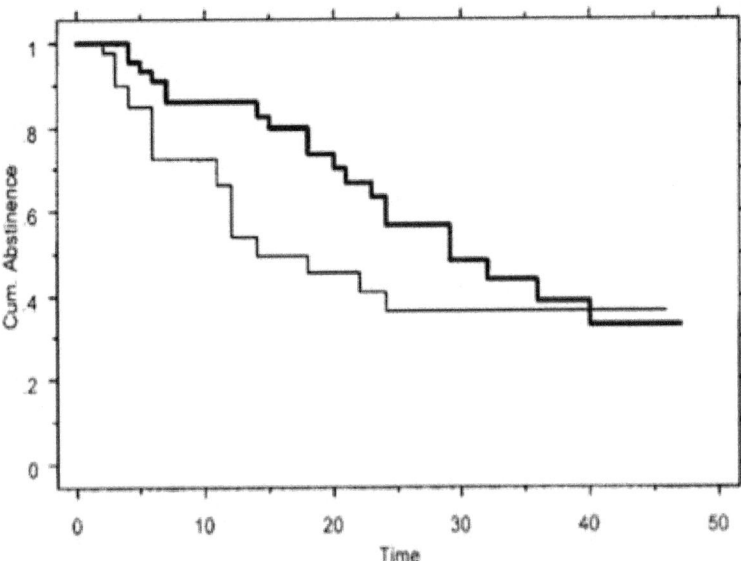

Kaplan–Meier curve showing length of post–transplantation abstinence in patients with (bold line) and without (thin line) ALD (time is shown as months post–transplant)

Printed with permission: Mackie, J., *et al. Liver Transpl.* 2001; 7(5):418-27.

"Your greatest invention lies in your hands, it is your future."

Apoorve Dubey

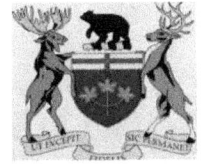

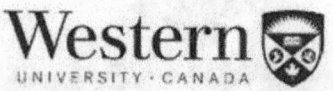

THERAPEUTIC PROCEDURES

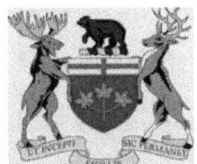

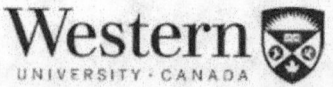

The Amazing New Era of HCV Therapy

Bandar Al-Judaibi

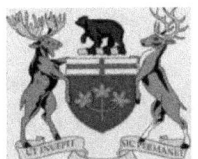

The Prevalence of HCV in different countries

➢ Demography

- o Prevalence of HCV is higher in countries located in Asia (2.1%, 83 millions) and Africa (3.2%, 28 millions), while a lower prevalence is found in North America, Europe and Australia (Asselah, T., *et al. Liver Int.* 2014; 34(10):1447-51).

- o HCV Burden of Disease in Canada:
  - – ↑ medical burden due to progression of liver deterioration
  - – HCV by disease stage, estimated for 2016 (x1000)
    - ▪ F_0, F_1, F_3 45
    - ▪ F_2 55
    - ▪ Cirrhosis   25

Cost of Untreated HCV Rises Significantly with Advanced Disease

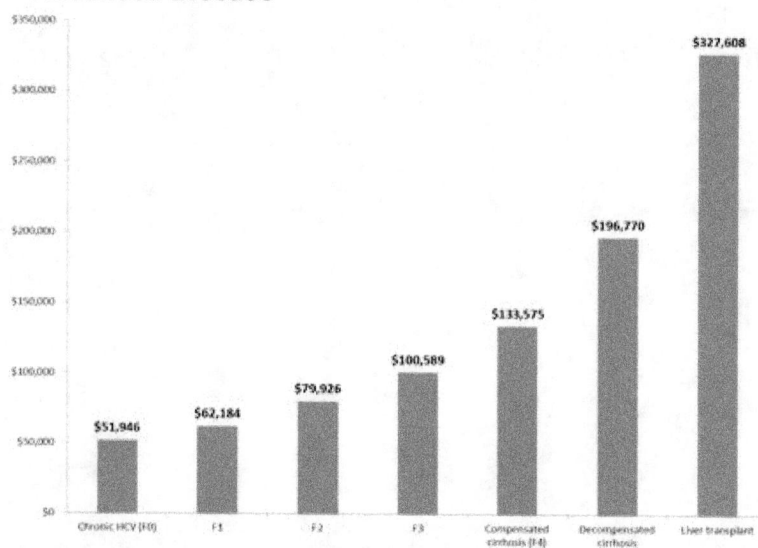

Adapted from: Myers, R.P., *et al. Can J Gastroenterol.* 2014; 28(5):243-50.

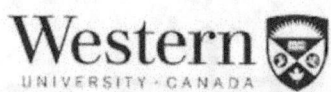

Achieving Sustained Virologic Response (SVR) Effectively Halts HCV–Disease Progression

- o For the patient
    - – Reduced disease sequelae
    - – Improved quality of life
    - – Prolonged life

- o For the healthcare system
    - – Reduced costs

- o For society
    - – More productive population

- o Mortality (approximate) at 10–year rate

	SVR	No SVR
– All–cause	8%	25%
– Liver–related or LT	2%	25%

Abbreviation: SVR, sustained virological response

Van der Meer, A.J., *et al. JAMA.* 2012; 308(24):2584-93.

- o Antiviral therapy must be maximized to make an impact

Davis, G.L., *et al. Gastroenterology.* 2010; 138(2):513-21, 521.

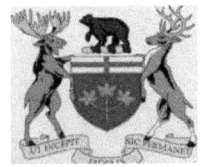

Other Issues with PI–Based Therapy

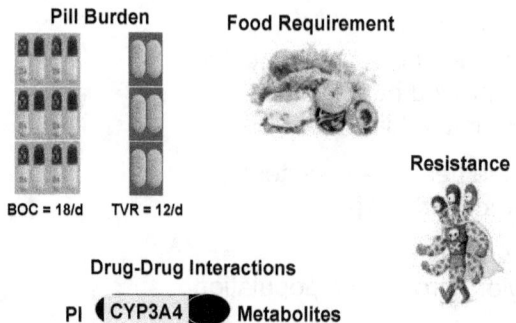

Pill Burden

Food Requirement

Resistance

BOC = 18/d   TVR = 12/d

Drug-Drug Interactions

PI ❰ CYP3A4 ❱ Metabolites

Phase 3 QUEST-1 and QUEST-2: Primary Endpoint: Over–all Virologic Response

SVR12

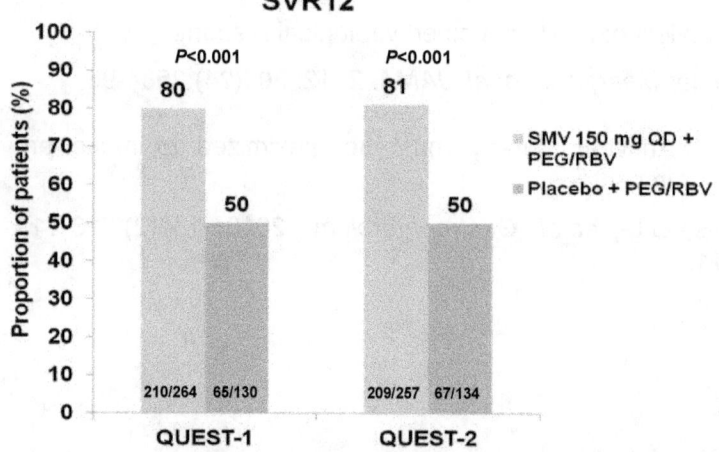

Baseline Q80K had an impact on treatment for G1a

Jacobson, I., *et al. EASL.* 2013. Amsterdam.   #1425.; Manns, M., *et al. EASL.* 2013. Amsterdam, The Netherlands. Oral #1413.

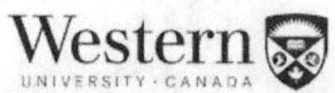

Retreatment of HCV GT 1 Treatment-Experienced Patients: Interim Analysis

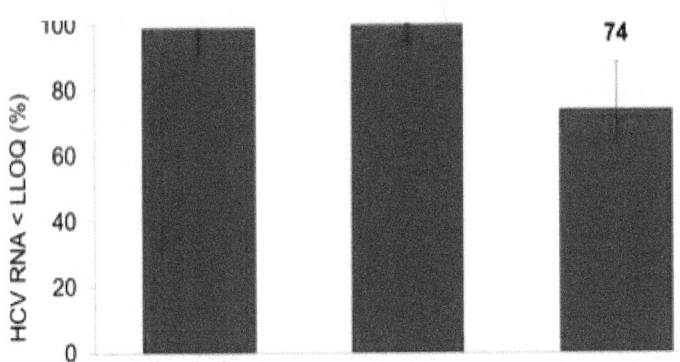

- o No clear impact of previous treatment failure on response
- o High SVR rates achieved despite presence of RAVs
- o Virologic failure only due to relapse
- o No discontinuations due to AEs

Error bars represent 95% confidence intervals

What Does HCV Treatment Look Like *Currently*?

Evolution of Hepatitis C Therapy to Date

	1st Gen PI (BOC/TVR)	2st Gen PI (SMV)	DAA (SOF)
Pill Burden	12/6 *bid/tid*	OD	OD
DDI	Many	Few	Nil
Multi–genotype	G1 only	G1 (2,4,5,6)	G1,4,5,6,2,3
Resistance Mutations	Yes	Q80K (G1a)	Nil
Duration of Therapy / RGT	24-48 weeks / YES	24/48 weeks / YES	12 weeks / NO

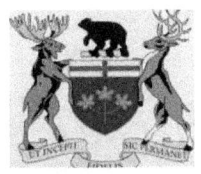

	1st Gen PI (BOC/TVR)	2st Gen PI (SMV)	DAA (SOF)
AEs	Many	Few	Fewer
Capacity	Low	Med	High
Adherence	60-80%	24 weeks PEG	12 weeks PEG
Costs / AEs	+30%	Neutral	Trivial
Good for F4s	15-60%	58-65%	80%
SVR	70%	80%	90%

Abbreviations: AEs, adverse effects; DDI, drug–drug interactions; RGT, response–guided therapy; SVR, sustained viral response

Evolution of SVR Rates in HCV Genotype 1

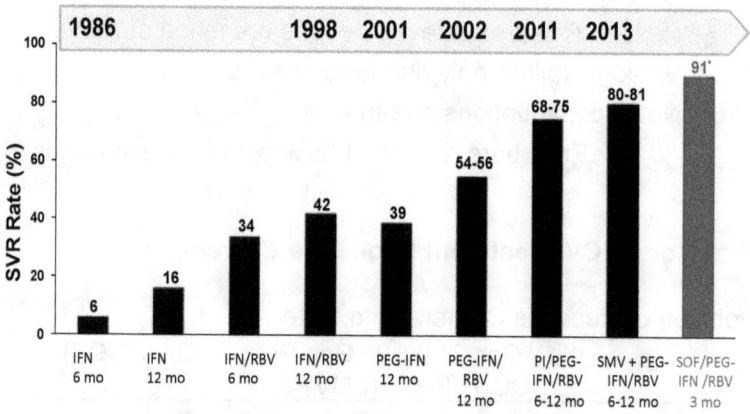

*SVR12 rate of 90% among GT 1 patients in the Phase 3 NEUTRINO trial (12 weeks of SOF+PEG-IFN+RBV)

Adapted from: Strader, D.B., et al. Hepatology. 2004; 39:1147-71.; INCIVEK [PI]. Cambridge, MA: Vertex Pharmaceuticals; 2013. VICTRELIS [PI]. Whitehouse Station, NJ: Merck & Co; 2014.; Jacobson, I., et al. EASL. 2013. Amsterdam. The Netherlands. Poster #1425.; Manns, M., et al. EASL. 2013. Amsterdam. The Netherlands. Oral #1413.; Lawitz, E., et al. APASL. 2013. Singapore. Oral #LB-02.

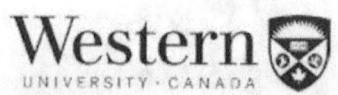

Sub–Optimal SVR Rates in HCV GT1 Patients with Bridging Fibrosis–Cirrhosis

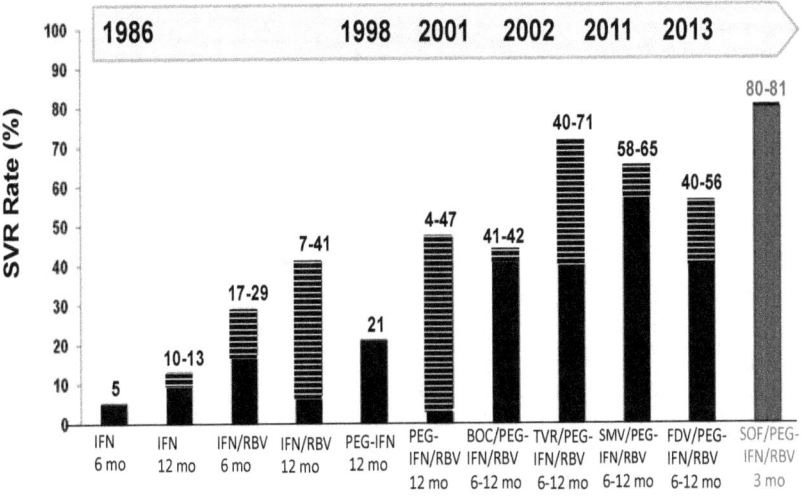

*Year of presentation/publication of SMV-, FDV-, and SOF-based regimens in HCV GT 1-3 patients with bridging fibrosis-cirrhosis

Adapted from: Strader, D.B., *et al. Hepatology.* 2004; 39:1147-71. INCIVEK [PI]. Cambridge, MA: Vertex Pharmaceuticals; 2013. VICTRELIS [PI]. Whitehouse Station, NJ: Merck & Co; 2014.; McHutchison, J., *et al. NEJM.* 1998; 339:1485-92.; Poynard, *T., et al. Lancet.* 1998; 352:1426-32.; Manns, M., *et al. Lancet.* 2001; 358:958-65.; Fried, M., *et al. NEJM.* 2002; 347:975-82.; Hadziyannis, S., *et al. Ann Intern Med.* 2004; 140:346-55.; McHutchison, J., *et al. NEJM.* 2009; 361:580-93.; PEGASYS [PI]. Hoffmann-La Roche Inc; 2013. PEGINTRON [PI]. Whitehouse Station, NJ: Merck & Co; 2013.; Jacobson, I., *et al. EASL.* 2013.; Manns, M., *et al. EASL.* 2013.; Ferenci, P., *et al. EASL.* 2013.; Fontaine, H., *et al. EASL.* 2013.; Amsterdam. #60; Lawitz, E., *et al. EASL.* 2013.; Amsterdam. Oral #1411; Lawitz, E., *et al. N Engl J Med.* 2013 May 16.

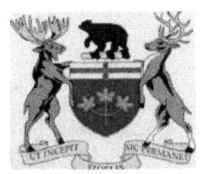

Key Elements of an Ideal HCV Regimen

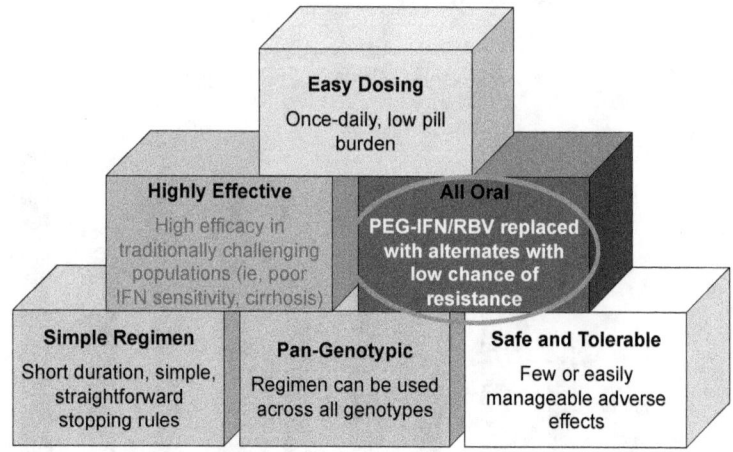

What's in the Future?

❖ Pipeline of direct–acting antivirals (DAA)

Faldaprevir	Samatasvir	ABT-333
Asunaprevir	ACH-2928	ABT-072
ABT-450/R	GSK2336805	Filibuvir
	BMS-824383	Setrobuvir (ANA-598)
Narlaprevir	PPI-461	Deleobuvir (BI-207127)
Danoprevir/R	PPI-667	BMS-791325
Vaniprevir	AZD-7295	Tegobuvir
Sovaprevir	ACH-3102	Lomibuvir (VX-222)
ACH-2684	MK-8742	VX-759
MK-5172	ABT-530	VX-916
GS-9451		TMC-649128
ABT-493		MK-3281
VX-500		INX-189
IDX 320		IDX-375

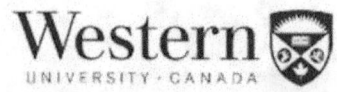

COSMOS Study: Simeprevir plus Sofosbuvir ± RBV in Naïve and Null–Responder G1 Patients

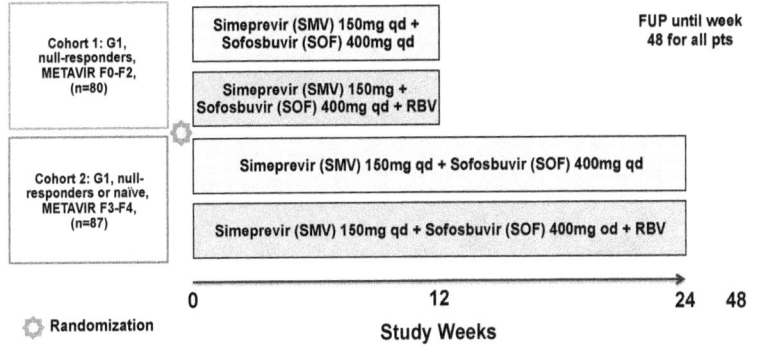

Cohort 1 was stratified by G1 subtype and IL28B, and Cohort 2 by G1 subtype and prior treatment status

Adapted from: Sulkowski, *et al*. *EASL*. 2014. Oral (O7).; Lawitz, *et al*. *EASL*. 2014. Oral (LB O165).

COSMOS Study: Simeprevir plus Sofosbuvir ± RBV in F0–F2 Null–Responder G1 Patients – SVR

Efficacy n/N (%)	SMV+SOF 12wk, N=14	SMV+SOF +RBV 12wk, N=27	SMV+SOF 24wk, N=13	SMV+SOF +RBV 24wk, N=21
SVR12 (ITT)	13/14 (92.9)	26/27 (96.3)	13/13 (100.0)	19/21 (90.5)
G1a	9/10 (90.0)	20/21 (95.2)	10/10 (100.0)	15/17 (88.2)
G1a; Q80K	5/6 (83.3)	8/9 (88.9)	3/3 (100.0)	8/10 (80.0)
G1a; no Q80K	4/4 (100.0)	12/12 (100.0)	7/7 (100.0)	7/7 (100.0)
G1b	4/4 (100.0)	6/6 (100.0)	3/3 (100.0)	4/4 (100.0)

Sulkowski, *et al*. *EASL*. 2014. Oral (O7).

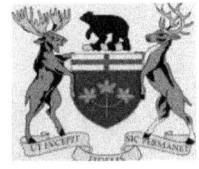

Safety and Efficacy of SOF–Containing Regimens for HCV

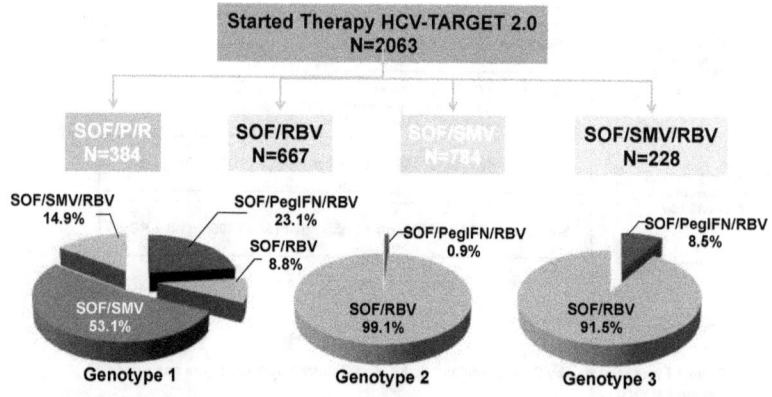

Real-world observational study of 2,063 patients treated with DAAs at academic (n=38) and community medical centers (n=15) in North America and Europe

Jensen, *AASLD*. 2014. Oral #45.

Demographics

n (%)	SOF+PegIFN +RBV n=384	SOF+RBV n=667	SOF+SMV n=784	SOF+SMV +RBV n=228	Total n=2063
Male	253 (66.2)	422 (63.6)	478 (62.0)	147 (65.3)	1300 (63.7)
Mean age, y (range)	53.9 (23 - 79)	56.9 (21 - 82)	59.5 (20 - 83)	58.8 (29 - 80)	57.6 (20 - 83)
Caucasian	270 (70.3)	539 (80.8)	584 (74.5)	177 (77.6)	1570 (76.1)
Black	68 (17.8)	37 (5.6)	96 (12.5)	33 (14.7)	234 (11.5)
Treatment Status					
Naive	211 (54.9)	371 (55.6)	318 (40.6)	82 (36.0)	982 (47.6)
Experienced	172 (44.8)	296 (44.4)	465 (59.3)	144 (63.2)	1077 (52.2)
PI Failure	47 (27.3)	25 (8.4)	76 (24.8)	45 (31.3)	193 (17.9)
Cirrhosis	120 (31.3)	302 (45.3)	440 (56.1)	137 (60.1)	999 (48.4)
Hx Decompensation	12 (11.4)	136 (49.5)	167 (44.8)	60 (50.8)	375 (43.1)
MELD >10	18 (17.1)	120 (43.6)	122 (32.7)	34 (28.8)	294 (33.8)
Liver Cancer	25 (6.5)	66 (9.9)	88 (11.2)	32 (14.0)	211 (10.2)
Liver Transplant	27 (7.0)	57 (8.5)	111 (14.2)	32 (14.0)	227 (11.0)
HIV	14 (3.6)	18 (2.7)	8 (1.0)	7 (3.1)	47 (2.3)

78% (253/323) of GT 1, non–cirrhotic, naïve has a baseline HCV RNA < 6 million IU/mL

Jensen, AASLD. 2014. Oral #45.

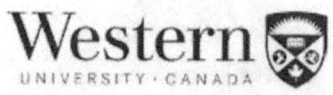

Efficacy and Safety of SOF–Containing Regimens

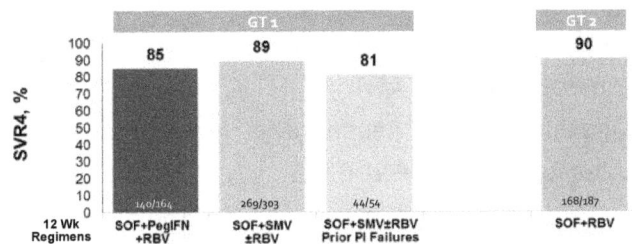

SVR4/SVR12 Concordance: 94.4–98.2% PPV

n (%)	SOF+PegIFN+ RBV n=384	SOF+SMV ±RBV n=228	SOF+SMV n=784	SOF+RBV n=667	Total n=2063
Completed treatment	332 (86.5)	189 (82.9)	663 (84.6)	429 (64.3)	1613 (78.2)
Ongoing treatment	41 (10.7)	32 (14.0)	101 (12.9)	205 (30.7)	379 (18.4)
D/C Prematurely*	11 (2.9)	7 (3.1)	20 (2.6)	33 (4.9)	71 (3.4)
AE	6 (1.6)	5 (2.2)	16 (2.0)	17 (2.5)	44 (2.1)
Death	1 (0.3)	2 (0.9)	6 (0.8)	3 (0.4)	12 (0.6)

*Not all premature D/C are summarized. Full list available in final slides.

Jensen, *AASLD*. 2014. Oral #45.

Daclatasvir (NS5A) + Sofosbuvir ± RBV in GT1 Patients With Prior Treatment Failure on TVR or BOC (non–cirrhotic)

- o Primary endpoint analysis of randomized, open–label phase IIa study

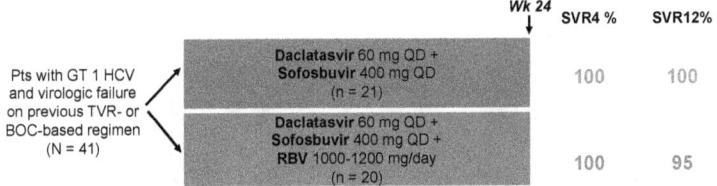

- o 45 – 48% had TVR/BOC resistance mutations, median 2.4 years since previous therapy
  - – No difference in response by the absence or presence of resistance mutations

- o Both regimens well–tolerated; 1 serious AE; no discontinuations due to AEs

Sulkowski, M.S., *et al. EASL*. 2013. Abstract 1417.

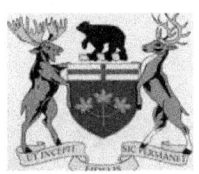

Direct–Acting Antivirals

Classes	Drugs	Dosing
NS3/4A protease inhibitor	ABT-450/RTV	150/100 mg
NS3 protease inhibitor	Asunaprevir	100 mg *bid*
NS3/4A protease inhibitor	MK-5172	100 mg *qid*
NS3/4A protease inhibitor	Simeprevir	150 mg *qid*
NS5B nonnucleoside polymerase inhibitor	Dasabuvir	250 mg *bid*
NS5B nucleotide polymerase inhibitor	Sofosbuvir	400 mg *qid*
NS5A inhibitor	Daclatasvir	60 mg *qid*
NS5A inhibitor	GS-5816	25 or 100 mg *qid*
NS5A inhibitor	Ledipasvir	90 mg *qid*
NS5A inhibitor	MK-8742	20 or 50 mg *qid*
NS5A inhibitor	Ombitasvir	25 mg *qid*

Ledipasvir+Sofosbuvir as the First HCV Single Tablet Regimen (STR)

2011-2013   2014

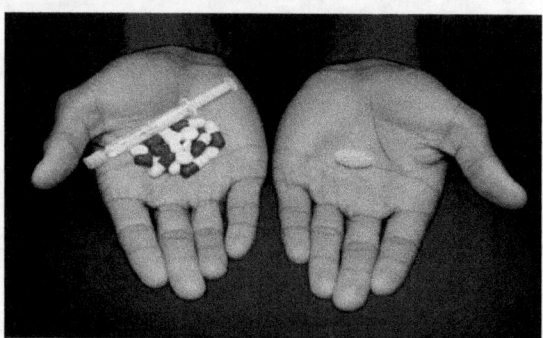

HARVONI ® [PI]. Gilead Sciences, Inc. Foster City, CA October 2014.

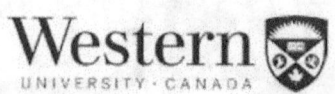

STR of LDV/SOF Phase 3 Results

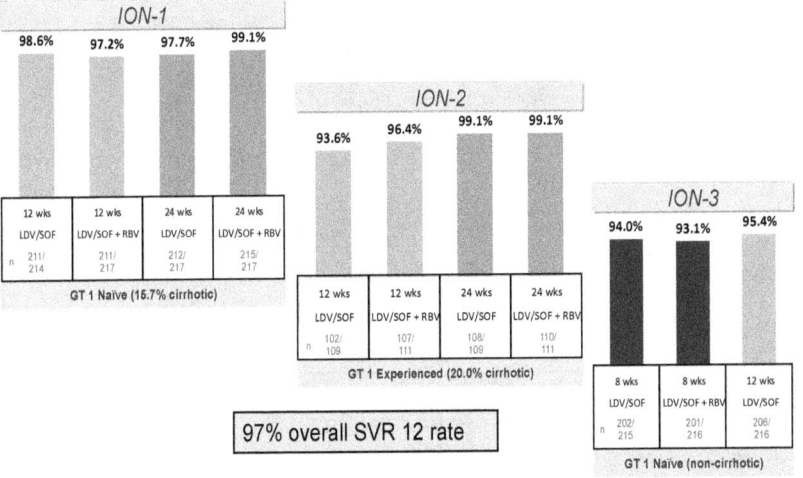

97% overall SVR 12 rate

Percentages represent SVR12 rates.

Afdhal, N., *et al. N Engl J Med.* 2014; 370:1889-98.; Afdhal, N., *et al. N Engl J Med.* 2014; 370:1483-93.; Kowdley, K., *et al. N Engl J Med.* 2014; 370:1879-88.

ION-1

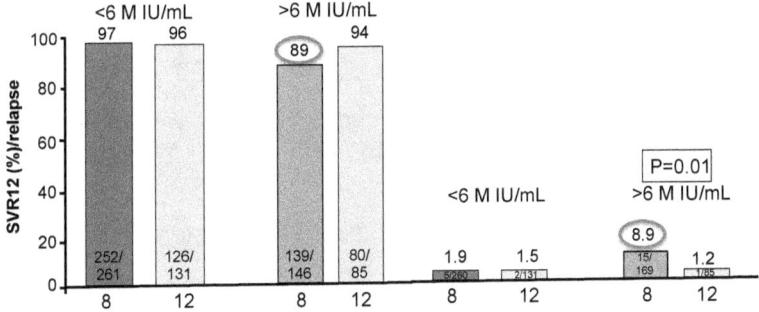

Depends how concerned we are about relapse...

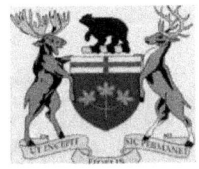

SVR12: Absence of Cirrhosis vs. Cirrhosis (ITT Analysis)

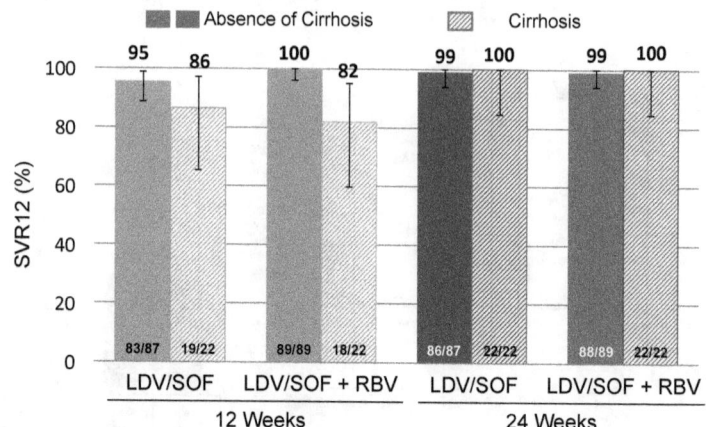

HARVONI ® [PI]. Gilead Sciences, Inc. Foster City, CA October 2014.

Afdhal, N., *EASL. 2014.* O109.; Afdhal, N., *et al. N Engl J Med.* 2014; 370:1483-1493.

Discontinuations Due to Adverse Events Were 1% or Less in Subjects Treated with LDV/SOF

0%	<1%	1%
LDV/SOF	**LDV/SOF**	**LDV/SOF**
8 Weeks	12 Weeks	24 Weeks
N=215	N=539	N=326

The most common adverse reactions (≥ 10%) were fatigue and headache in subjects treated with 8, 12 or 24 weeks of LDV/SOF.

HARVONI ® [PI]. Gilead Sciences, Inc. Foster City, CA October 2014.

Afdhal, N., *et al. N Engl J Med.* 2014; 370:1889-1898.; Afdhal, N., *et al. N Engl J Med.* 2014;370:1483-1493.; Kowdley, K., *et al. N Engl J Med.* 2014;370:1879-1888.

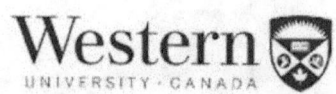

Ledipasvir–Sofosbuvir (*Harvoni*): **Indications and Usage**

Genotype 1 Patient Populations	Treatment Duration*
Treatment naïve with or without cirrhosis	12 weeks
Treatment experienced** without cirrhosis	12 weeks
Treatment experienced** with cirrhosis	24 weeks

*Consider treatment duration of 8 weeks in treatment–naïve patients without cirrhosis who have a pretreatment HCV RNA less than 6 million IU/mL

**Treatment–experienced patients who have failed treatment with either (a) peginterferon alfa plus ribavirin, or (b) HCV protease inhibitor plus peg–interferon alfa plus ribavirin

Source: *Harvoni* Prescribing Information. Gilead Sciences.

Ledipasvir–Sofosbuvir (*Harvoni*): **Estimated Cost of Therapy**

Estimated Cost of Ledipasvir–Sofosbuvir Based on Treatment Duration

Duration of Treatment	Estimated Cost*
8 Weeks	$63,000
12 Weeks	$94,500
24 Weeks	$189,000

*Estimated cost based on Wholesaler Acquisition Cost in United States of $1125 per pill

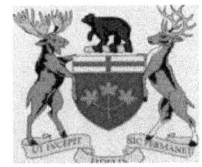

LDV/SOF in Cirrhotic Patients Who Previously Failed PI–Based Triple Therapy

Double–blind, placebo–controlled study in cirrhotic GT1 patients who failed both Peg–IFN+RBV and PI+Peg–IFN+RBV regimens in France (null or partial responders)

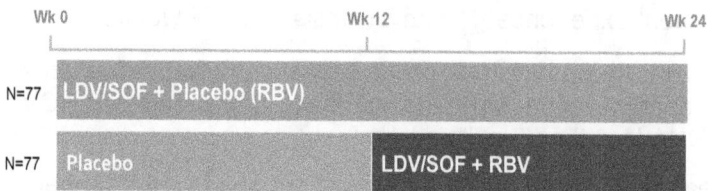

- ○ 30% of patients were previously enrolled in the CUPIC cirrhotic study
  - – RBV dosing was weight–based (< 75 kg = 1000 mg; ≥ 75 kg = 1200 mg)
- ○ Randomization was stratified by:
  - – HCV genotype
    - ▪ 1a *vs* 1b (mixed or other GT 1 results stratified as GT 1a)
  - – Prior HCV therapy treatment response
    - ▪ Never achieved HCV RNA < LLOQ *vs* Achieved HCV RNA < LLOQ
- ○ Cirrhosis was determined by biopsy, Fibroscan > 12.5 kPa, or FibroTest® score of > 0.75 and an AST of platelet ratio index (APRI) of > 2

Bourliere, *AASLD*. 2014. Oral #LB-6.

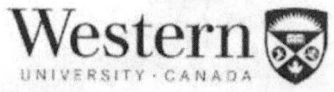

Demographics

	Placebo 12 weeks > LDV/SOF + RBV 12 weeks (n=77)	LDV/SOF + Placebo RBV 24 weeks (n=78)
Mean age, y (range)	56 (39–74)	57 (23–77)
Male, n (%)	58 (75)	56 (72)
White, n (%)	76 (99)	75 (96)
Mean BMI, kg/m^2 (range)	27.9 (19.6–47.1)	26.3 (19.1–39.8)
IL28B non-CC, n (%)	73 (95)	72 (92)
Genotype 1a	48 (62)	50 (64)
Mean HCV RNA, log10 IU/mL (range)	6.5 (5.3–7.7)	6.5 (3.9–7.5)
Mean MELD (range)	7 (6-16)	7 (6-12)
Varices, n (%)	16 (21)	25 (32)
Mean platelets (range)	153 (54–316)	141 (59–278)
Platelets, < 100 x 10^3/μL	14 (18)	13 (17)
Mean albumin, g/dL	3.9 (3.2–4.6)	3.9 (3.0–4.9)
Albumin, < 3.5 g/dL, n (%)	6 (8)	14 (17)
Mean INR (range)	1.1 (0.9–2.4)	1.1 (0.9–1.4)
Mean bilirubin, mg/dL (range)	0.8 (0.3–2.5)	0.8 (0.3–1.8)

Bourliere, *AASLD. 2014*. Oral #LB-6.

LDV/SOF in TE Cirrhotic Patients: SVR12

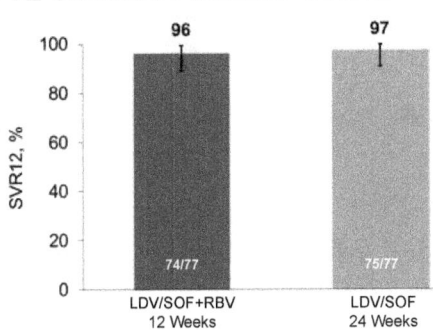

Error bars represent 95% confidence intervals

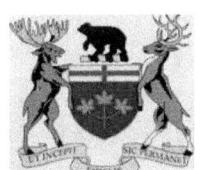

TE cirrhotics had a similar response to LDV/SOF+RBV for 12 weeks and LDV/SOF for 24 weeks

Bourliere, *AASLD*. 2014. Oral #LB-6.

Results: Safety Summary

| Patients, n (%) | Placebo 12 Weeks → LDV/SOF + RBV 12 weeks | | | LDV/SOF 24 weeks | |
		Placebo 12 Wk n=77	LDV/SOF + RBV 12Wk (n=76)	Overall Period n=77	First 12 Wk n=78	Overall Period n=78
Overall Safety	AEs	63 (82)	66 (87)	74 (96)	66 (85)	68 (87)
	Grade 3-4 AEs	1 (1)	5 (7)	6 (8)	2 (3)	10 (13)
	SAEs	1 (1)	3 (4)	4 (5)	3 (4)	8 (10)
	Treatment Related SAEs	0	1 (1)	1 (1)	0	0
	Treatment D/C due to AEs	1 (1)	0	1 (1)	0	0
	Death	0	0	0	0	0
	Grade 3-4 lab abnormalities	18 (23)	8 (11)	24 (31)	11 (14)	15 (19)
	Hb < 10 g/dL	1 (1)	1 (1)	2 (3)	0	1 (1)
	Hb < 8.5 g/dL	1 (1)	1 (1)	2 (3)	0	0

- Related event was anemia attributed to study treatment

- Treatment discontinue due to adverse effects: bacterial arthritis; decompensated cirrhosis (placebo period)

Bourliere, *AASLD*. 2014. Oral #LB-6.

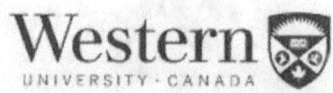

Results: Adverse Events ≥ 15%

Preferred term, n (%)	Placebo 12 Wk → LDV/SOF + RBV 12 Wk			LDV/SOF 24 Wk	
	Placebo 12 Wk n=77	Second 12 Wk n=76	Overall Period n=77	First 12 Wk n=78	Overall Period n=78
Asthenia	24 (31)	29 (38)	45 (58)	28 (36)	35 (45)
Headache	16 (21)	13 (17)	21 (27)	27 (35)	31 (40)
Pruritus	14 (18)	11 (14)	22 (29)	4 (5)	7 (9)
Insomnia	9 (12)	7 (9)	17 (22)	11 (14)	13 (17)
Nausea	8 (10)	8 (11)	14 (18)	7 (9)	8 (10)
Fatigue	3 (4)	5 (7)	7(9)	13 (17)	15 (19)
Dry skin	6 (8)	5 (7)	12 (16)	4 (5)	4 (5)
Arthralgia	5 (6)	0	6 (8)	6 (8)	12 (15)
Bronchitis	1 (1)	4 (5)	4 (5)	4 (5)	13 (17)

o   Most AEs are mild or moderate in severity

Bourliere, *AASLD*. 2014. Oral #LB-6.

LDV/SOF + RBV for HCV Patients with Decompensated Cirrhosis

Prospective, multicenter study of 12 or 24 weeks of LDV/SOF + RBV in TN and TE HCV GT 1 and 4 patients with CTP B (N=59) or CTP C (N=49) clinically decompensated cirrhosis

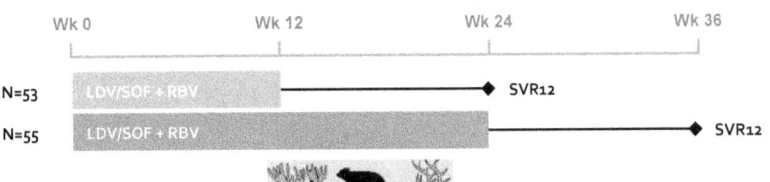

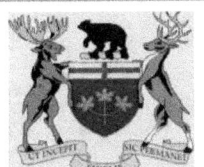

- o 108 patients randomized 1:1 to 12 or 24 weeks of treatment
- o Stratified by CTP class B [7 – 9] or C [score 10 – 12]*
- o Broad inclusion criteria:
  - – No history of major organ transplant, including liver
  - – No hepatocellular carcinoma (HCC)
  - – Total bilirubin ≤ 10 mg/dL, hemoglobin ≥ 10 g/dL
  - – CrCl ≥ 40 mL/min, platelets > 30,000
- o RBV dosing: dose escalation, 600 – 1200 mg/d

Flamm, *AASLD*. 2014. Oral #239.

Demographics

	CTP B		CTP C	
	12 wks n=30	24 wks n=29	12 wks n=23	24 wks n=26
Median age, y (range)	60 (28-69)	58 (35-69)	58 (41-71)	59 (48-68)
Male, n (%)	22 (73)	18 (62)	14 (61)	18 (69)
White, n (%)	29 (97)	26 (90)	21 (91)	24 (92)
BMI ≥ 30 kg/m^2, n (%)	10 (33)	10 (34)	13 (57)	9 (35)
Mean HCV RNA, $\log_{10}$ IU/mL (range)	5.9 (4.3-6.7)	5.8 (3.2-7.1)	5.6 (4.1-6.5)	5.8 (3.7-6.9)
GT 1a, n (%)	19 (63)	22 (76)	15 (65)	18 (69)
IL28B non-CC, n (%)	26 (87)	23/28 (82)	17 (74)	19 (73)
Prior HCV treatment, n (%)	22 (73)	19 (66)	11 (48)	18 (69)

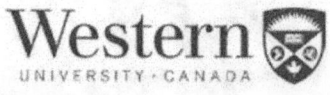

	CTP B		CTP C	
	12 wks n=30	24 wks n=29	12 wks n=23	24 wks n=26
MELD score, n (%)				
< 10	6 (20)	8 (28)	0	0
10–15	21 (70)	16 (55)	16 (70)	13 (50)
16-20	3 (10)	5 (17)	7 (30)	12 (46)
21-25	0	0	0	1 (4)
Ascites, n (%)	17 (57)	17 (59)	22 (96)	25 (96)
Encephalopathy, n (%)	20 (67)	16 (55)	21 (91)	23 (88)

Flamm, *AASLD*. 2014. Oral #239.

Results: SVR12

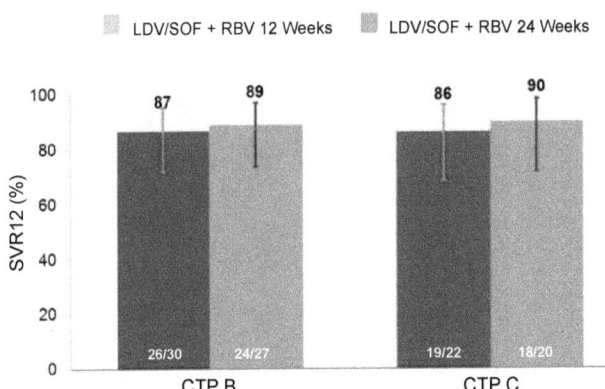

Error bars represent 90% confidence intervals

- o SVR rates were similar with 12 or 24 weeks of LDV/SOF + RBV

Flamm, *AASLD*. 2014. Oral #239.

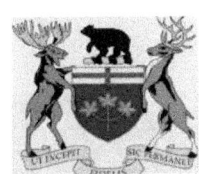

Results: Overall Safety Summary

Patients, n (%)	CTP B		CTP C	
	12 wks n=30	24 wks n=29	12 wks n=23	24 wks n=26
Any AE	29 (97)	27 (93)	23 (100)	26 (100)
Grade 3/4 AE	2 (7)	8 (28)	6 (26)	11 (42)
SAEs	3 (10)	10 (34)	6 (26)	11 (42)
Treatment–related SAEs	2 (7)	0	0	2 (8)
D/C due to AE	0	1 (3)	0	2 (8)
Death	1 (3)	2 (7)	2 (9)	1 (4)

- Related severe adverse events (SAEs): anemia (2), hepatic encephalopathy, peritoneal hemorrhage
- Early discontinuations: sepsis, hepatic encephalopathy, peritoneal hemorrhage
- Deaths: septic shock (2), multi–organ failure and septic shock (2), oliguric renal failure, cardiac arrest
- Patients continue to be followed for 5 years for long term outcomes

Flamm, *AASLD*. 2014. Oral #239.

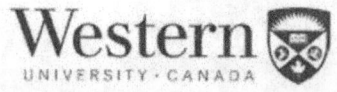

C–WORTHY: Grazoprevir + Elbasvir ± RBV x 12 or 18 weeks in GT1 HCV Patients

Randomized phase IIb trial

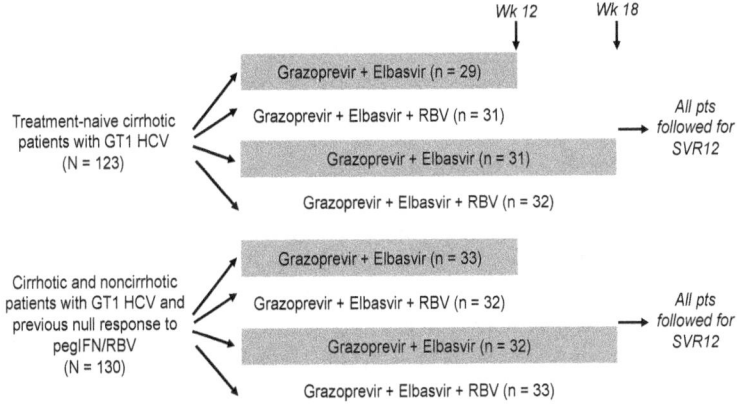

Grazoprevir 100 mg once daily; elbasvir 50 mg once daily; weight-based RBV 800, 1200, or 1400 mg daily.

Lawitz, E., *et al. AASLD*. 2014. Abstract 196.

C–WORTHY: Efficacy of Grazoprevir + Elbasvir ± RBV x 12 or 18 weeks

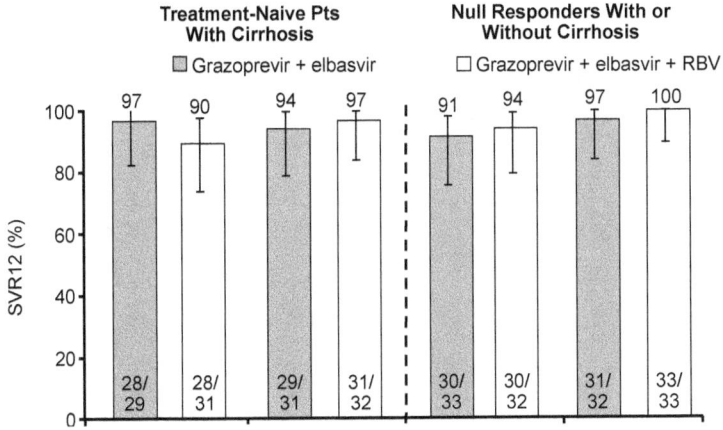

Lawitz, E., *et al. AASLD*. 2014. Abstract 196.

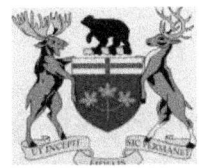

Treatment G1

- ○ Cirrhotic, null responder
    - – Harvoni for 24 weeks
    - – Harvoni + RBV for 12 weeks
    - – PEG–IFN, Sovaldi and RBV for 12 weeks
    - – Simeprevir and Sovaldi for 12 weeks (SVR 79% in CTP B,C)

- ○ Naïve, non–cirrhotic
    - – Harvoni
        - ▪ 8 weeks (viral load < 6 logs)
        - ▪ 12 weeks (viral load > 6 logs)
    - – Sovaldi and RBV (24 weeks)
    - – PEG–IFN, Sovaldi and RBV for 12 weeks
    - – Simeprevir and Sovaldi for 12 weeks

- ○ Naïve, cirrhotic
    - – Harvoni (12 *vs* 24 weeks, SVR 86% *vs* 93%)

FISSION Study (G2&3)

Response during and after treatment period (HCV RNA < 25 IU/mL – no. / total no. [%])

Response	NEUTRINO Study	FISSION Study	
	SOF + PEG +RBV for 12 wk	SOF + RBV for 12 wk	PEG + RBV for 24 wk
	(N = 327)	(N = 253)	(N = 243)
At 4 wk	321 / 325 (99)	249 / 250 (> 99)	158 / 236 (67)
At 12 wk	295 / 327 (90)	170 / 253 (67)	162 / 243 (67)

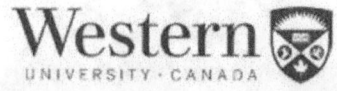

Fission Study (G2&3)

- o Response rates in the sofosbuvir–ribavirin group are lower among patients with genotype 3 infection than those with genotype 2 infection (56% vs. 97%)

- o Objective
  - – VALENCE (NCT01682720) is a Phase 3 study conducted in Europe assessing safety and efficacy of SOF + RBV administratered for

    12 weeks in patients with HCV GT2

    24 weeks in patients with HCV GT3

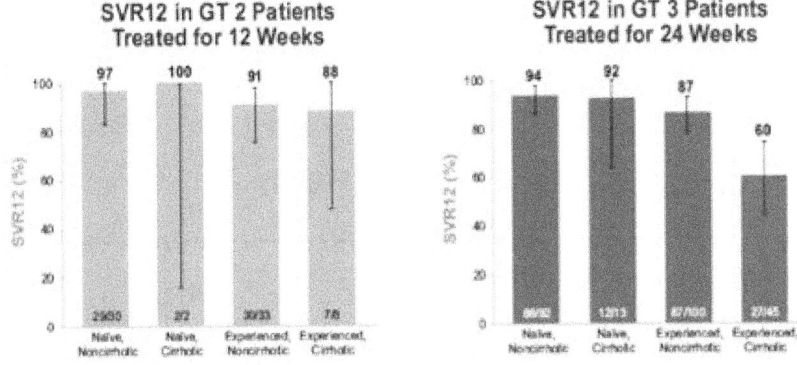

http://www.natap.org/2014/HCV/022114_02.htm

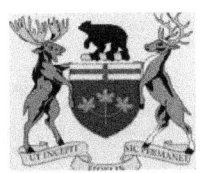

Retreatment with SOF Regimens for HCV GT 2 or 3 Who Failed Prior SOF+RBV Therapy: Interim Analysis

Open–label study offered to n=107 GT 2 or 3 treatment failures from FISSION, POSITRON and FUSION who received SOF+RBV

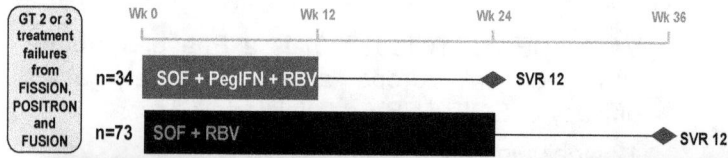

	SOF + PegIFN + RBV n=34	
Mean age, y (range)	53 (31–70)	53 (38-63)
Male, n (%)	26 (77)	63 (86)
Black, n (%)	1 (1%)	0
Mean BMI, kg/m² (range)	29 (22–39)	28 (20-41)
Cirrhosis* n (%)	14 (41)	25 (34)
Genotype 2, n (%)	6 (18)	5 (7)
Genotype 3, n (%)	28 (82)	68 (93)
Mean baseline HCV RNA, log$_{10}$ IU/mL (range)	6.3 (4.8-7.8)	6.6 (4.4–7.6)

Esteban, R. *EASL*. 2014. O8.

Retreatment with SOF Regimens for HCV GT 2 or 3 Who Failed Prior SOF+RBV Therapy: Interim Results

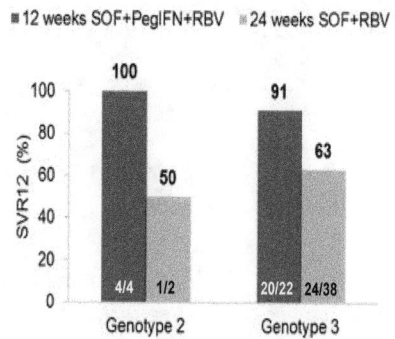

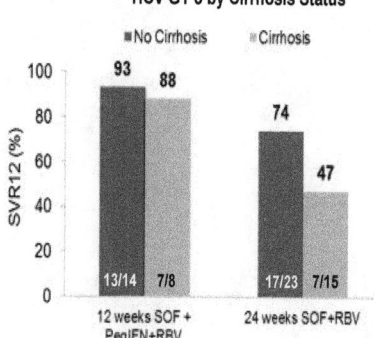

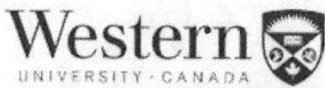

- o Retreatment with SOF–based regimen was successful in GT2 or GT3 patients who previously failed SOF–containing regimens

- o 12 weeks of SOF+Peg–IFN+RBV had higher overall SVR rates, including in patients with cirrhosis

- o The 24–week IFN–free regimen was safe and well–tolerated and offers a retreatment option for those ineligible to receive IFN

- o No discontinuations due to AEs

Esteban, R. *EASL*. 2014. O8.

LDV/SOF + RBV for 12 Weeks for HCV GT 3 Treatment–Experienced

Two–center, open label study in New Zealand

Wk 0	Wk 12	Wk 24

| n=50 | LDV/SOF + RBV | SVR12 |

- o Demographics

– Mean age, y (range)	52 (28–66)
– Male, n (%)	39 (78)
– White, n (%)	40 (80)
– Asian, n (%)	3 (6)
– Mean BMI, kg/m^2 (range)	26.0 (17.5–34.5)
– *IL28B* non–CC, n (%)	32 (64)
– Cirrhosis	22 (44)
– Mean HCV RNA, log$_{10}$ IU/mL (range)	6.3 (4.5–7.3)
– HCV GT 3a, n (%)	49 (98)

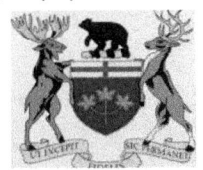

LDV/SOF + RBV for 12 Weeks for HCV GT 3 Treatment–Experienced

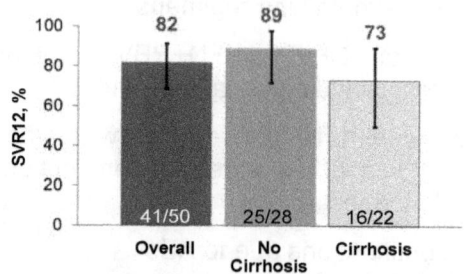

- LDV / SOF + RBV for 12 weeks resulting in high SVR rates in TE GT3

Gane, *AASLD*. 2014. Poster #LB-11.

SOF–Based Regimens for HCV GT 3

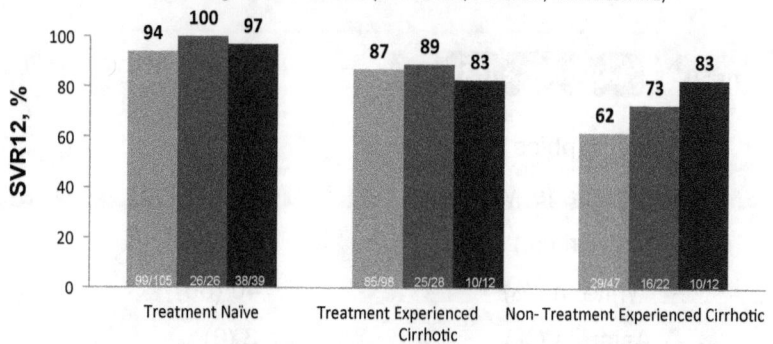

- SOF–based regimens resulted in similar SVR12 rates in TN and TE HCV GT 3

Zeuzem, S., *et al. NEJM*. 2014.; Gane, *EASL*. 2014. Oral #6.; Gane, E., *et al. NEJM*. 2013; 368:34-44.; Lawitz, E., *et al. Lancet Infect Dis*. 2013; 13:401-8.; Gane. *AASLD*. 2014. Poster #LB-11.

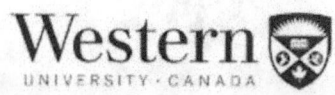

ALLY–3: SOF + DCV x 12 Wks in GT3 HCV Patients

o Primary endpoint: SVR12

o Inclusion criteria
- 18 years of age or older with GT3 HCV and HCV RNA ≥ 10,000 IU/mL
- Treatment naïve or experienced (no previous NS5A inhibitor use is allowed)

o Cirrhosis in 19% of naïve patients, 25% experienced patients

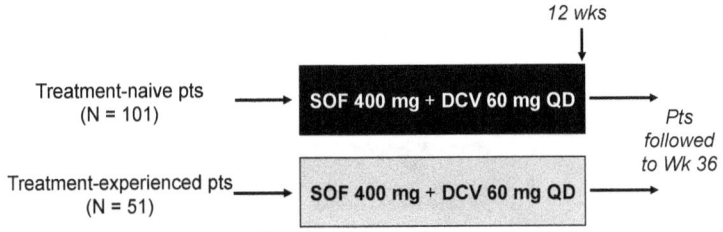

Nelson, D.R., *et al. AASLD*. 2014. Abstract LB-3.

ALLY–3: SVR12 With SOF + DCV x 12 Weeks in GT3 HCV Patients

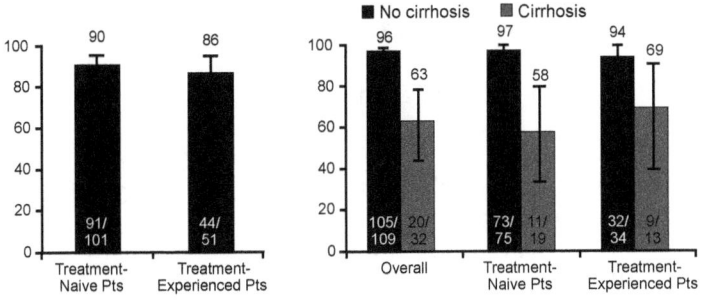

o Of 16 patients with relapse, 11 had cirrhosis

o 1 of 16 relapses occurred between post–treatment weeks 4 and 12

o RAVs emerging at relapse: NS5A Y93H emerged in 9 of 16 patients

Nelson, D.R., *et al. AASLD*. 2014. Abstract LB-3.

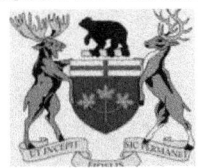

ELECTRON–2: SOF + GS-5816 ± RBV x 8 Weeks in Non–cirrhotic Patients With GT3 HCV

- ○ Randomized, open–label phase II trial
- ○ Primary endpoint: SVR12

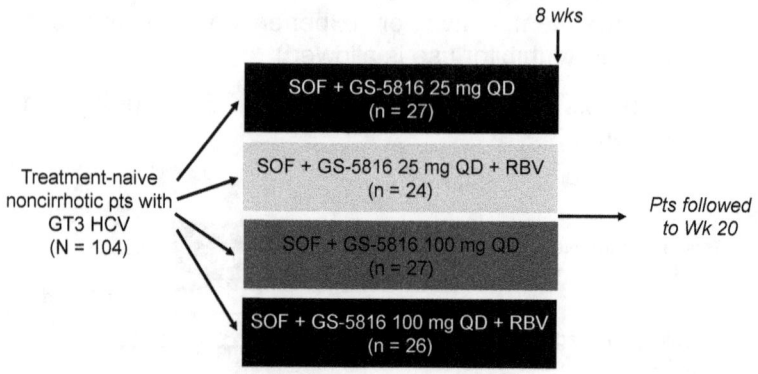

Gane, E.J., *et al. AASLD*. 2014. Abstract 79.

ELECTRON–2: SVR12 With SOF + GS-5816 ± RBV x 8 Weeks in Noncirrhotic GT3 Patients

SVR12, GT3 Non-cirrhotic Patients
% (n/N)

	SOF + GS-5816 25 mg (n = 27)	SOF + GS-5816 25 mg + RBV (n = 24)	SOF + GS-5816 100 mg (n = 27)	SOF + GS-5816 100 mg + RBV (n = 26)
Overall	100	88	96	100

- ○ Baseline NS5A RAVs had no effect on efficacy

Gane, E.J., *et al. AASLD*. 2014. Abstract 79.

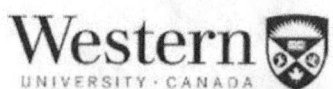

Treatment for G2

- o   Sovaldi and RBV
- o   PEG–IFN and RBV
- o   PEG–IFN, Sovaldi and RBV

Treatment for G3

- o   Naïve, non–cirrhotic
  - –   Sovaldi and RBV for 24 weeks
  - –   Harvoni+RBV for 12 weeks

- o   Others
  - –   PEG–IFN, Sovaldi and RBV

Hepatitis C Therapy

	1st Gen PI (BOC/TVR)	2st Gen PI (SMV)	DAA (SOF)	STR (LDV/SOF)
Pill Burden	12 / 6 *bid/tid*	*Od*	*od*	*od*
DDI	Many	Few	Nil	Nil
Resistance Mutations	Yes	Q80K (G1a)	Nil	Few
Duration of Therapy / RGT	24-48 wks / YES	24/48 wks / YES	12 wks / NO	8-12 wks/No
AEs	Many	Few	Fewer	Fewest
Capacity	Low	Med	High	Highest
Adherence	60-80%	24 wks PEG	12 wks PEG	No PEG No RBV
Costs / AEs	+30%	Neutral	Trivial	Minuscule
Good for F4s	15-60%	58-65%	80%	≥ 90%
SVR	70%	80%	90%	97%

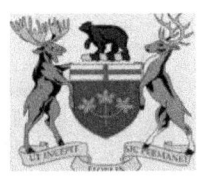

SOF+RBV for GT 4 HCV

Randomized, open–label, single–center study conducted in the US of the safety and efficacy of all–oral SOF + RBV in patients of Egyptian ancestry with HCV GT 4 – 23 – 24% cirrhotics; 52 – 55% treatment–experienced

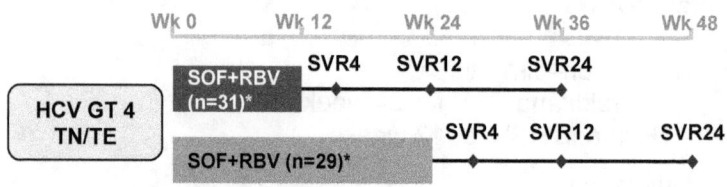

*SOF 400 mg/d; RBV 1000–1200 mg/d

- o SOF+RBV was well–tolerated for up to 24 weeks of treatment
  - – No discontinuation due to AEs
  - – No Grade 4 AEs or lab abnormalities were reported
- o No SOF resistance mutation S282T was found in any patient with virologic failure

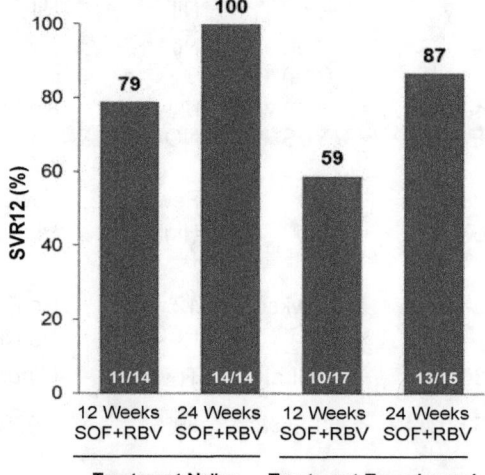

*1 patient had RBV discontinued after day 35 due to AE of dyspnea and completed SOF 24 weeks

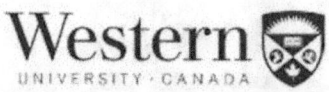

All–Oral Treatment for GT 4 with LDV/SOF

- o Interim results from a single center, open–label, Phase 2a trial of LDV/SOF in HCV GT 4

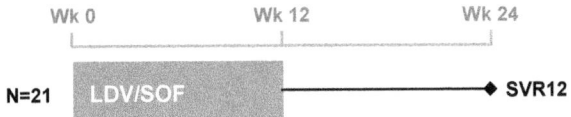

Demographics

–	Age	55 ± 10
–	Male, n (%)	14 (67)
–	Black, n (%)	9 (43)
–	Country of Origin	
	• Egypt, n (%)	6 (29)
	• United States, n (%)	5 (24)
	• Ethiopia, n (%)	4 (19)
	• Cameroon, n (%)	3 (14)
–	HCV RNA > 800,000 IU/mL, n (%)	13 (62)
–	Treatment Experienced, n (%)	8 (38)
–	Cirrhotic, n (%)	7 (33)

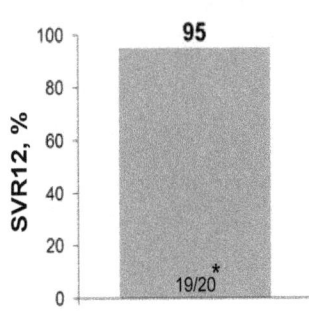

95% SVR12 with LDV/SOF for GT 4 HCV

No patient discontinued due to AE

*1 patient has not reached SVR12 timepoint yet

Kapoor. *AASLD*. 2014. Oral #240.

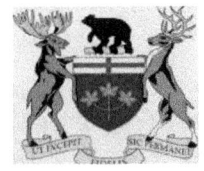

HCV G4

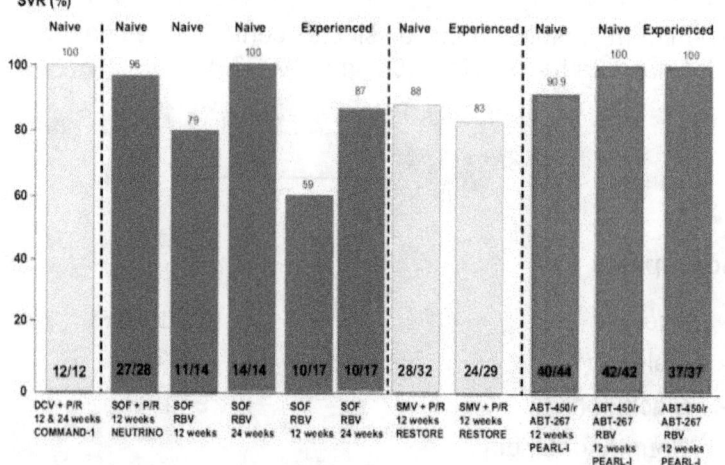

Results of treatment with direct–acting antivirals (DAAs) for HCV genotype 4 infection

Abbreviations: DCV, daclatasvir; PR, pegylated interon/ribavirin; SMV, simeprevir; SOF, sofosbuvir

Treatment G4

- o Cirrhotic, null responder
  - – Harvoni for 12 weeks
  - – PEG–IFN, Sovaldiand RBV for 12 weeks
  - – Sim (12 weeks), PEG–IFN and RBV (48 weeks)
- o Naïve, non–cirrhotic
  - – Harvoni for 12 weeks
  - – **Sovaldi & RBV (24 weeks)**
  - – PEG–IFN, Sovaldi and RBV for 12 weeks
  - – Simeprevir (12 weeks), PEG and RBV (24 weeks)
- o Naïve, cirrhotic
  - – Harvoni for 12 weeks
  - – PEG–IFN, Sovaldi and RBV for 12 weeks
  - – Simeprevir (12 weeks), PEG and RBV (24 weeks)

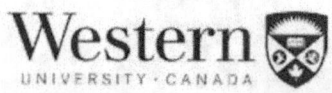

Simeprevir–based therapy (HCV G4)

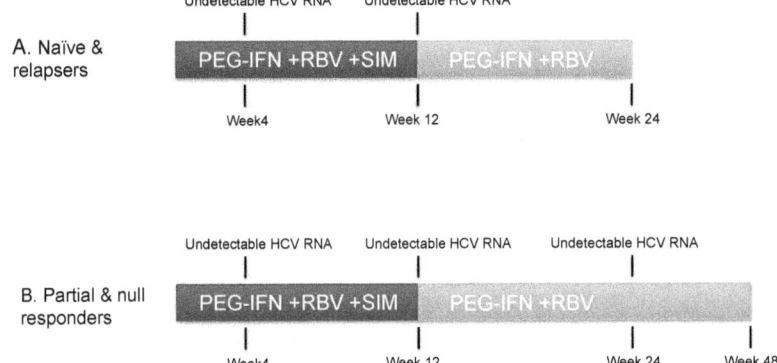

Duration of therapy using response–guided therapy guidelines in patients treated with simeprevir–based triple therapy

Patient	HCV RNA result			Action
	Week 4	Week12	Week24	
Treatment naïve and prior relapse	Undetectable	Undetectable	———	Stop simeprevir at week 12 and then continue PEG-IFN and RBV for until week 24
	Undetectable	Detectable	———	Stop therapy
	Detectable	———	———	Stop therapy
Partial and null responders	Undetectable	Undetectable	Undetectable	Stop simeprevir at week 12 and then continue PEG-IFN and RBV for until week 48
	Detectable	———	———	Stop therapy
	Undetectable	Detectable	———	Stop therapy
	undetectable	undetectable	Detectable	Stop therapy

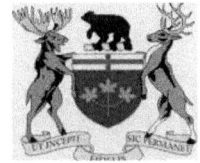

LHSC Experience Sofosbuvir/Ledipasvir +/- Ribavirin

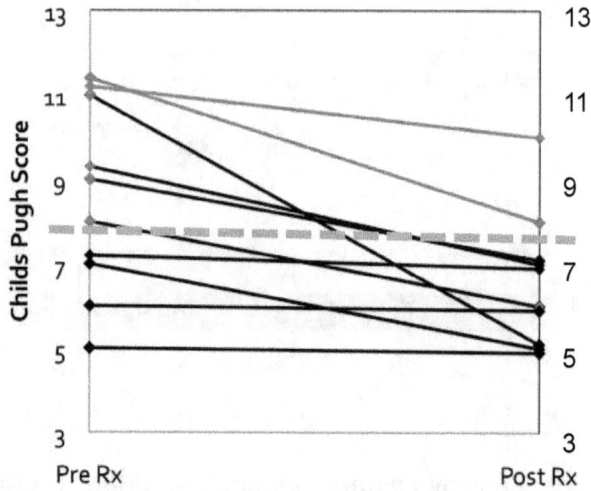

LHSC Experience Sofosbuvir/Ledipasvir +/- Ribavirin

Baseline CPS	Current CPS	Transplant Status
9	7	LIST – HOLD
11	8	LIST – HOLD
9	7	LIST – OFF
11	5	LIST – OFF
8	6	LIST – OFF
7	5	POST
11	10	POST
7	7	POST
5	5	POST
6	6	POST
40% Waitlisted Patients on HOLD		60% Removed from Waitlist

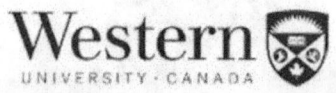

SOF + RBV in Patients with Severe Renal Impairment

Study Rationale: Prior studies in renally impaired patients without HCV demonstrated higher exposures of SOF and GS–331007[1]

Phase 2b, efficacy, PK, and safety of SOF + RBV in patients with HCV GT 1 and GT 3 with eGFR < 30 mL/min (Stage 4 CKD)

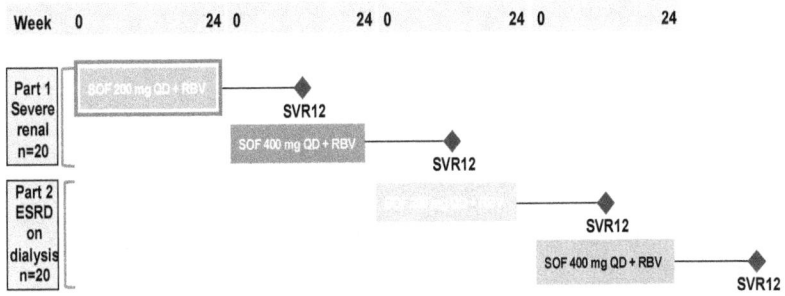

o   The cause of renal disease was not defined for participation; medical history of patients included HCV, diabetes, hypertension and lupus nephritis

Cornpropst, M., *et al. EASL*. 2012. Poster 1101.; Gane, *AASLD*. 2014. Poster #966.

SOF + RBV in Patients with Severe Renal Impairment

o   Similar rapid virologic decline observed to those with normal renal function
o   SVR4 and SVR12: 40%

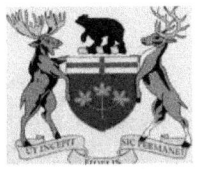

SOF and GS–331007 Pharmacokinetics

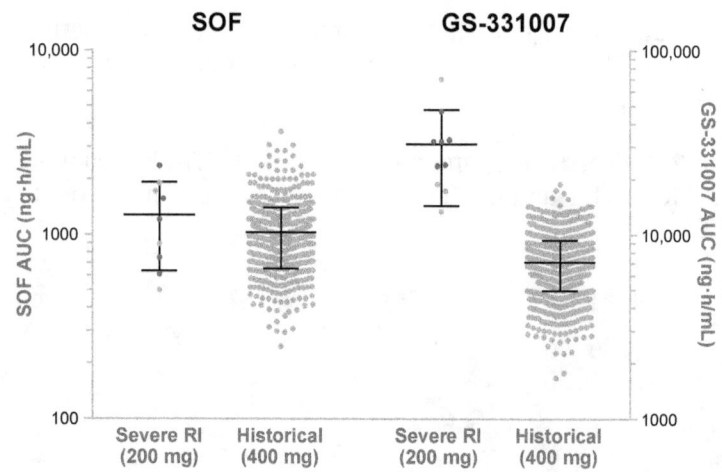

Dots indicate patients with SVR4 (blue dots) or viral relapse (red dots).

○ Comparable SOF and ~ 4–fold higher GS–331007 exposures compared with historical HCV-infected population

Adverse Events	SOF 200 mg + RBV N=10
– Anemia	5
– Headache	4
– Pruritus	3
– Rash	3
– Muscle spasms	2
– Hypoesthesia	2
– Insomnia	2
– Irritability	2

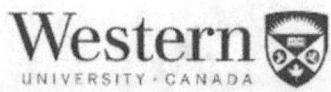

o   Mean eGFR change from baseline to EOT (week 24): -3.12 mL/min

o   No treatment–emergent clinically significant ECG results

o   SOF 200 mg + RBV was safe and relatively well tolerated in patients with severe renal impairment with exacerbation of anemia via RBV–induced hemolysis as primary AE

Gane, *AASLD.* 2014, Poster #966.

ION–4: Ongoing study of LDV/SOF in HCV/HIV Co–infection

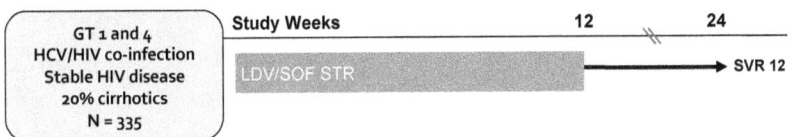

Inclusion Criteria:

o   HCV treatment naïve and experienced (including PI failures)

o   HCV GT 1 and 4

o   HIV–1 virologic suppression for at least 6 months prior to screening

o   Stable, protocol approved ARV regimen for ≥ 8 weeks prior to screening
    – FTC/TDF plus EFV or RPV or RAL

o   CD4 T–cell count > 100 cells/mm^3 at screening and no opportunistic infection within 6 months prior to screening

o   Canada, New Zealand, USA

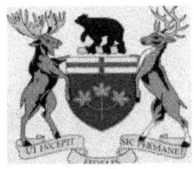

Sofosbuvir with peginterferon–ribavirin for 12 weeks in previously treated patients with hepatitis C genotype 2 or 3 and cirrhosis

- They assessed the efficacy and safety of sofosbuvir plus peginterferon and ribavirin (SOF+Peg–IFN+RBV) administered for 12 weeks to treatment-experienced patients with HCV genotypes 2 and 3, with and without cirrhosis

- 47 patients were enrolled in this open–label

- Rates of SVR12 were higher in patients with genotype 2 than in those with genotype 3 (96% *vs* 83%)

- Rates of SVR12 were similar in patients with and without cirrhosis for genotype 3 (83%)

"An alcoholic is a person who drinks more than his physician!"

Don't believe it:

TRUST, BUT VERIFY.

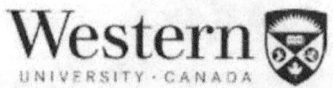

The Bright and Dark Side of Transarterial Chemoembolization (TACE)

Neel Malhotra

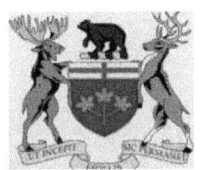

Overview

- ○ Transarterial Chemoembolization (TACE) uses catheter to deliver both chemotherapy and allows embolization of material into the blood vessels that lead to the tumor
- ○ HCC receives its blood supply from the hepatic artery
- ○ TACE is considered one of two palliative forms of therapy to treat HCC

Abbreviation: HCC, hepatocellular cancer

A Real Case

- ○ 72–year old man from Windsor with known HCC in setting of HCV infection
  - Received TACE 6 months prior without complication
  - Lesion measured 3.5 cm in left lobe (unchanged)
  - Repeat TACE as recommended as possible bridge to surgical intervention

- ○ Procedure Note
  - 5 French catheter was advanced to celiac artery
  - Angiogram demonstrated adequate catheter position
  - Microcatheter was advanced into the left hepatic artery; could not be advanced distally due to the presence of spasm (despite nitroglycerin)
  - Additional angiogram demonstrated known to be HCC in left lobe
  - Doxorubicin (DC bead) 70 mg were given by slow infusion with no evidence of "non–target embolization" to adjacent organs

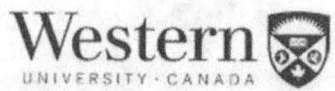

- o Outcome
  - – Persistent N/V post procedure and required admission for 48 hours
  - – Treated successfully with anti–emetics
  - – 72 hours later, readmitted with acute onset of hematemasis
  - – EGD
    - ▪ Multiple irregular gastric ulcers
    - ▪ Biopsies taken to rule out metastases disease
    - ▪ Treatment with both epinephrine and clips (Forest 1b)

Sessile Polypoid Lesion Seen on EGD

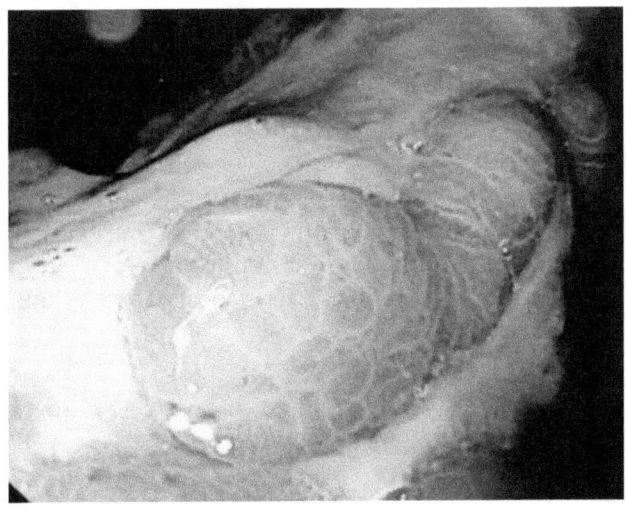

TACE

- o Once the catheter is positioned for treatment: arteriography is used to locate all the feeding arteries of a tumor

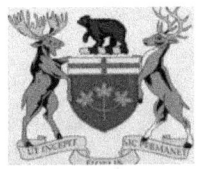

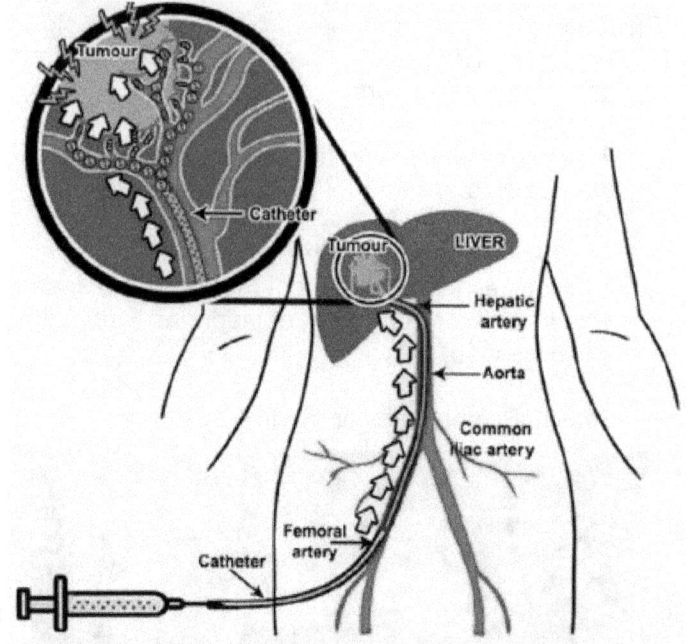

- May see cystic, right gastric or falciform arteries arising from the target hepatic artery
- May see guide–wire–induced spasms in the target arteries

o Goal
- Visualize the complete blockage of the tumor–feeding branch

CASL Statements

o TACE is standard of care for patients with large single HCC who are not candidates for resection or ablation; also used for multifocal HCC without evidence of portal vein invasion or extrahepatic spread (level 1A)

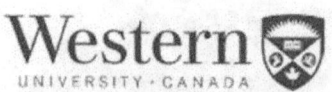

- o TACE can be used to bridge patients to liver transplantation (level 4)

- o TACE should be avoided in patients with main portal vein thrombus and in patients with decompensated cirrhosis (level 5)

- o Compared with conventional TACE, drug–eluting beads provide a more standardized technique with a better safety profile

Abbreviations: HCC, hepatocellular cancer; TACE, transarterial chemoembolization

Burak, K.W., et al. Can J Gastroenterol. 2015; 29(4):178-184.

Complications of TACE

- o Complications at puncture sites
  - – Hematoma
  - – Pseudoaneurysm
  - – AV distula

- o Hepatic artery injury
  - – Arterial Spasm
  - – Dissection
  - – Thrombosis
  - – Reduce risk with the following:
    - ▪ Microcatheters
    - ▪ Vasodilators

- o Variceal Bleeding
  - – Further ↑ portal pressures in those with coexisting portal hypertension

- o Non–target embolization

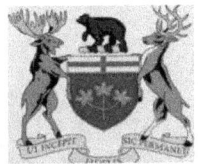

Non–target Embolization

- o Reflux of chemoembolic agents back along the catheter during delivery
- o Failure to recognize arterial supply to non–hepatic structures
- o Incidence is unknown
- o Result
  - Mucosal ulceration
  - Perforation
- o Vessels involved
  - Left hepatic *vs* left gastric artery
    - Effervescent granules given to patient to distend the stomach and see the left gastric course the lesser curve
  - Right gastric artery
    - Can arise from the proper hepatic artery, common hepatic or right hepatic artery
    - Need to visualize catheter beyond the vessel
  - Gastroduodenal artery
    - Mucosal ulceration
    - Perforation
  - Pancreaticoduodenal artery
    - Pancreatitis
  - Cystic artery
    - Chemical cholecystitis, with gallbladder thickening
- o Pulmonary embolization
  - Occurs through AV shunting or portovenous shunting
  - Might be diagnosed incidentally on subsequent imaging *vs* chemical pneumonitis
  - Issue lipiodol more so than smaller particles and microspheres
- o Post–embolization syndrome
  - Occurs in ~ 90% of patients
  - Fever, Malaise, RUQ pain, N/V

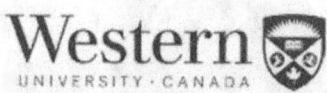

- Treatment
  - Analgesics
  - Antiemetics
  - Fluid replacement as needed
- o Infection
  - Biloma, with subsequent hepatic abscess
  - Ischemic injury to peribiliary capillary plexus
  - Bacteremia and sepsis
  - Consider prophylactic antibiotics
- o Renal Failure:
  - Incidence: up to 9% (creatinine > 150)
  - Causes and associations
    - Repeated TACE procedures
    - Diabetes
    - Chemotherapeutic agent
    - Post–embolization syndrome (volume depletion)
  - Treatment: periprocedural hydration
- o Liver failure after TACE
  - Risk factors
    - Those identified at high risk of liver failure following TACE:
      - Lactate dehydrogenase (LDH) > 425
      - AST > 100
      - Bilirubin > 34
      - Tumor burden > 50% of liver volume
  - Consensus*: No TACE in the following
    - Child–Pugh C liver disease
    - Portal vein thrombosis (high risk for liver failure)
    - UNLESS: known sufficient collateral flow
    - Consider using reduced amounts of chemoembolic mixture

*Based on single unpublished series of patients (unproven)

Abbreviations: N, nausea; RUQ, right upper quadrant; V, vomiting

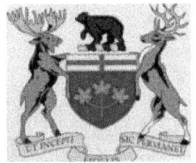

➤ Pathology

   o Histologic appearance
       – Basophilic microspheres on the background of
          purulent exudate and necrotic debris

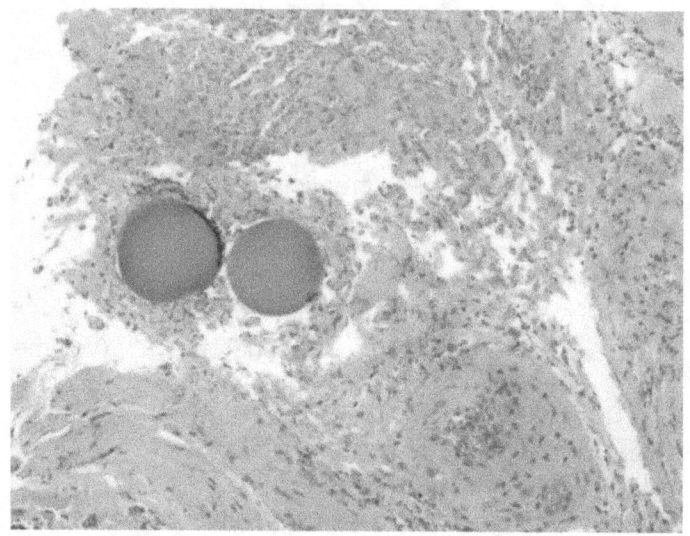

➤ Diagnosis

   o Gastric ulcers secondary to drug–eluting beads (non–
      target embolization)

➤ Treatment

   o In the setting of known non–target embolization:
       – Stomach
           ▪ No standard of care for the treatment or
              prevention of gastroduodenal injury
           ▪ Monitor patient for symptoms
       – GI bleed
           ▪ EGD to look for and treat ulceration
           ▪ PPI infusion where appropriate (Forrest Ib,
              IIa, after EHT)

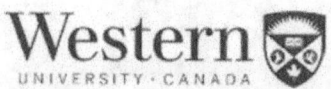

Conclusion

- ○ Infrequent non–target embolization is a known but complication of TACE

- ○ Knowledge of hepatic anatomy and non–hepatic arteries originating from hepatic arteries will help avoid complications

- ○ Slow infusion of chemotherapeutic material will minimize reflux into adjacent vessels

- ○ Yet to be proven if PPI therapy post–TACE procedure helps ↓ risk of erosive or ischemic gastritis

"Play a crucial and critical role in finding your own humility and humanity."

Grandad

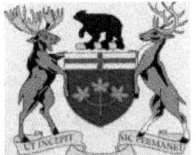

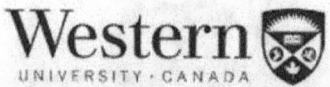

INDEX

Note: Page number followed by f and t indicates figure and table respectively.

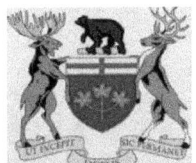

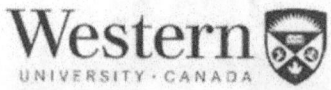

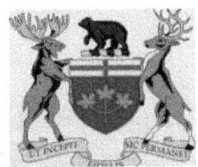

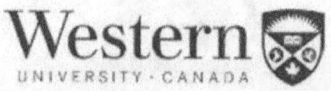

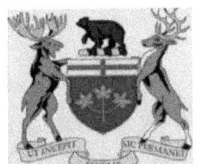

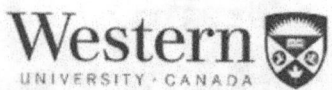

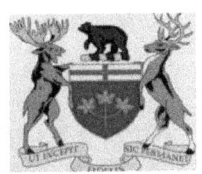

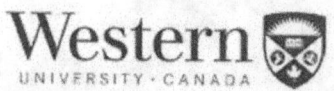

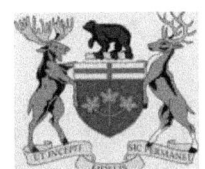

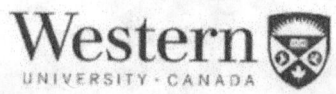

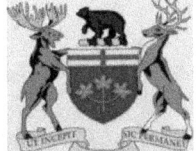

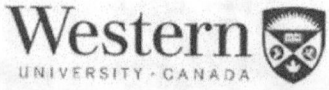

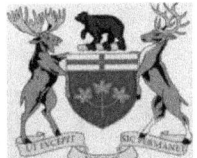

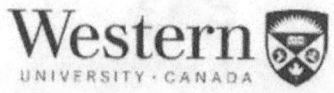

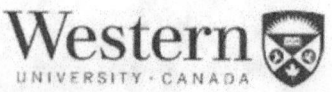

treatment, 113

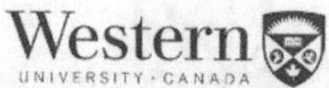

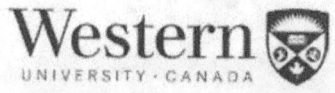

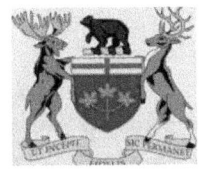

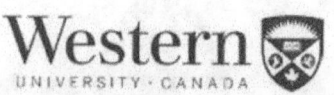

OWRD. *See* Osler-Weber-Rendu disease

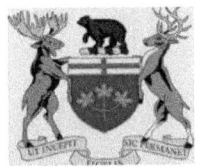

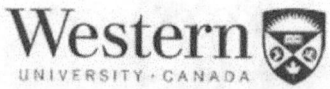

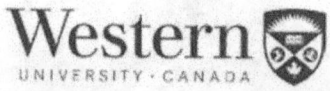

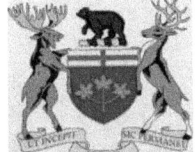

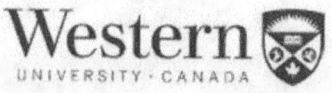

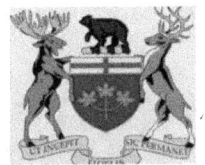

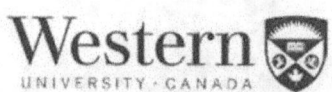

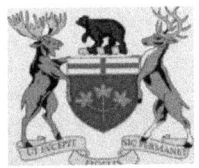

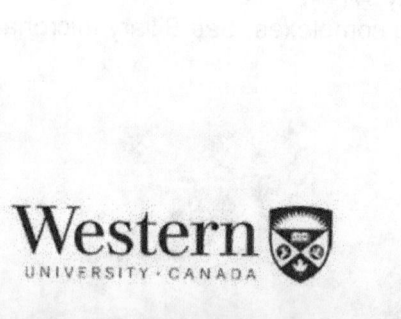

www.ingramcontent.com/pod-product-compliance
Lightning Source LLC
Chambersburg PA
CBHW051620170526
45167CB00001B/7